The Prosperous Dental Practice

A Guide to Building Financial Success

Anthony S. Feck, D.M.D.

The Prosperous Dental Practice

A Guide to Building Financial Success

edra
PUBLISHING

This edition first published 2022

ISBN: 978-1-7371261-5-7
eISBN: 978-1-957260-93-8

edra
PUBLISHING

Edra Publishing US LLC
3309 Northlake Boulevard,
Suite 203,
Palm Beach Gardens,
FL, 33403
EIN: 844113980

info@edrapublishing.com
www.edrapublishing.com

Printed in Italy by Editoriale Bortolazzi-STEI S.r.l. – San Giovanni Lupatoto (VR)

I dedicate this work to the memory of my son, Travis Feck. To this day, I am in awe of his courage, humility, demonstration of love, and outlook on life. This has been his legacy to me, inspiring me to excel in all walks of my life.

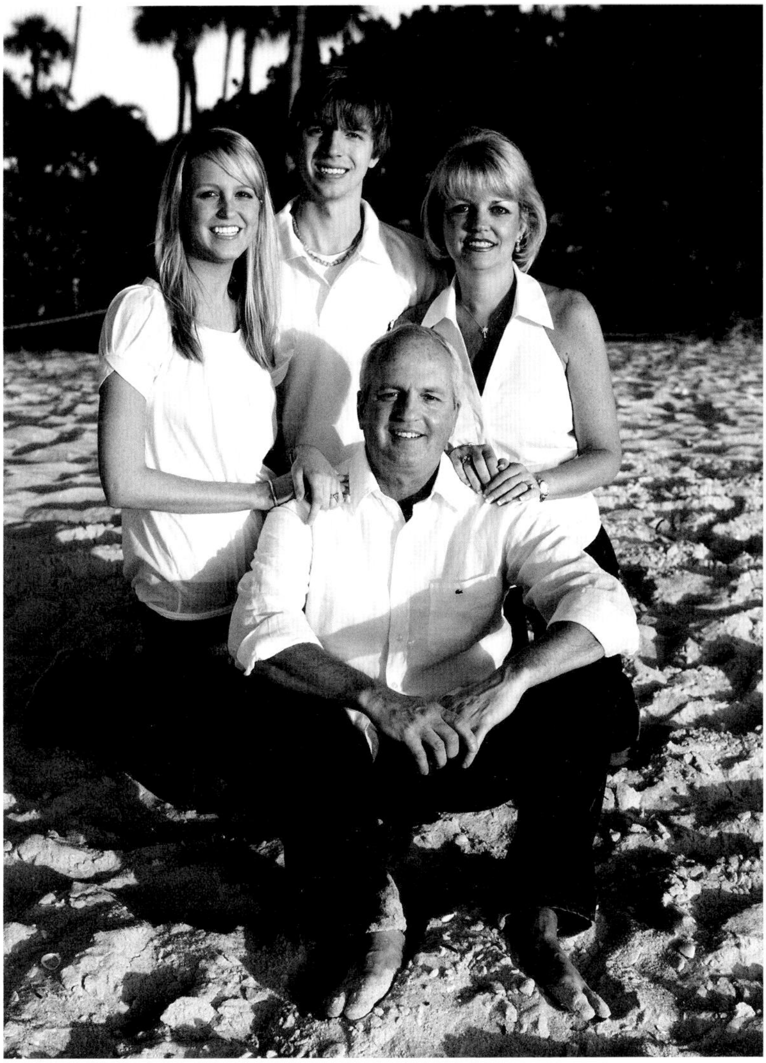

Preface

For years I considered writing a book. Several of my colleagues often inquired as to why I hadn't done so already. I responded by saying, "that's a lot of work for very little return." After all, I had repeatedly told my dentist clients before making any decision involving their resources to always consider the return on investment of those resources, especially their time.

Now that I'm in the autumn of my career, the temptation to put into words much of what I've learned and created over four decades of practicing, teaching, consulting, and coaching is just too compelling. I am humbled by the opportunity and sincerely hope that those who read this book will enjoy a fruitful and enduring return on the investment in resources they devote to it.

My path to this point started as a teenager, while visiting a dentist for a filling. I was impressed by the experience: the dentist in his white smock, the smell of the office, the cuspidor (spittoon), the feeling of being numb for the first time, the belt-driven handpiece, and the vibrations from the slow-moving bur. I was smitten, and whenever someone asked me what I wanted for a career, I said I wanted to be a dentist. How blessed I was to know my vocation at a young age! I've never regretted that decision. Sure, there are days when I want to be anything but a dentist but, all things considered, dentistry has been the best profession in the world for me.

Perhaps my love of science, the enjoyment of working with my hands, my independence, and my entrepreneurial nature led me subconsciously to that decision. Still, as I was building my practice, an inner voice kept telling me that practicing dentistry was not the end, but the means to an end. It wasn't until after I had built a successful practice that I realized I didn't know what my true purpose was. A good friend, colleague, and client, Dr. David Pier, shared with me a short book titled, *The On-Purpose Person: Making Your Life Make Sense*, by Kevin McCarthy. Finding my true purpose changed my life immeasurably. I learned that once you discover your purpose, contentment in your professional life follows along with real success – enjoying what you do, making a difference in the lives of others, and leaving a legacy.

I learned that my purpose was to create wealth for dental practice owners. I don't mean wealth in its most primitive sense of accumulating a lot of money, but wealth resulting from an abundance of resources – money certainly, but also time, skills, and knowledge that can benefit others and, in the process, provide financial and lifestyle independence for the creator of that wealth. This book is merely another expression of living that purpose.

Along this multi-decade journey of pursuing my purpose, I've had the honor to educate, consult, and coach tens of thousands of dentists and dental team members. I've also been on the receiving end of these encounters, with each one becoming a lesson adding another layer of knowledge that, in turn, I can share with others.

This book is the culmination of that knowledge. Within these pages are the secrets to building a prosperous dental practice and enjoying all the benefits that accompany that accomplishment. A Buddhist proverb says, "When the student is ready, the teacher will appear." It is my sincerest hope that the reader is ready and that the lessons in this book will be the difference between owning an ordinary practice and enjoying an extraordinary one.

Table of Contents

Introduction to The Prosperous Dental Practice

The Prosperous Dental Practice is a practice that generates extraordinary levels of profitability and allows the realization of ambitious professional and personal goals. These goals include:

Professional – Significant practice growth in terms of size of the patient base, quality of the practice personnel and their professional development, technological advances, and over-the-top patient care.

Personal – Substantial advancement toward financial and lifestyle independence by a desired date.

Admittedly, the above definitions are general in scope. We will define the specifics of phrases like "extraordinary levels of profitability," "ambitious professional and personal goals," and words like "significant" and "substantial" as we proceed through each chapter of *The Prosperous Dental Practice.*

THE TWO PARTS OF *THE PROSPEROUS DENTAL PRACTICE*

A Successful Clinical Practice - The purpose of which is to take exceptional care of patients

A Successful Business - The purpose of which is to create exceptional profitability

While the purposes of both are different, they are inseparable - one cannot exist without the other. The prosperous dental practice has both.

The key to realizing both parts is:

"A ***Great Team*** Implementing ***Great Systems*** in the presence of ***Great Leadership***"

This book is about the Key Principles of the Successful Business and will be organized into the following chapters: The Team, The Systems (Production, Financial, Growth, and Profitability), The Leadership, and The Transition Options. They will be presented separately, but they must be developed simultaneously. Throughout the book, Key Concepts – core principles that support *The Prosperous Dental Practice* – will be defined and illustrated.

The Most Essential Ingredients of the Prosperous Dental Practice – Persistence and Determination

The prosperous dental practice owner must have a big dream, a relentless drive to accomplish that dream, and an entrepreneurial spirit. You simply cannot accomplish anything this big without taking considerable risks. This is not a goal for the faint of heart. If it were easy, prosperous dental practices would be everywhere, and there wouldn't be a need for this book. The fact that the prosperous dental practice as defined here is very uncommon means that the qualities that make up the prosperous dental practice owner are uncommon. This is true despite those qualities having little to do with talent, genius, or education, and everything to do with two things all of us can access – Persistence and Determination.

THE KEY CONCEPT

The Key Concept of Persistence and Determination – Calvin Coolidge once said, "Nothing in this world can take the place of persistence. Talent will not; nothing is more common than unsuccessful men with talent. Genius will not; unrewarded genius is almost a proverb. Education will not; the world is full of educated derelicts." When it comes to success, nothing can replace persistence and determination.

Chapter 1
The Team

THE ORGANIZATION

A high-quality team starts with a plan. And a high-quality plan starts with a vision. What you want to accomplish will guide you in deciding what your team will consist of before you begin assembling it. The number of team members, their roles, and their job descriptions should be clear before you begin your search for team members.

The Size of Your Team

You should staff for both now and the future. The concept of "build it and they will come" applies here. The size and floor plan of the facility will have an impact on your ultimate success. Your basic staff will include team members from the business office, dental hygiene, and dental assistant departments. When in doubt, it is better to err toward being slightly overstaffed, rather than slightly understaffed. The additional manpower will come in handy during times of extra demand, or when the practice is expectedly – or unexpectedly – without a team member.

Dental Business Office – The key roles of the business office are three-fold – Reception, Scheduling, and Collections. This is *the most under-staffed* department of any dental practice. Clearly defined roles in the business office are critical. Still, each member of the business office team should be cross trained in the other roles of the department. All team members should not only be accountable for their individual role's job description, but also responsible for their fellow team members' job descriptions.

THE KEY CONCEPT

The Key Concept of Responsibility Versus Accountability – Within a team, a designated individual should be assigned and accept primary accountability for the outcome of a key system. Accountability makes for a deeper commitment on the part of the designated individual, while allowing more efficient management of the assigned system. Responsibility in this context refers to sharing in the outcome of key systems.

Dental Hygiene Department – The key roles of the hygiene department are data collection, education, prevention, prophylaxis, periodontal treatment, case presentation, and acceptance. Because most hygienists only fulfill these roles to a fraction of their potential, this department is *the most under-producing* department of any dental practice.

THE KEY CONCEPT

The Key Concept of Leverage – By expanding a team member's role, efficiency and effectiveness are enhanced.

Dental Assistant Department – The key roles of the dental assisting department are chairside support of the doctor, expanded duties when allowed, disinfection and sterilization, laboratory liaison, clinical supply control, case presentation, and case acceptance. This department is *the most under-utilized* department of any dental practice.

THE KEY CONCEPT

The Key Concept of Delegation – Any role that a team member can legally perform to the standards set by the practice owner should be delegated to that team member.

Each department may have specialized roles such as an administrative coordinator in the business office, a patient care specialist and hygiene assistant in the hygiene department, and a sterilization or lab assistant in the assistant department. Management and leadership roles will be covered in the Leadership chapter.

The Job Description

Right after the top three reasons why employees change jobs (compensation, appreciation, and path to growth) is "not receiving feedback about job performance and not knowing what's expected." The job description serves as a blueprint of expectations as well as a guide to selection and appraisal of a team member. Samples of job descriptions for hygiene, assistant, business office, lab department, plus leadership roles, can be found in the Glossary.

Compensation Range

Compensation (salary/hourly wage, benefits, incentive pay) for each role within the office is primarily a function of wage ranges for the area; marketplace supply and demand; existing compensation within each department of the practice; and the experience, qualifications, and qualities of the individual. Secondarily, the compensation package for individual roles should fit within the total practice budget for gross salaries and employee benefits. It is usually best to have a range of compensation rather than a specific amount; this gives the employer the capability to acquire the best team members available and negotiate when appropriate. More information about compensation can be found in the Leadership chapter.

The Office Policy Manual

Along with not having a practice budget and job descriptions, the biggest mistake dental practice owners make is not having an updated office policy manual. Whenever a dentist contacts me with a potential or actual employee dispute, my first question is, "What does your Office Policy Manual say?" More times than not, the response is "I don't have one," or "It hasn't been updated in a long time," or "That isn't covered in my manual." Office policy must be mapped out in the Office Policy Manual; documented, understood and agreed to in writing by all practice personnel; and updated on a regular basis (every two years or more often if major changes are made). It will be an invaluable reference for Human Resources questions, and it will prevent as well as resolve employee disputes.

THE INDIVIDUAL

Now that you know the details of the role, you can develop an image of the individual you need to fill that role. Be as specific as possible when it comes to characteristics such as experience, training, personality type, knowledge, and skills. This way you will recognize the right candidates when they interview.

Qualities - The Three As

When it comes to any hire, consider the most important qualities of a potential team member: Aptitude, Ability, and Attitude.

EXCELLENCE IN HIRING & EVALUATION - The Three As

Aptitude – This is a person's knowledge and skills. These can be acquired through training and experience. The employer has some control over the future development of aptitude.

Ability – This is a person's potential. It involves intelligence, physical ability, and other genetic traits. Much of a person's ability is programmed into them by their DNA. The employer has little control over ability.

Attitude – This is a person's view of the world. It is the culmination of experiences, teaching, and choices. It includes how the individual was brought up, their childhood, young adulthood, and educational experiences. It is also what they go home to every day. Despite common misconceptions, the employer has very little control over attitude.

Of the Three As, the most important is attitude, followed by ability, and then aptitude. You should look for all three, but if you can't have all three, you must have attitude and ability. These are the two things the employer has the least ability to alter, so it is critical to find someone who doesn't require change in these two areas.

The Search

Now that you know *who* and *what* you want, you must find them. Two things will make your search more successful: the message (the *why*) and the range of the search (the *where*).

The Message - Notice that I didn't say "offer." The offer usually refers to details of the working relationship such as compensation, but the message needs to be more than what you are willing to pay. The message is just like the marketing message for attracting new patients. And just like the patients with the most value already have a dentist, the team members with the most value already have an employer. In both cases, your message to attract them must be all about what makes you unique as an employer, and what gives them something they are not getting from their current employer. That message will include compensation (although not necessarily specifically), but will also include growth potential, culture, appreciation, and convenience, among others. It will also include qualifiers such as experience, accreditation, and schedule. Finally, the search should request that all interested, qualified applicants send a resume to a specific location. Here's an example of such an advertisement:

> ***Full-Time Dental Assistant***. *We are looking for someone special who shares our passion for providing the best care to our patients in a friendly, positive, and fast-paced environment. This person wants to learn, grow, and advance in their career. Our team has very little turnover, so we're looking for someone who wants to stay and play a part in continuing to build the best dental practice in the region. Our team culture is built upon winning as individuals and as a team. We appreciate and reward excellent performance excellently which is reflected in our compensation/benefit package. We require two years experience as an expanded-duty dental assistant. Visit our website at <practice website address> to learn more about us. If you feel you're the one we've been looking for, we would love to hear from you. Please send your resume along with a narrative describing your qualifications and what makes you the special person we are looking for. Send to <practice mailing address>. All inquiries are treated confidentially.*

The Search Range – Because you want as many qualified candidates as possible to choose from, you need to cast a wide net. The concern that you will have to wade through multiple non-qualified candidates will be eased somewhat by the qualifiers contained in your message. The search network should include local, regional, and in some cases national online sites. The search should also include word-of-mouth promotion through existing team members and others in the local dental community. In cases where the job market requires it, you should consider using a headhunter. If the response is low, you should reconsider both the message and the range of search.

The Selection

Screening Applicants – The initial screening process can be delegated to a highly qualified team member or handled personally by the practice owner. Either way, the initial screening entails reviewing the resume for the quality of the document as well as the qualifications of the applicant. Is the resume professional-looking and organized? Do the applicant's qualifications match the practice needs for that role? Does the applicant's job experience reflect stability or frequent employment changes?

All applicants who pass the resume review should have a telephone screening interview using a list of questions designed to get the best picture possible of how the applicant stacks up against the Three As. The key here as throughout the selection process is to not compromise.

THE KEY CONCEPT

The Key Concept of Team Member Quality - Decide on a scale of 1-10, with 10 being the best, what quality of practice and business you want. Then realize that, whatever number you've chosen, the quality of each team member on a similar scale cannot be less than the number you've chosen for your practice.

TELEPHONE SCREENING INTERVIEW FOR APPLICANTS INQUIRING ABOUT A POSITION WITH <NAME OF PRACTICE>

Name of Applicant ______________________ Date ______________________

Position ____

Team Member Performing Screening Interview ______________________

Qualifications of the position:

Education ____

Credentials ____

Experience ____

Skills ____

Knowledge ____

Days, Hours ____

Other requirements ____

Is there a resume? If so, quality of the resume (check all boxes that apply):

- ☐ Professional
- ☐ Well-written
- ☐ Comprehensive

Notables of Resume – Does the applicant appear to meet the requirements of the position?

____

Questions to ask:

What about the advertisement for this position motivated you to contact us?

____

Are you currently employed? ____

(If so, all inquiries are confidential outside of the management team of the practice.)

Why are you interested in leaving your present position? ______________________

____

Ask about and confirm the applicant's qualifications for the position (education, credentials, experience, skills, knowledge, availability for days and hours needed, and any other special requirements). Does the applicant meet the following requirements for the position?

- ☐ Education ____________________
- ☐ Credentials ____________________
- ☐ Experience ____________________
- ☐ Skills ____________________
- ☐ Knowledge ____________________
- ☐ Days, hours ____________________
- ☐ Other ____________________

If the applicant does not meet the minimal requirements, then politely inform them and thank them for their inquiry. Otherwise, ask if they have any questions regarding the position. (Unless otherwise directed, any questions regarding compensation will be addressed through the in-person interview process.)

Impressions

- ➤ Voice ____________________
- ➤ Language skills ____________________
- ➤ Eagerness ____________________
- ➤ Meets qualifications ____________________
- ➤ Other ____________________

Next Steps

- ☐ Schedule in-person interview – Date, Time ____________________
- ☐ Discover additional information and follow-up with applicant (social media, etc.)
- ☐ Decline

If the applicant meets all the qualifications as well as at least the two most important As (Attitude and Ability), then schedule an in-person interview.

In-Person Interview – The in-person interview should be held at the office and conducted by the practice owner or in appropriate situations by a key team member(s). A job description for the role being hired for should be available, as well as the screening interview form and resume. The applicant's appearance, demeanor, communication skills, and answers to pertinent interview questions should be evaluated. The applicant should be directed toward doing most of the talking through open-ended questions.

THE KEY CONCEPT

The Key Concept of Controlling the Conversation – You dominate a conversation by talking – You control a conversation by asking questions.

PROSPECTIVE TEAM MEMBER INTERVIEW

Name ______________________ Date ______________________

Position Applying For ______________________ Interviewer ______________________

Initial Impression (check all that apply)

- ☐ Dressed appropriately for interview
- ☐ Neat, well-kept, professional appearance
- ☐ Appearance reflects overall health and wellness
- ☐ Healthy, attractive-looking smile

Questions (Interviewer should ask follow-up questions as needed):

1. Tell me about your background as it relates to the position you are applying for.
2. Share with me the scope of your current position (if employed).
3. What do you like most about your current position?
4. What do you like least about your current position?
5. What is the ideal work environment for you?
6. Do you consider yourself a team player, and if so, why?
7. What do you bring to this position that would make this practice better?
8. What would be the most ideal work schedule for you?
9. What requirements do you have for employment (days, hours, pay, time off, etc.,)?
10. If hired, when would you be available to begin?
11. May we contact your references?

Interviewer's Impressions

Attitude

- ☐ Appears motivated and ambitious
- ☐ Has a friendly demeanor
- ☐ Uses positive sounding language

Aptitude

- ☐ Meets educational requirements
- ☐ Meets experience requirements
- ☐ Currently has the skills to perform at practice standards
- ☐ Well-spoken (uses language appropriately)

Ability

- ☐ Expresses ideas and thoughts well
- ☐ Is alert and attentive
- ☐ Asks intelligent questions
- ☐ Has good comprehension of what the position entails and what is expected

Personality (DISC) ____________ (This is not explained yet. See Chapter 2: Production Systems – Case Acceptance)

Overall impression as to the match of the person with the position

____

____

Can this individual make our team better?

____

Other Comments:

____

____

____

Next step

- ☐ Offer position or recommend hiring to practice owner
- ☐ Keep this person as a potential hire, but continue to interview
- ☐ Acquire more information
- ☐ Decline the applicant

I have found that personality and cognitive ability tests are very useful in discovering how a potential team member views the world, their mental ability (important for performing most tasks efficiently and effectively as well as problem solving), and their capability to work independently. For example: business office personnel, due to the nature of their role, must be able to multi-task, tolerate interruptions, and be able to return to their task without missing a beat.

I prefer the *DISC Personality Profile* for personality typing. (This test is explained in detail in the *Production Systems* section on *Case Acceptance*). This test categorizes people into four categories. No one category is "best," but some categories indicate that an individual will perform better at certain positions. These categories will be referred to as each of these positions are covered in more detail. Each team member, plus the practice owner(s), should have a DISC Personality Profile on file. An individual's DISC Profile is unlikely to change over time.

The prototypical cognitive ability test is the Wonderlic Test. It consists of fifty multiple choice questions to be answered in twelve minutes. The score is calculated as the number of correct answers given in the allotted time. A score of twenty indicates average intelligence.

The test I prefer over the Wonderlic Test is the *Caliper Personality Profile*. Results from this test provide information about the way an individual sees the world and about their ability. This test is especially useful in selecting team members who will be in high-level positions of accountability such as office managers, chief operating officers, associates, and partners of the practice. The Caliper Profile is explained in more detail in the *Associate Selection* section of the Transitions chapter.

The question often comes up about how best to address the compensation question at the interview. First of all, it is not inappropriate, nor is it necessarily a sign that the applicant is the wrong person, if the applicant brings up the issue. It is considered negative only if the applicant asks about it early in the interview, or if it appears to be their primary focus. The employer should have a compensation package in mind and be open to adjusting that package based on the quality of the applicant. If the applicant doesn't ask, the employer should turn the question around and ask the applicant the compensation they are looking for. Whoever mentions a number first is at a disadvantage. This is a negotiation, and the goal of any negotiation involving a future team member isn't to win, but to create a win-win.

The Culture – In addition to evaluating the individual's qualifications and qualities, they should be evaluated as to how they "fit" within the culture of the team (more on culture in the Leadership chapter). This is often referred to as "chemistry." Some personalities clash, while others blend harmoniously. The owner and team should have training on personality types – what kinds, what they need to succeed, which ones fit best when it comes to a role, and which ones fit best when it comes to working closely with other personalities on the team. But chemistry is more than the right blend of personalities. Essentially, it is about the commitment that team members must have in order to work together to accomplish the collective vision of the practice.

The Offer

Compensation – Compensation within a range is determined prior to the interview, just like the job description.

THE KEY CONCEPT

The Key Concept of the Law of Compensating for Quality (aka "You get what you pay for") – Henry Ford said, "In industry, there is only one rule: achieve the highest possible quality of products at the lowest possible costs and pay the highest salaries."

Salary or Hourly Wage? – The decision to pay a salary or hourly wage comes down to weighing the pros and cons of each.

Advantages and Disadvantages of Salary Pay versus Hourly Wage Pay		
	Salary	**Hourly**
Pros	Employer and employee can reliably plan for income/expense	Employee gets paid for actual time worked – advantageous when they work more than usual time
Pros	Employer may not have to pay additional wages when employee works additional time	Employer pays for actual time worked – advantageous when employee works less than usual time
Cons	Employer may pay for time employee doesn't work	Employee may not be able to plan for a predetermined pay/pay period
Cons	Employee may not get paid for additional time worked	When employee works additional hours, employer may not be able to plan for salary expenditures

For small businesses like dental practices, hourly wage has more potential to be a win-win for employer and employee.

Benefits – Benefit packages may mean as much as, if not more than, salary/hourly wages. These benefits may include insurance (health, life, disability, supplemental health), retirement, paid holidays, paid vacation, paid sick/wellness time, dental care, uniform allowances, signing bonuses, and bonus plans, among others.

In constructing an employee benefit package, the employer must consider the cost of the benefit in both dollars as well as time. For instance, paid vacation extracts more of a cost while the employee is on vacation than the salary that would be paid if they were working in the practice. Not only is that team member being paid during their absence, but their absence is likely affecting productivity of the practice.

The benefit package should be tailored to the individual needs of the team member and should not be activated until the team member has successfully completed a 90-day trial employment period.

Rewards – Often referred to as Bonus Systems or Incentives, rewards systems are a popular method of rewarding team members for reaching goals tied to performance metrics such as production or collections. There are many systems in use, and the decision regarding which system is best for you, if any, will be covered in more detail in the Leadership chapter.

The Employee Contract

The details of the agreed-upon working relationship should be spelled out in the form of an employee contract. An employee contract ensures that both employer and employee are on the same page regarding employment terms and it helps prevent potential misunderstandings.

SAMPLE EMPLOYMENT CONTRACT

<Practice Name>

<Date>

Employee Agreement for <Employee Name>

Welcome to our office. This contract of employment serves as an agreement regarding your terms of employment. The terms of employment are meant to be confidential and are not to be shared with other employees of the office.

Office Policies

The office has an employee handbook detailing all office policies. All employees are required to read and sign a document stating they have read the handbook, resolved any questions they have regarding policies, and agree to abide by the policies in the handbook. Specifics regarding wages and benefits are outlined herein:

Wages

$ <$ amount>/hr.

Performance and compensation will be evaluated annually. Adjustments to compensation level will be based upon level of performance and profitability of the practice.

Benefits (Full-time*)

1. Vacation. One week of vacation will be granted on the anniversary date of your first year of employment. Two weeks of vacation will be granted on the anniversary date of your second year of employment. Vacation hours must be used in the year they are given and are not allowed to be carried over into a following year. You must notify the office manager or <Practice Leader> 90 days in advance of anticipated vacation time. The exception to this would be a legitimate family emergency, or the use of two or fewer days of vacation, in which less notice is satisfactory. As the office cannot function smoothly with more than one member of a department away at a time no guarantee can be given that a requested vacation time will be granted, although every effort will be made to accommodate your selected dates. In any year your employment terminates, any remaining vacation pay will be paid on a pro-rated basis.

2. Retirement Plan. You will be eligible for the office 401K plan after one full year of employment. The rules and regulations are determined by federal law. More information concerning this can be obtained by request from <Practice Leader>.

3. Sick Leave. Six sick days will be available per calendar year. These are to be used for your personal illness only. Any sick days you do not use in a calendar year will be paid to you at the end of the year, or any time before then at <Practice Leader>'s discretion.

4. Paid Holidays. You will be paid your regular workday hours for each major holiday: New Year's Day, Memorial Day, Independence Day, Labor Day, Thanksgiving Day, and Christmas Day.

5. Health Insurance. Coverage for you is available, and other members of your family can be covered at an additional cost. A maximum of $<Dollar Amt.>/month will be allocated for this coverage, with any additional premium balance to be deducted on a monthly basis from your compensation.

Benefits (Full-time and Part-time*)

1. Monthly Bonus. This is a profit-sharing plan from the profits of the office. A bonus will be paid only on months the office meets or exceeds a certain profit level. The terms of the bonus are established by <Practice Leader> and are subject to change as conditions change. If you are not a full-time employee (see definition below of "full-time"), you will be paid a pro-rated portion of the full-time bonus.

2. Free Dental Care. Free dental care is available for you and your immediate family: spouse and children living in your residence. This does not include outside expenses such as laboratory fees and products.

3. Continuing Education. This shall be paid for by the office, at the discretion of <Practice Leader>, when related to office functions.

*Full-time is defined as averaging 32 or more hours per week during the previous six months. Vacation hours taken during those months can be used in the calculation of this average. Part-time is defined as any amount of hours less than the full-time minimum amount.

There is a 90-day probationary period in which no benefits will be provided other than uniforms health insurance, and hourly wages. During this time either you or <Practice Leader> may terminate the working relationship without notice. At the end of this period, a determination will be made about whether your employment will continue; if so, you will be eligible for the remaining benefit package based on the number of hours you work (part-time or full-time). By signing this contract, you agree that you have read the above agreement and believe it to be accurate. You agree to abide by this covenant until your employment terminates or a new agreement supersedes this one.

____

<Employee Name> Date

____

<Authorized Practice Signature> Date

Termination of a Team Member

Terminating an employee is often a stressful, anxiety-filled event. Any practice owner (or other designated individual) dreads confronting an employee on this issue. But that dread can often cause the termination to be delayed long after it should have happened.

While certain events (for example, acting unprofessionally or in a way that endangers themselves, other team members, or patients) can result in the immediate termination of a team member, termination is usually the result of choosing the wrong person or not creating an environment in which the right person can succeed. Either way, the responsibility for the failed working relationship falls on the leader, the practice owner. I have talked about choosing the right person in this section, and I will address creating the right environment for team members to succeed in the Leadership chapter.

The best way to end a working relationship is to approach it with the right attitude. The individual in question is failing, and as a result the practice is failing with this individual. Terminating the relationship not only allows the practice a better opportunity to succeed, but it also creates a situation where the terminated employee can succeed – somewhere else. The termination takes a lose-lose situation and creates a win-win situation. The termination does a favor for both the employer and the employee.

The right time for the employer to terminate the working relationship may not be the right time for the employee. Typically, when an employee resigns, they give two weeks notice and they already have found replacement employment. They likely spent more than two weeks finding that replacement job. When they give notice, it will likely take the employer more than two weeks to find their replacement. Because of this, the employer is justified in finding an employee's replacement *prior to terminating* their employment (barring some act that warrants immediate termination).

Termination should be handled in a respectful manner. As soon as the practice owner knows that they will be terminating the employee's employment (and when possible, they have a replacement employee), they should act. The best time of the week is at the beginning; the best time of day is at the end. This enables the practice owner to reduce the disruption and control the fallout to the rest of the team.

The termination should occur in a semi-private location, allowing for only selected individuals to be within sight or earshot. These individuals should be the practice owner, or team leader, office manager, or COO. In addition to the employee being dismissed, there should always be two individuals to witness the conversation.

Any remaining pay for time worked, benefits, or severance pay should be prepared in advance and ready to deliver to the employee at the time of dismissal. Letters of reference, if appropriate, should be prepared upon request. Most practices reside in "at will" states, meaning they can terminate employment at will without reason. The employee can interpret a reason that can be construed to be discriminatory or an unfair work practice, so the employer should be brief and to the point. The tendency of the well-meaning person terminating the employee's employment is to try and make them feel better. The employee can interpret this language as if it is the employer's fault. There should be no apology. Keep in mind that anything said might be used against the employer. The words can be as simple as, "The decision has been made to let you go, effective immediately. We need to collect any practice property from you before you leave."

If the employee asks why, or whether there is anything they can do to change your mind, a simple, "After careful consideration, we believe this is the right move," or "The decision is final," are effective responses. Resist being drawn into an antagonistic discussion; it is better to walk away, even if the employee pleads or cries. While this may seem cold-hearted, it is ultimately in the best interest of the employer – and the terminated employee, as well.

Team Member Resignation

Just as often, the tables are turned. It's the employee that gives what is often unwelcome news to their employer. It is imperative to be prepared in advance for this inevitable consequence of owning a business. The practice owner should have contingency plans for the loss of every member of the team. These plans include cross training of members of each department, having a list of potential employees for each role in the office, and, whenever possible, being overstaffed. While it may sound counter to good principles of overhead maintenance and profitability to be overstaffed, the additional personnel are always performing productive tasks, and are ready to step in at short notice when someone needs to be out of the office or resigns. Once more, it is better to be overstaffed than to be understaffed.

If staff turnover happens frequently, then the practice owner needs to look at team systems and leadership. Nothing is more important to the success of the practice than its team. Exit interviews should be performed on all departing team members and carefully reviewed for patterns that may indicate a culture and/or environment that leads to the loss of quality team members.

THE EXIT INTERVIEW

1. Why did you begin looking for a new job?
2. What ultimately led you to accept the new position?
3. What could we have done better?
4. Did you feel that you were equipped to do your job well?
5. How would you describe the culture of our practice?
6. What could we have done for you to remain employed here?
7. Did you share your concerns with anyone at the office prior to leaving?
8. If you could change anything about your job here or the practice, what would you change?
9. Were you satisfied with the way you were managed?
10. Were you comfortable talking to your team leader?
11. Did we provide you with clear goals and objectives?
12. Do you feel your job description changed since you were hired? How?
13. Did you feel like a valuable part of the practice?
14. Did you receive constructive feedback to help you improve your performance?
15. How can our practice improve training and development programs?
16. What qualities do you think we should look for in your replacement?
17. What was the best part of your job?
18. What was the worst part of your job?
19. How would you improve employee morale?
20. Would you consider coming back to work here in the future? In what area or function? What would need to change?

SUMMARY OF KEY POINTS FROM CHAPTER 1 – THE TEAM

1. A high-quality team starts with a plan. Decisions about the number of team members, their roles, and their job descriptions should precede the search for team members.
2. You should staff for both now and for the future. When in doubt, it is better to err toward being slightly overstaffed rather than slightly understaffed.
3. The business office is *the most under-staffed* department of any dental practice. The hygiene department is *the most under-producing* department of any dental practice. The assistant department is *the most under-utilized* department of any dental practice.
4. A job description for each role in the office is essential. It serves as a blueprint of expectations as well as a guide to selection of and appraisal of a team member.
5. Compensation (Salary/Hourly Wage, Benefits, Rewards) for each role within the office is primarily a function of wage ranges for the area; marketplace supply and demand; existing compensation within each department of the practice; and the experience, qualifications, and qualities of the individual. Compensation packages for individual roles should fit within the total practice budget for gross salaries and employee benefits.
6. One of the biggest mistakes dental practice owners make is not having an updated office policy manual. The manual is an invaluable reference for human resources questions and can resolve and prevent employee disputes.
7. The most important qualities of a potential team member are Aptitude, Ability, and Attitude.
8. When hiring, keep in mind that the individual you are looking for is most likely already employed. Your message must give them a compelling reason to change employers: your unique qualities, and something they are not getting from their current employer.
9. The details of the agreed-upon working relationship should be spelled out in an employment contract.
10. Terminating a working relationship that is failing not only allows the practice a better opportunity to succeed, but it creates a situation where the terminated employee can succeed – somewhere else.
11. The practice owner should have contingency plans for the loss of every member of the team.

Chapter 2
The Systems

Systems are methods of accomplishing an objective. In order for any system to be as effective as possible, that objective should be well-defined. Since the purpose of the business part of the prosperous dental practice is profitability, all business systems should have objectives that are measured against the standard of increasing profitability.

THE PROFITABILITY FORMULA

Business principles are simple, but many insist on making them complex. The simpler a concept is, the easier it is to communicate and perform, and the more likely a predictable, successful outcome will be achieved. It is the same with profitability.

Profitability, simply put, is:

Production (P) X Collection Rate (CR) - Expenses (E) = Profit ($)

Any individual desiring to own and grow a prosperous dental practice must maximize production and collection rate, while decreasing expenses, or overhead. In this book, business systems will be organized according to these three variables.

But before we delve into these systems, we must first define what the specific profitability objective is for the dental practice in question. The profitability objective is arrived at through the budget tool.

THE BUDGET

In my work with dentists over the years, I continue to be amazed at how few of them have a budget for their business. And when the few who say they have a budget are asked to provide that budget in the form of a document or a spreadsheet, they can't because it's "in their head." For the few who can, their accountant either produced it with little involvement on the owner's part, or it is a poor representation of what a budget should accomplish.

The reasons I hear for this lack of having a very basic, yet essential, business function include "I don't know how," "It's too much trouble," "It isn't necessary," and "I don't want to be limited by it," among others. None of these excuses are valid. A good budget is simple to construct, requires less than three hours in the beginning to create, and requires less than an hour each month to review and update.

A budget is essential for goal setting, and goals are required for consistent success. In addition, a budget is a fluid instrument that can be modified as circumstances dictate. And while it is a plan that should be accompanied by commitment on the part of the owner, it is not written in stone.

BENEFITS OF THE PRACTICE BUDGET

1. **Goal Setting** – The practice budget is the starting point for production, collection rate, and overhead goal setting, among others.
2. **Forecasting** – The budget allows the business owner to look ahead at anticipated expenses and make projections regarding profitability.
3. **Buying Decisions** – Every major buying decision should answer the question, "Does this purchase bring me closer to or farther away from my profitability goal?" The budget brings objectivity to that decision-making process.
4. **Tracking Results** – The budget defines the desired end point numerically. Comparing actual results with this budgeted end point allows the practice leader to not only tell how they're doing, but also whether midstream adjustments are needed.

Budget Example

Doctor Budget & Financial Goals	Doctor:	2021	Collection Rate Factor*	1.14
Line Item Expense	**Budgeted Expenses**	**Actual YTD Expenses**	**YTD Difference**	**Average MTD Difference**
Fixed Expenses				
Business Insurance	$ 36,428.08	$ 35,027.00	$ 1,401.08	$ 116.76
Dues	$ 4,283.76	$ 4,119.00	$ 164.76	$ 13.73
Equipment Lease	$ 84,774.56	$ 81,514.00	$ 3,260.56	$ 271.71
Fixed Miscellaneous	$ 305.76	$ 294.00	$ 11.76	$ 0.98
Janitorial	$ 7,672.08	$ 7,377.00	$ 295.08	$ 24.59
Loan Payments	$ 30,316.00	$ 29,150.00	$ 1,166.00	$ 97.17
Phone	$ 8,593.52	$ 8,263.00	$ 330.52	$ 27.54
Rent	$ 49,920.00	$ 48,000.00	$ 1,920.00	$ 160.00
Service Contracts	$ 14,459.12	$ 13,903.00	$ 556.12	$ 46.34
Taxes	$ 49,403.12	$ 47,503.00	$ 1,900.12	$ 158.34
Utilities	$ 7,046.00	$ 6,775.00	$ 271.00	$ 22.58
Variable Expenses				
Advertising	$ 49,632.96	$ 47,724.00	$ 1,908.96	$ 159.08
Bank Charges	$ 19,279.52	$ 18,538.00	$ 741.52	$ 61.79
Business Supplies	$ 14,904.24	$ 14,331.00	$ 573.24	$ 47.77
Charitable Contributions	$ 4,380.48	$ 4,212.00	$ 168.48	$ 14.04
Clinical Supplies	$ 203,075.60	$ 195,265.00	$ 7,810.60	$ 650.88
C.E. Doctors	$ 11,512.80	$ 11,070.00	$ 442.80	$ 36.90
C.E. Team	$ 25,695.28	$ 24,707.00	$ 988.28	$ 82.36
Employee Benefits	$ 51,572.56	$ 49,589.00	$ 1,983.56	$ 165.30
Equipment Purchase	$ 11,975.60	$ 11,515.00	$ 460.60	$ 38.38
Equipment Service	$ 21,027.76	$ 20,219.00	$ 808.76	$ 67.40
Gross Associate Salaries/Wages	$ 83,235.36	$ 80,034.00	$ 3,201.36	$ 266.78
Gross Salaries/Wages	$ 624,738.40	$ 600,710.00	$ 24,028.40	$ 2,002.37
Laboratory Fees	$ 194,549.68	$ 187,067.00	$ 7,482.68	$ 623.56
Legal/Professional	$ 58,970.08	$ 56,702.00	$ 2,268.08	$ 189.01
Office Improvement	$ 23,064.08	$ 22,177.00	$ 887.08	$ 73.92
Postage	$ 4,519.84	$ 4,346.00	$ 173.84	$ 14.49
Refunds	$ 13,973.44	$ 13,436.00	$ 537.44	$ 44.79
Travel/Entertainment	$ 12,290.72	$ 11,818.00	$ 472.72	$ 39.39
Variable Miscellaneous	$ 34,828.56	$ 33,489.00	$ 1,339.56	$ 111.63
Practice Reserve & Contingency	$ 156,000.00	$ 150,000.00	$ 6,000.00	$ 500.00
Total Practice Budget	**$ 1,912,428.96**	**$ 1,838,874.00**	**$ 73,554.96**	**$ 6,129.58**
Personal Expenses				
Living Expenses	$ 361,920.00	$ 348,000.00	$ 13,920.00	$ 1,160.00
Retirement	$ 15,080.00	$ 14,500.00	$ 580.00	$ 48.33
Contingency	$ 15,600.00	$ 15,000.00	$ 600.00	$ 50.00
Tax Account	$ 208,000.00	$ 200,000.00	$ 8,000.00	$ 666.67
Long-Term Goals	$ 33,280.00	$ 32,000.00	$ 1,280.00	$ 106.67
Vacation/Discretionary	$ 6,240.00	$ 6,000.00	$ 240.00	$ 20.00
Total Personal Expenses of Doctor/Owner	**$ 640,120.00**	**$ 615,500.00**	**$ 24,620.00**	**$ 2,051.67**
Total Collections from Business	**$ 2,552,548.96**	**$ 2,454,374.00**	**$ 98,174.96**	**$ 8,181.25**
Total Annual Production from Business	**$ 2,909,905.81**	**$ 2,797,986.36**	**$ 111,919.45**	**$ 9,326.62**
Monthly Production Needed from Business	**$ 242,492.15**	**$ 233,165.53**	**$ 9,326.62**	**$ 777.22**
Practice Goals				
Practice Providers	**Monthly Goals**	**Daily Goals**	**Actual YTD Production**	**Actual Avg. Mo. Production**
Dr. #1	$ 147,030.00	8,700.00	$ 869,835.00	$ 72,486.25
Dr. #2	$ 50,700.00	3,000.00	$ 348,873.98	$ 29,072.83
Dr. #3	$ 67,600.00	4,000.00	$ 274,614.31	$ 22,884.53
Dr. #4	$ 12,000.00	1,200.00	$ 144,000.00	$ 12,000.00
Hygienist #1	$ 33,800.00	2,000.00	$ 225,163.00	$ 18,763.58
Hygienist #2	$ 33,800.00	2,000.00	$ 232,780.00	$ 19,398.33
Hygienist #3	$ 33,800.00	2,000.00	$ 232,780.80	$ 19,398.40
Hygienist #4	$ 33,800.00	2,000.00	$ 254,997.60	$ 21,249.80
Hygienist #5	$ 33,800.00	2,000.00	$ 184,416.00	$ 15,368.00
Totals	$		**2,767,460.69**	**$ 230,621.72**

*Collection Rate Factor = 1.00 minus (Practice Collection Rate/100), plus 1.00

The first step in the budget process is to establish the owner's vision for their professional and personal goals. As with any plan, the planner must start with the end in mind and work backwards. Personal goals will dictate professional goals.

Personal Goals

These goals comprise the financial vision of the practice owner and reflect every aspect of their personal economic situation. These will usually include:

1. **Living Expenses** – Often referred to as "Lifestyle Expenses," this is money regularly spent to satisfy lifestyle desires and obligations. This includes mortgage or rent payments, utilities, transportation, debt retirement, food, entertainment, among others.

2. **Retirement** – Any form of regular contributions toward retirement savings (for example, IRA, 401K, pension).
3. **Contingency** – Money set aside for unexpected financial emergencies.
4. **Tax Account** – Money set aside for income and other personal taxes.
5. **Long-Term Goals** – Savings account for tuition, home or car purchase, or other big-ticket items.
6. **Vacation/Discretionary** – Savings for vacation, holiday/special-occasion gifts, luxury items, among others.

The prosperous dental practice owner should account for each of these personal financial goal items and set up separate banking accounts to fund each of them on a regular basis, up to a personally defined maximum.

Most dentists struggle with personal projections, limiting themselves by their past or their fear of change and failure.

Prosperous dental practice owners, on the other hand, dream big. They realize that they are unlikely to achieve anything big unless they first envision it.

THE KEY CONCEPT

The Key Concept of The Law of Attraction – loosely based on the quote by Paul J. Meyer, the Law of Attraction says: "Whatever you can vividly imagine, ardently desire, earnestly believe in, and expectantly act toward, with God's help, must inevitably come to pass. That which you are seeking, is seeking you."

Professional Goals

These budget line items account for two types of practice expenses: *Fixed Expenses* that occur on a regular basis and are largely independent of the amount of production, and *Variable Expenses* that are mostly dependent on the amount of production.

FIXED EXPENSES

Fixed Expenses include the following:

- Business Insurance
- Professional Dues
- Equipment Lease
- Fixed Miscellaneous – fixed recurring expenses not covered in other line-item descriptions
- Janitorial
- Loan Payments – any loan related to the practice, regardless of whether the loan is in the name of the practice or an individual
- Phone
- Rent
- Service Contracts
- Taxes –property taxes on the facility, consumer use taxes, governmental taxes on equipment, and other practice taxes not related to personal income
- Utilities

VARIABLE EXPENSES
Variable Expenses include the following: • Advertising • Bank Charges –credit card fees and other management fees • Business Supplies • Charitable Contributions From The Practice • Clinical Supplies • Continuing Education Owners –tuition, learning materials, travel, lodging, food, and any other expense related to continuing education for the owner(s) • Continuing Education Team - tuition, learning materials, compensation pay, travel, lodging, food, and any other expense related to continuing education for the team and associate(s) • Employee Benefits –all employee benefit costs not related to wages or continuing education, including insurance, uniforms, retirement contributions, and other • Equipment Purchase • Equipment Service • Gross Associate Salaries/Wages – gross wages before deductions for the associate(s) excluding employee benefits. For the purposes of the budget, associates are considered employees of the practice, but their salaries/wages are tracked separately. • Gross Team Salaries/Wages – gross wages before deductions for all team members excluding employee benefits and owner wages. Owner wages are not considered a practice expense, but rather are paid out of practice profit. • Laboratory Fees • Legal/Professional – legal and accounting, plus consulting/coaching costs • Office Improvement • Postage • Practice Reserve & Contingency – unexpected and/or emergency practice needs such as large equipment replacement, legal expenses, or work stoppages. It should be a periodic recurring expense (funded every one to three months as necessary) held in a separate account until a balance of three months total practice expenses is accumulated, at which time regular payments are discontinued until the fund balance is below the three-months level. • Refunds – considered an expense because money is collected and then paid back. This does not include discounts. • Travel/Entertainment • Variable Miscellaneous - variable expenses not covered in other line-item descriptions

Making Budget Projections

Budget projections are determined by history, industry norms, and the owner's vision for the next twelve months of the practice.

The starting point for the coming year's projections are last year's numbers for each expense line item. With fixed expenses, there is likely to be very little, if any, change.

With variable expenses, whether personal or professional, the owner's desire for increase, intended changes, and industry norms related to dental inflation and other circumstances need to be taken into consideration.

For example, if the practice owner desires to add capacity in the form of additional team members or treatment rooms, the anticipated costs should be reflected in gross team member salaries, employee benefits, continuing education for the team, office improvement, as well as most other expense categories related to the expected increased production.

When in doubt about the amount of increased expense for the coming year's budget, it is safe to increase the line item by the cost of dental inflation. Dental inflation reflects the increase in cost due to rising costs, which in the dental industry is often one to two points above the change in the consumer price index (the standard in the United States general economy for measuring inflation).

Determining Collections Needed from Budget

Once all the projected personal and professional expense line items for the coming year are determined, they are added together to determine the amount of money needed to be collected.

Determining Production Needed from Budget

Multiplying the needed collection amount by the **Collection Rate Factor (CRF)** for the practice determines the approximate amount of production needed. The CRF is determined by the following formula:

CRF = 1.00 minus (Practice Collection Rate divided by 100), plus 1.00

The Practice Collection Rate is the percentage of net collections divided by gross production.

EXAMPLE of Determining Production Needed

A practice that needs to collect $1,000,000/yr. to satisfy its budget and has a collection rate of 90% needs to produce $1,100,000.

1,000,000 X ((1.00 - 90/100)) + 1.00), or
1,000,000 X (.1 + 1.00), or
1,000,000 X 1.1
= 1,100,000 of needed production

The accuracy of the CRF in this equation increases with the scale (the number of digits to the right of the decimal point, also called the fractional part). For instance, in the above example the Production Needed is more accurate if the number used for the CRF is 1.1111111 rather than 1.1.

Once you determine the annual amount that needs to be produced, you can calculate the monthly production by dividing by twelve.

Setting Production Goals for Providers

To determine the production goal per provider (i.e., doctors and hygienists), use the production based on history (last twelve months) and future potential (e.g., change in number of days, training, support, treatment rooms utilized, treatment mix, fees, etc.) of each provider. If the total annual production goals do not exceed past production, or if it is determined that the goals do not match the producer's estimated potential, you can make adjustments to the personal and professional expense line-item projections in the budget spreadsheet, and adjust the provider's goals.

Monthly and daily production goals for each provider can be determined by dividing the annual goal by twelve to determine the monthly goal, and by dividing each monthly goal by the planned number of days worked by provider to determine the daily goal.

MONITORING PERFORMANCE

In addition to having a well-defined objective, systems must have a method of measuring the performance of the dental team in accomplishing those objectives. This is not only key to evaluating performance, but it is also a key management and leadership concept that will be covered in much more detail in the Leadership chapter.

Practice statistics are snapshots in time that reveal past annual, monthly, and daily performance. The more current the metrics being measured, the more valuable the data is. Daily dashboards are near real-time information about key practice statistics. The important parameters to measure are shown here:

KEY PRACTICE MONITORS

Production

- Days Worked/Time Period YTD, Monthly, & Month to Date (MTD)
  - Compared to Plan
- Practice Production YTD, Monthly, & MTD
  - Compared to Historical
  - Compared to Goal
  - Monthly Trends
- Departmental Production (Doctor, Hygiene) YTD, Monthly, & MTD
  - Compared to Historical
  - Compared to Goal
  - Monthly Trends
- Percentage of Production by Department YTD, Monthly, & MTD
- Provider Production YTD, Monthly, & MTD
  - Compared to Historical
  - Compared to Goal
  - Monthly Trends

– cont'd

KEY PRACTICE MONITORS – cont'd

Financial

- Practice Collections YTD, Monthly, & MTD
  - Compared to Historical
  - Compared to Goal
  - Monthly Trends
- Collection Rate YTD, Monthly, & MTD
- Accounts Receivable Aged 0-30, 31-60, 61-90, and over 90 days
- Accounts Receivable Trend
- Accounts Receivable/Monthly Production Ratio

Growth

- New Patients YTD, Monthly, & MTD
- Annual & Monthly by Source
- Annual Value of a New Patient by Practice and Doctor Provider
- Annual & Monthly by Estimated Gross Production by Source

Profitability

- Adjustments Annual, Monthly, & MTD
  - Total & by Category
- Practice Expenses Annual, Monthly, & MTD
  - Broken Down by Line-Item Category (Fixed & Variable)
- Practice Overhead % - Annual, Monthly, & MTD
- Practice Profitability - Annual, Monthly, & MTD

Companies such as Sunrise Dental Solutions® (annual and monthly) and Dental Intel® (daily dashboard) produce reports that contain this information and more. Examples of the Sunrise Dental Solutions® Monthly Monitors can be found in the Glossary.

Interpretation of Monitors

The Key Practice Monitors are divided into four categories: Production, Financial, Growth, and Profitability. While they impart valuable information about practice performance, the real value of these metrics is when the monitors indicate a performance gap between goals and results, pointing the practice owner to specific systems that may not be working as designed.

As an example, if practice production is less than the production goal, then the systems that impact production need to be examined. Determining which production systems need to be reviewed and possibly modified by the practice are in turn identified by specific monitors.

PRODUCTION SYSTEMS

Early in my consulting career, I found a repeating pattern of systems that were essential to a dental practice having a successful and productive schedule. Since all of these systems were interrelated in their impact on the schedule, it occurred to me that this relationship was like a wheel with the schedule being the hub, and the production systems the spokes.

The 12 Systems – The Production Wheel

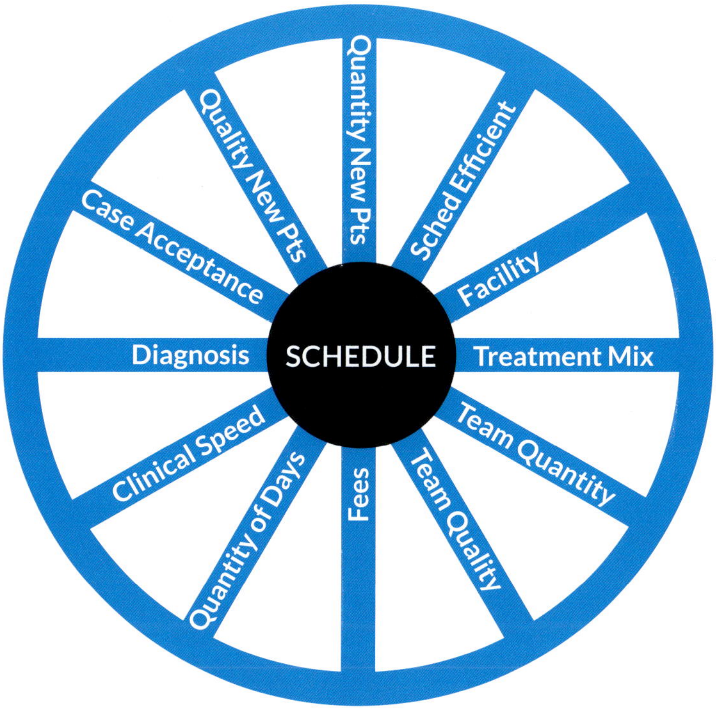

Production System #1 – Diagnosis

You must find it to produce it. You can't schedule it until the patient says yes, and *the patient can't say yes until the opportunity is identified and presented.* Continuing education to expand practice offerings, as well as sharp focus by the dental team, leads to more elective, as well as non-elective, care being presented.

Diagnosis Philosophy

Each dentist must establish a philosophy of diagnosing treatment. What constitutes treatment that should be recommended is not always black and white, but rather shades of gray. The practitioner needs to establish standards that reduce as much as possible the shades of gray, be committed to those standards, and apply them to everyone without prejudice.

Here's what I mean by treating everyone the same. One of the questions that I usually ask a new client is what they would do in the following two scenarios:

Scenario 1 – A *new patient* comes into the practice and tells you they recently received a new crown six months ago from their previous dentist. They are asymptomatic and appear pleased with the results. You do an exam and find that the margins of that crown are rough and not up to your standards. What do you tell the patient, and what do you recommend, if anything?

Scenario 2 – You see *your existing patient* for their bi-annual exam and prophylaxis and notice that the crown you placed six months ago has a rough margin and is not up to your standards.

The patient is asymptomatic and appears pleased with the result. What do you tell the patient, and what do you recommend, if anything?

What I often find is that in Scenario 1 dentists will tell the patient the crown margins could be better, and that they will "keep an eye" on this, because it may become a problem in the future. In Scenario 2 those same dentists don't even blink an eye before saying that they will replace the crown as soon as possible at no charge.

Why the different approach between Scenarios 1 and 2? Because most dentists have low confrontational tolerance – they want to tell patients what they want to hear. They equate giving unwelcome news with making a bad impression. Another factor here is that dentists often hold themselves to a higher standard than their colleagues. A big part of excelling at diagnosis is being honest with the patient and treating them just like you would want to be treated – in other words, having high standards. When dentists accept this, they diagnose a lot more dental care.

MONITORS FOR DIAGNOSIS

- Value of a new patient
- Production
- Collections
- Overhead %
- Practice profitability

Production System #2 – Case Acceptance

They must accept it before you can produce it. Case acceptance is quite often the most overlooked and most substantial weakness of all the production components in the dental office. While many dentists lament the low number of new patients entering the practice, they fail to capitalize on increasing the net value of the new patients they do receive. If patients are to accept recommended treatment, the practice must have good communication skills, a sincere belief in what they are recommending, and tools for approaching case acceptance (listening, finding the what and the why behind what patients want, having answers to objections, storytelling, building trust, and making treatment as affordable as possible).

Case Acceptance Tools

The ability to effectively communicate with a patient is a game changer for the dental practice owner desiring to be a prosperous dental practice owner. Dentists often ask me, "How can I sell more dentistry?" Before I answer I let them know they are asking the wrong question. No one wants to be sold, and frankly not many of us want to sell. The connotation is that the seller has more to gain from the transaction than the buyer.

The reason commonly-taught selling techniques in dentistry don't work is that many of the procedures performed in dentistry people really don't want, and people don't buy what they don't want.

Therefore, the question should be, "How do I help people want more of the dentistry they need?"

If you give people what they want, you will never have to sell dentistry again.

How do you know what they want? You ask.

THE KEY CONCEPT

The Key Concept of Asking – In the New Testament Bible Jesus taught the message of asking – "Ask and it shall be given. Knock and the door will be opened to you" (Matthew 7:7,8). In fact, there are more than a hundred Bible verses with the message – "You have not because you ask not.". The key is to ask. Asking is the first step in seeking knowledge (remember the acronym A-S-K – Always Seeking Knowledge), and knowledge is essential to influencing others.

Finding Out What the Patient Wants

Now that you know you must ask to get, you need to know what questions to ask. This can be as simple as, "What would you like us to do for you?" Or the question could have more structure. "SWOT," an analytic tool often used by businesses to assess their needs and form the basis for a strategic plan, can also be used to interview patients and determine what they really want. SWOT is an acronym for the following questions:

S – Strengths. "*What do you like about your smile?*"
W – Weaknesses. "*What do you not like about your smile?*"
O – Opportunities. "*If there was nothing standing in your way, what would you like your smile to look like?*"
T – Threats. "*What is standing in the way of you having the smile of your dreams?*"

It is important that the interviewer listen carefully to the answers to these questions. But while this is important information, these answers are not the key to case acceptance. Rather, they are the path to the key.

The key to case acceptance lies in the emotion behind what the patient wants.

For example, a patient may say they want porcelain veneers, but what they really want is the life-changing effect they believe those veneers will bring.

THE KEY CONCEPT

The Key Concept of Emotional Decision-Making – While it's logical for people to make big decisions based on logic, that is the exception rather than the rule. Ask yourself, "What are the biggest decisions I've ever made?" They are likely to be marriage, purchasing a home, choosing a career path, and so on. More than likely, these decisions were emotionally charged. You may have used logic to justify the emotional decision, but if you had done it the other way around, you likely would not have decided to move forward.

This same principle applies to case acceptance of dentistry, especially larger cases.

Finding Out the Why Behind the What – The Dominant Buying Motive

More likely than not, your patient will make an emotional decision, which is the "why" behind the "what" they want. We call the "why" the Dominant Buying Motive (DBM).

You get to the DBM by asking leading questions such as, *"How would this make you feel?" or "What difference would this make in your life?"* or *"If this were to happen, what could you do that you can't do now?"*

Sometimes uncovering the DBM stimulates a deeply personal and emotional response on the part of the patient. This is when the DBM becomes the patient's *"Emotional Treasure."* As with the DBM, the key here is to ask the right questions, until the why is discovered. Given that people buy on emotion, the stronger the emotion, the greater the motivation to proceed with treatment.

While asking SWOT and DBM questions, you have been listening not only to what the patient says, but also to how they say it. This is where you learn about the patient's *Personality Type.*

Personality Types

The patient's personality type reflects how they see the world around them and respond to it. Understanding this is key to how best to communicate with them.

For years, authors and teachers have used personality typing systems to place people into groups based on certain characteristics. One of the most common personality type systems places patient into one of four groups. Of these systems, the one that we use and teach to our clients is the *DISC Personality Profile.* The letters in DISC represent the following four personalities:

THE FOUR DISC PERSONALITY PROFILES
D - Dominance – The "D" personality values time and control and is usually direct and short in communication. They often appear insensitive and unfriendly. They don't shy away from confrontation. In the dental office they respond well to a no-nonsense approach. They want action and they want it now. They fear losing control and being taken advantage of, so involving them in decision-making and building trust is imperative with the D personality type.
I - Influence – The "I" personality is outgoing, friendly, and positive. Gregarious in nature, they make friends easily and are not afraid of rejection. They like to be heard; they don't like to be ignored. In the dental office, these individuals need time to talk, and should not be interrupted. Allowing them to be the center of attention goes a long way in developing a positive relationship. They tend to be good starters, and can thrive in a less organized environment, but often don't respond to deadlines and need others to finish projects for them.

– cont'd

THE FOUR DISC PERSONALITY PROFILES – cont'd
S - Steadiness – The "S" personality values harmony, and fears conflict and rejection. They like to be liked, and desire sincere friendship, so taking the time in the dental office to learn about what they care about is important in developing rapport. Because of their friendly nature, they may not share their true feelings, especially if the feelings are not positive. They place less value on time and organization than they do on relationship building.
C - Conscientiousness – The "C" personality thrives in an organized, structured environment where they are allowed to do things their way. Their thinking is logical and analytical, and often place more value on the means than the end. In the dental office they need details, and those details need to make sense to them. They may not be visionaries, but they are good at developing and fulfilling the plan for the vision. These people are good at getting things done but may lack the people skills to solicit the help they may not realize they need.

Belief Windows

In addition to the patient's personality type, the way the patient views the world is shaped by their background, their lifestyle, their occupation, their age, and other factors that define them. The way an individual sees the world is their *Belief Window*. We can use a patient's belief window to enhance communication.

A person's occupation can provide insight into their belief window. For example, if we know that a patient is a fire fighter, then we can use words, phrases, and analogies that the patient can easily understand, such as "preventing a fire" and "putting out hot spots."

Putting It All Together to Gain Case Acceptance

The information we need to properly present treatment and achieve the highest rate of case acceptance is:

1. Chief Complaint
2. SWOT
3. DBM
4. DISC Profile
5. Belief Window

In my practice as well as in many other practices I work with, this information is acquired by a highly trained team member, the Patient Care Specialist, and transferred to the doctor prior to meeting with the patient. The job description for the Patient Care Specialist can be found in the Glossary.

After greeting the patient and making friendly conversation, the doctor confirms the preliminary treatment information with the patient. This lets the patient know that the doctor understands them, as well as allows the patient to add any additional pertinent information.

Next, the doctor can perform an examination, obtain additional clinical data, and create a treatment plan. At this point another critical mistake in the case presentation process is commonly made: *the patient is presented with too many treatment options.*

This is an easy mistake to make when the practitioner feels an obligation to give a patient all their options. However, presenting multiple plans can stymie the decision-making process. The case presenter must not let minutiae get in the way of what is truly important – that the patient's needs and desires are met. Because the doctor and team have listened to the patient, performing both a clinical and emotional exam, they can recommend the best course of treatment for the patient with confidence. When necessary, a second option can be also be presented. At the very most, there should never be more than three options for the patient to choose from. It is perfectly appropriate for the practitioner to recommend one option over another.

Case Presentation Technique

I'm often asked about the language I recommend when presenting a case to a patient. I prefer not to script the presentation or use the same words with every patient. Rather I recommend an approach to case presentation that consists of five parts:

THE FIVE STEPS TO SUCCESSFUL CASE PRESENTATION

1. Remind the patient of their DBM.
2. Present the recommended treatment.
3. Address any questions/objections, while referring to their DBM.
4. Present financial arrangements.
5. Address any objections (including financial), and remind them of their DBM.

This approach to case presentation reflects the emotional basis for case acceptance by weaving the DBM throughout the process. Notice that it starts with the DBM and repeats the DBM at each point where obstacles to case acceptance are most likely to pop up – after treatment is presented, and after finances are discussed.

Objections to case acceptance are most likely to be one of four things:

OBJECTIONS AND SOLUTIONS TO CASE ACCEPTANCE
1. **Money** – Patient says, "I can't afford it." Responses: • "Treatment will never be more affordable than right now as treatment will become more extensive as your condition worsens." • "We have payment options to help make the dentistry you want more affordable." • "Would you like to look at other options that might fit your budget better?" • Don't forget to use belief windows and storytelling.

– cont'd

OBJECTIONS AND SOLUTIONS TO CASE ACCEPTANCE – cont'd

2. **Trust** – Patient says, "I'll think about it."

Responses:

- "Do the problems I see, and the treatment I recommend, make sense?"
- "May I show you with our intraoral camera, scan, or x-ray what I am seeing?"
- Don't forget to use belief windows and storytelling.

3. **Sense of Urgency or Time** – Patient says, "I'll wait on that."

Responses:

- "That is your choice, but because these things get worse with time, tomorrow's solution may be more invasive and costly compared to treatment undertaken now."
- "Taking care of this problem now before it begins to bother you will prevent an emergency visit to deal with discomfort in the future, which always happen at an inconvenient time."
- Don't forget to use belief windows and storytelling.

4. **Fear** – Patient says, "I'm too anxious to do that." Money, trust, and sense of urgency often mask the objection of fear, so the patient could also say "I can't afford it" or "I'll think about it" or "I'll wait on that."

Responses:

- "We have solutions that allow you to have what you want performed comfortably, will little or no memory of the appointment."
- "Your comfort is our first concern. We won't do anything unless you're completely comfortable."
- Don't forget to use belief windows and storytelling.

The Role of Storytelling in Case Acceptance

Perhaps there is no better way to make a case for any point than telling a story. A story is much more effective in making the case for moving forward with treatment than simply enumerating the advantages and disadvantages of accepting treatment. The narrator creates a movie picture in the mind of the listener and draws the listener in to an account of a previous individual who made a decision like the listener is contemplating.

THE KEY CONCEPT

The Key Concept of Storytelling – Telling a story is an excellent way to make a point. People are drawn into an account of someone like them who faced a similar challenge and overcame it. Every good story has a hero, a plot, and a point to be made. The point can precede the story or follow the story. Make a point, tell a story – tell a story, make a point.

Here's an example of storytelling in the context of case acceptance:

"Mrs. Jones, I know this is a big decision for you. I also know, based on what you've told me, that having a healthy, attractive smile will make a big difference in your life. I'm reminded of a patient

of ours who recently had a similar situation as you have and faced a similar decision. He decided to move forward with the recommended treatment, and it turned out great. I can show you some pictures of his case, and you can hear his testimonial. When his treatment was completed, he said what we hear all too often, 'I wish I had done this sooner.'"

Case Acceptance is Team Driven

Everyone on the practice team plays a vital role in a patient moving forward with treatment. Any weak link along the way can become an obstacle to successful case acceptance. All team members who interact with the patient must be committed to the patient saying yes to treatment that will make the patient healthier and happier with their oral condition. Larger practices may employ the Patient Care Specialist (PCS) covered in the system, "Quality of New Patients" (system #3 of the 12 Production Systems). The PCS specializes in new patient interaction and plays a large part in case acceptance with those who have the most production potential for the practice.

Not All Case Presentations End in Acceptance

When it comes to case acceptance, no one has a 100% acceptance rate. The presenter needs to adopt an attitude of realizing the word "No" sometimes means "not now" rather than "never." Case presentations are often seeds that the presenter sows that eventually bear fruit.

The Morbidity & Mortality (M&M) Meeting

This meeting is held once a month and is attended by the owners, the scheduling coordinator(s), the team leaders of each department, and the patient care specialist (if applicable). The purpose of the meeting is to analyze those case presentations that did not result in case acceptance (i.e., treatment not scheduled). In this instance, the M&M term, borrowed from the medical profession that describes undesirable outcomes, is applied to the most undesirable outcome of case presentation – treatment not scheduled.

The scheduling coordinator (or the PCS if applicable) facilitates the meeting and prepares a spreadsheet called the Case Acceptance Tracking (CAT) form (see next page for an example). This form lists all new patients seen in the office since the last M&M meeting, the amount of treatment presented, the amount of treatment scheduled, and comments related to why any treatment is not scheduled. The scheduling coordinator reviews each patient who has not scheduled, and anyone who has direct knowledge of the patient can comment and ask questions.

The ultimate goal of the meeting is to determine why treatment was not accepted, what could have been done differently, and what might still be done to recapture the unscheduled dentistry. Everyone in attendance should leave with an action plan designed to improve their department's case acceptance systems, as well as what they can still do to gain acceptance with the patients mentioned in the meeting.

MONITORS FOR CASE ACCEPTANCE

- Value of a new patient
- Production
- Collections
- Overhead %
- Practice profitability

Case Acceptance Tracking Spreadsheet

SUNRISE DENTAL SOLUTIONS **CASE ACCEPTANCE TRACKING (CAT)** SUNRISE DENTAL SOLUTIONS

Johnstown Center Dental Care | **Dr. Williams** | **JANUARY NEW PATIENT CAT 1-31-20**

	PATIENT	INS	DR.	REFERRAL	NPE DATE	TXPLAN$	SCHED $	APPT. DATES	COMPL $	ACTION ITEM / COMMENTS
1	Patient #1		MW	Patient	04/01/20	$ 6.750	$ 4.400	1- 4 H, 1- 4 D	$ 4.400	
2	Patient #2	SJC	MW	Gift Card	04/01/20	$ 8.120	$ 1.340	1-11 D	$ 1.340	
3	Patient #3		MW	Gift Card	05/01/20	$ 3.390	$ -	-	$ -	LMOC, spoke with mom
4	Patient #4	SJC	MJC	TV	05/01/20	$ 2.596	$ 2.596	1-13 H, 1-13 D	$ 2.596	
5	Patient #5		MW	Reactivated	06/01/20	$ 19.556	$ 4.200	1-11 H	$ 4.200	sedation paperwork completed
6	Patient #6		MW	Reactivated	11/01/20	$ 20.140	$ 10.556	1-19 D	$ 10.556	lower veneers & bridge
7	Patient #7	IBM	MW	Internet	11/01/20	$ 42.314	$ 22.226	2-14 D	$ -	
8	Patient #8	UMR	MW	Internet	11/01/20	$ 1.250	$ 1.250	1-11 H	$ 549	
9	Patient #9		MW	Gift Card	12/01/20	$ 4.750	$ 1.750	1-19 H	$ 1.750	
10	Patient #10		MW	Internet	12/01/20	$ 5.126	$ 1.390	1-20 H, 1-21 D	$ 1.390	
11	Patient #11		CAW	Reactivated	12/01/20	$ 17.765	$ -	-	$ -	LMOC
12	Patient #12		MW	Patient	13/01/20	$ 29.000	$ 21.751	2-3 D	$ -	
13	Patient #13	Mlife	MW	Gift Card	13/01/20	$ 6.652	$ 1.426	1-20 D	$ 1.426	
14	Patient #14	SJC	MW	Professional	14/01/20	$ 10.629	$ 10.629	1-21 D	$ 10.629	
15	Patient #15		MW	Internet	14/01/20	$ 23.565	$ 1.400	2-2 H	$ -	
16	Patient #16	NAA	MW	Internet	18/01/20	$ 1.900	$ 1.900	2-15 D	$ -	
17	Patient #17		MW	Internet	18/01/20	$ 6.552	$ 650	1-18 H	$ 650	spoke with wife, he will sched. Perio & resins
18	Patient #18	Mlife	MW	Patient	19/01/20	$ 8.146	$ 7.504	2-2 H, 2-9 D	$ -	
19	Patient #19		MW	Internet	19/01/20	$ 6.806	$ 2.700	3-5 D	$ -	
20	Patient #20	Hum	MW	Gift Card	20/01/20	$ 2.502	$ 2.037	2-4 D	$ -	
21	Patient #21	SJC	MW	Internet	20/01/20	$ 4.440	$ 2.244	2-19-D	$ -	
22	Patient #22	Mlife	MW	TV	21/01/20	$ 7.188	$ -		$ -	6MS, $$ issue
	TOTALS				22	$ 239.137	$ 101.949		$ 39.486	
	Scheduled Case Acceptance Percentage				**43%**	Measures Case Acceptance by Treatment Scheduled to Date				
	Treated Case Acceptance Percentage				**17%**	Measures Case Acceptance by Treatment Completed to Date				

SCHEDULED CASE ACCEPTANCE

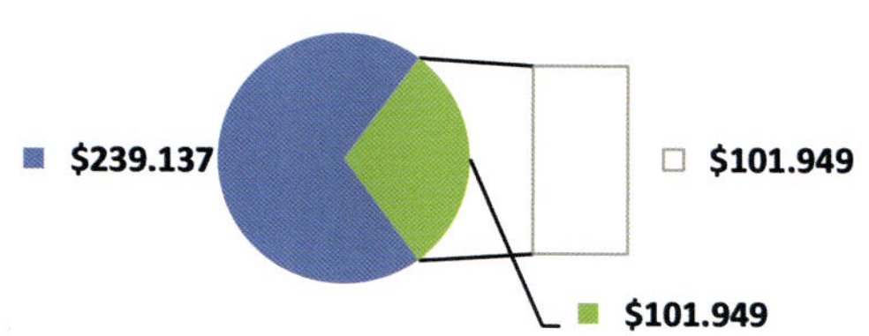

TREATED CASE ACCEPTANCE

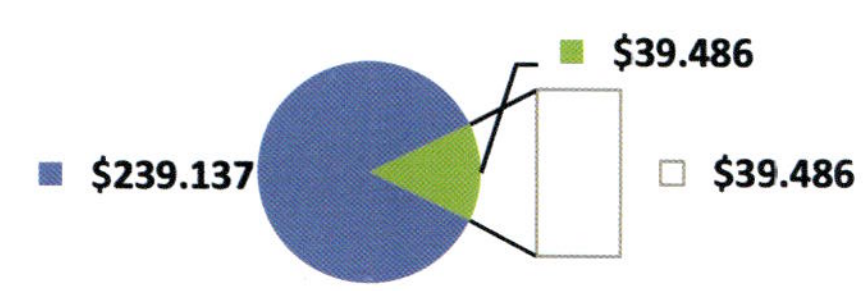

Production System #3 – Quality of New Patients

They must want it before you can produce it. Even in the presence of good diagnosis and case acceptance technique, if patients need, want, or can afford very little, then their value to the production of the practice is small. Given that the lion's share of production per patient is performed during a patient's first nine months after they enter the practice, *having more new patients with a higher production value is a key to being highly productive.* Practice location, local market conditions, the kind of dentistry offered, and marketing will all affect the quality of new patients.

Patients who have the potential to become high quality patients have one or more of the following characteristics: 1. They don't have a dentist because they are new to the area, 2. They have a dentist and are receiving regular care, but are under-treated because their dentist doesn't provide services they need and/or want, or 3. They haven't been receiving dental treatment because the dental team didn't know how to lead the patient from "need" to "want" (case acceptance).

THREE WAYS TO INCREASE THE NUMBER OF HIGH-QUALITY NEW PATIENTS

1. **Provide highly productive services.** These are procedures that many dentists don't provide, yet a high percentage of the population wants and needs. This includes full-mouth rehabilitation, replacement of teeth with implant solutions, cosmetic dentistry, and treating the highly-anxious patient who has not received professional care for years.
2. **Market for highly productive services.** The formula for effective marketing is the right message, to the right people, the right number of times. The most effective marketing message for any dental practice is what makes them different from anyone else. If that difference involves providing highly productive services, and that message is directed to a population who are most likely to need and be able to afford those services, then the best results can be achieved. Targeting that population involves internal marketing within the practice through patients who have received that care, and external marketing utilizing demographics such as income, age, and education.
3. **Increase the quality of the new-patient experience.** The directly proportional relationship between the quality of the new patient experience and the quality of the new patient is often overlooked. Because of this, some practices invest in a new patient "specialist" within the office who is accountable for making the patient's first visit to the practice "over the top."

The Patient Care Specialist

Many dentists cite the ability to afford dentistry as the number one characteristic that defines a high-quality new patient, but the new-patient experience can define the high-quality patient, too. The new-patient experience is also critically important to internal marketing for the practice. Because of this, some practices invest in a new patient or patient care specialist.

The Patient Care Specialist (PCS) contacts the new patient the day before their visit to welcome them, ask if they have any concerns, and inquire about what the practice could do to make their first visit special.

On the day of the first visit, the PCS greets the patient when they arrive at the office and gives them a tour, highlighting the team and other unique attributes of the practice. The PCS performs an emotional exam, gathering their chief complaint, SWOT (strengths, weaknesses, opportunities, and threats), DBM (dominant buying motive), emotional treasure, DISC profile, and belief windows. The PCS may also gather clinical information such as charting existing restorations, decay, periodontal probing, and, when appropriate, prophylaxis. (This is one reason that many PCSs are hygienists.) While PCSs may not be qualified to diagnose dental disease, they may have the ability to suggest likely treatment recommendations by the dentist, setting the stage for case presentation and acceptance.

The PCS meets with the dentist prior to the dentist seeing the patient, providing the dentist with all of the pertinent information, so that the dentist's time with the new patient is efficient and effective. If a treatment plan is determined during this first visit, the PCS stays with the new patient during financial arrangements and scheduling, ready to assist the patient to stay committed in case any obstacles to following through with treatment are encountered.

Finally, the PCS facilitates the monthly M&M Meeting (see Production System #2 - Case Acceptance).

MONITORS FOR QUALITY OF NEW PATIENTS

- Value of a new patient
- Sources of new patients
- Production
- Collections
- Collection rate
- Adjustments
- Overhead %
- Practice profitability

Production System #4 – Quantity of New Patients

There must be enough opportunities for you to produce it. New patients are the lifeblood of any practice. Not only do the patients in the practice need to accept and follow through with treatment, but there also needs to be enough of them to ensure a productive schedule. It's a numbers game - the more new patients you have, the more opportunities you have to be productive.

A practice establishes a dominant market presence by creating a healthy flow of new patients and offering a unique experience that patients aren't likely to find anywhere else.

The flow of new patients into the practice always begins with a first encounter. What my experience from working with hundreds of dentists over three decades tells me is that the quality of that first experience with the office, whether it be a walk-in patient or a telephone call, is pivotal to new-patient flow into the practice. Unfortunately for many practices, that initial experience is often mishandled. The initial experience is a system. As with any good system, a designated individual accountable for the performance of that system makes a positive difference.

The Receptionist

This role, which is sometimes coupled with another role in the business office (scheduling coordinator, financial coordinator), or elevated in the larger practice to a practice concierge, is primarily accountable for patient intake. This person needs to be a "people-person," with a welcoming smile and a warm and friendly demeanor. In the DISC Personality Profile, they are the prototypical "S" personality. They need to remember names and be ready with a conversation that communicates caring for the patient as a person. They are the practice's designated chief officer of first impressions. They may also be responsible for other roles in the business office, including scheduling patients and collecting money. Their skill as communicators makes them the best team member to take and receive incoming and outgoing phone calls.

Telephone Etiquette

The telephone might be the most important piece of equipment in the dental office. The telephone conversation is the most often the first point of personal contact with incoming new patients, and it is a recurring interaction with existing ones. Telephone communication must be handled expertly if the impression on the patient is to be positive. Prospective patients can be lost at this critical juncture in the relationship-building process, and most dentists have no idea this is happening in their practice.

A GREAT TELEPHONE CALL CONSISTS OF THREE THINGS

1. **A real person answers within three rings**. Nothing says cold and impersonal like an automated message that makes the caller listen to a menu of choices that mostly have nothing to do with what the caller wants. If the phone cannot be answered within three rings, a voice message should say, "Thank you for calling <Practice Name>. All our team members are currently taking care of patients. However, your call is very important to us. Just as soon as someone is available, we will return your call. Please leave your name and a phone number so we can return your call just as soon as possible. Thank you for calling and we look forward to speaking with you soon."
2. **The caller is greeted by a "smiling voice."** There should be a mirror next to every phone in the business office, so that the team member answering the phone can look into the mirror and smile before picking up the phone receiver. That smile sets the tone for the voice that answers the call. For years we've used the greeting, "It's a great day at <Practice Name>. This is <Team Member Name>. I can help you." No matter what the caller is inquiring about, that greeting sets the tone.
3. **The call accomplishes a positive purpose**. On behalf of our dentist clients, we have recorded hundreds of incoming calls from people pretending to be prospective patients. Unfortunately, many of these calls never resulted in practice personnel asking the caller to make an appointment. Whatever the reason a patient or prospective patient calls the practice, the call should not end until a positive outcome is reached for both the caller and the practice.

MONITORS FOR QUANTITY OF NEW PATIENTS

- Production
- Collections
- Number of new patients
- Overhead %
- Practice profitability

Production System #5 – Schedule Efficiency

The day's potential must be maximized for you to produce more. Scheduling, like everything else that happens in a practice, can be reduced to a system.

You control the schedule, or the schedule controls you. Patients should be placed into the schedule primarily to accomplish one thing for the business – to accomplish the practice's daily goal.

To accomplish this, the scheduling coordinator must place emphasis on building the schedule around productive appointments. This requires training for the team and support on the part of the practice leader.

The Scheduling Coordinator

This may be the most important position in any dental practice because a practice cannot collect more than it produces and cannot produce more than it schedules. The scheduling coordinator is primarily accountable for scheduling each provider to reach their production goal. In larger practices with multiple doctors and hygienists, this role should be divided into scheduling coordinators for both the doctor and hygiene departments, and in even larger practices, multiple doctor scheduling coordinators.

In the DISC Personality Profile system, this individual should have a "D-C-I oriented profile" (in that order). They should take control of the schedule, be analytical enough to *schedule to a predetermined number*, and be influential enough to make people feel good about the appointment time the scheduling coordinator *has chosen for them*. How efficiently the scheduling coordinator schedules to goal is dictated by how well he/she manages the scheduling system.

Scheduling Systems

In my experience as a practice owner as well as a consultant, I have seen many types of scheduling systems. Most involve templates or "blocks" to ensure that certain types of appointments are reserved space in the schedule. These types of appointments may be a certain procedure, or a certain level of productivity based on dollar value. When it comes to levels of productivity, the concept of Rock, Sand, and Water is often applied.

THE KEY CONCEPT

The Key Concept of Rock, Sand, and Water - The rock, sand, and water metaphor has been applied to many aspects of life. The teaching exercise for the concept involves a jar, and a combination of three components to fill that jar - rocks, sand, and water. Rocks represent the most important things to accomplish the purpose of filling the jar. Sand, while necessary, has less value, and water which is also necessary, represents the least value of all. The basic premise is that in order to accomplish the most, and more importantly accomplish the most important first, rocks need to go into the jar first, followed by sand, and lastly by water. In terms of a dental practice, the jar represents the schedule, rocks represent highly productive appointments, sand represents less productive appointments, and water represents appointments that have no production when it comes to dollar value. Since the purpose of a schedule is to schedule to goal, then highly productive appointments (rocks) must go in first, followed by less productive ones.

Goal-Focused Scheduling

This is a term I coined years ago for a modified version of traditional template scheduling with rock, sand, and water. The modification involves two things:

1. Elimination of templates and blocks, since they often prevent the scheduling coordinator from accomplishing the ***true purpose of scheduling - to schedule to production goals arrived at by the budget process***.
2. A relentless mindset to scheduling to goal. Remember, ***the goal is not to make providers busy. It is not to fill all the openings in the schedule***. The focus must be single-minded in purpose - to schedule to goal.

This is where many practices go awry when scheduling. They place more focus on patient care or patient convenience. Do not misinterpret the meaning of the previous statement. Patient care is the ultimate purpose of the practice, and convenience is important to patient satisfaction, attraction, and retention. But assembling a daily schedule that reaches production goals does not have to come at the expense of patient care and convenience.

Most practices, in their effort to make the schedule all about taking care of the patient, lose total control over it. Either the patient controls the schedule, or the practice controls the schedule.

Patient care can be accomplished in a convenient manner, while creating a schedule that addresses business objectives.

Therefore, for a practice to schedule to goal, the first appointments that are placed in any day's schedule are highly productive ones (rocks). The numerical value of these appointments is determined by the budget-arrived-at goal, and should be at least forty percent of that daily goal. No less-productive appointments (sand) should be placed in that day's schedule until the daily goal is at least eighty percent full. No non-productive appointments (water) should be placed in that day's schedule until the day is scheduled to at least one hundred percent of its daily goal.

Scheduling coordinators are often anxious about implementing a system so highly dependent on highly productive appointments. This is where the leadership of the practice needs to affirm its commitment to the system and assure the scheduling coordinator that the ownership and team will take collective responsibility for generating those highly productive appointments (see production systems quantity and quality of new patients, diagnosis, treatment mix, and case acceptance).

Goal-focused scheduling, when fully implemented, is often responsible for a fifteen-percent or more increase in daily production.

THE FOUR REQUIREMENTS FOR THE GOAL-FOCUSED SCHEDULING SYSTEM TO BE SUCCESSFUL:

1. Understanding the why and how of the goal-focused system
2. Leadership in the form of commitment to and accountability for the success of the goal-focused system
3. A consistent number of highly productive appointments in the scheduling queue
4. Control of canceled and failed appointments

Controlling Canceled and Failed Appointments

While all the previous four components for the success of the goal-focused schedule are required, the fourth is the most common missing ingredient. The reason for goal-focused scheduling is obvious, it's a simple system and implementation is straightforward, and when new-patient flow and case acceptance is ample, the only thing left is for the patients to show up as scheduled. However, in practices all over the country, schedules consistently fall apart at the last minute, leading to loss of production and associated profit, along with frustration and even a feeling of hopelessness at the lack of control caused by this scheduling misadventure.

First, you must accept that canceled and failed appointments cannot be completely avoided. They will occur despite your best efforts and systems. Secondly, you need to understand that there are very good reasons for a patient to miss an appointment that are largely out of anyone's control. What you can do is control these scheduling misadventures enough so that they are an uncommon occurrence, especially when it comes to the most highly productive appointments. This requires an understanding of why they occur, as well as what can be done to reduce their occurrence.

The Six Reasons Why Canceled and Failed Appointments Occur and Their Solutions

1. **Not *requiring* patients to keep their appointment**. The mindset and actions of your team are more important than any other factor in enforcing practice policies regarding patients being held to a standard regarding keeping appointments. First, you must appreciate the value of the care you provide and communicate that. Policies need to be effectively conveyed verbally as well as in writing and need to be prominently displayed in the office. Secondly, you must understand the significance of missed appointments to the practice and business objectives. What is the cost to the practice? The practice owner should ask

his/her team this important question, because it often fails to register as a problem, and even is looked forward to by some team members who think the cost/benefit of a missed appointment is irrelevant to them whether the patient shows up or not.

That appointment time is valuable – to the patient, to the practice, and to everyone involved in the practice. Each time increment is worth something, as it is parcel of time that the practice could have provided care. If it is lost, it affects that patient, another patient that could have been seen during that time but is now lost, and the business, which ultimately affects all who benefit from the business, not just the owner.

There is another way to look at a scheduled appointment that is not as practical but rather more principled.

When an appointment is scheduled with a patient, a commitment is made by both parties. The practice makes a promise to set aside time and all that comes with that (including being on time), and in return the practice asks that the patient honor that promise as well. Not until each team member understands the critical importance of a patient honoring their appointment will the practice be able to control canceled and failed appointments.

2. **Not placing value on the appointment**. Can anyone imagine forgetting about or not showing up for their wedding? How about a date with someone special? Or an appointment to look at a house that they are excited about possibly buying? While these may seem like ridiculous analogies in comparison to keeping a dental appointment, they underscore an important element in the missed dental appointment dynamic:

   People place the most importance on those things that are important to them.

   It also highlights something else: the most important things have an emotional component tied to them.

   Therefore,

   You should not expect your patients to want to keep their appointment any more than you communicate to them the importance of doing so.

   This is most often a problem with hygiene appointments. When, you use words like "cleanings," especially since hygiene appointments occur on a recurring basis, you risk communicating the comparison to haircuts or car washes. When however, you use words and phrases like, "treating infection," "preventing the recurrence of infection, which leads to bone loss, tooth loss, bad breath, and other health problems," "it is important to keep you on a tight schedule of preventive and therapeutic treatment in order to address *your* disease so that you don't incur costly and preventable invasive treatment in the future," you convey importance. The idea is not to scare people, but to honestly communicate the associated risks and benefits of recommended care.

3. **Not establishing financial arrangements in advance**. It is not surprising that some patients reschedule or fail their appointment for financial reasons. By either paying in advance, not having an existing balance, or having clear financial arrangements made ahead of the appointment, the likelihood of canceling or missing an appointment is lessened.

All patients must pay for their treatment in advance or at time of treatment. When scheduling an appointment, the patient should be notified of their financial responsibility. If this involves insurance and the office accepts assignment of benefits, then the patient should be told that their cost at time of treatment is an estimate. The only exception to this is when the patient is rescheduled for hygiene recare. When appointments are made in person, financial arrangements should be made in writing and signed for all treatment over $300. When the appointment is made by any other means, financial arrangements should be signed prior to treatment.

The biggest impact advance financial arrangements can have on reducing missed appointments is when payment is made in advance. This one policy can do more to prevent last-minute schedule adjustments for highly productive appointments than anything else.

Payment in advance is recommended for all procedures that involve sedation (not counting nitrous oxide when used as the sole sedative agent), all procedures that are two hours in length or more, and all procedures involving more than $2,000 in treatment. The office may choose to collect from fifty percent to one hundred percent of the appointment value. All sedation appointments should be collected at one hundred percent. If the office accepts insurance assignment, then the patient's portion is the chosen percentage of the patient's estimated portion after insurance.

4. **Not confirming the appointment in advance**. I must admit that I've wrestled with this one for as long as I've been a practice owner. What I eventually decided was that I had to accept that my own values regarding keeping appointments are not that common in our modern-day culture.

   When I make an appointment, it goes into my calendar which I check daily. I don't miss appointments. I don't need anyone to contact me to remind me of my responsibilities. It would take a very good reason for me to miss an appointment, and it would mortify me to fail to show up for an appointment without adequate notice. But alas, those beliefs are not as common as they used to be. Therefore, for the sake of the practice schedule, *all appointments should be confirmed forty-eight hours in advance.*

   Patients should be given the option of having their appointment confirmed by email, text, phone call, or any combination of the three. Whatever the confirmation method, if not handled correctly it can be an invitation for the patient to cancel or reschedule. The language should not be in the form of a question – "Do you plan on keeping your appointment?" It should be a declaration – "This is a friendly reminder of your appointment with our office on _______ (date and time). We look forward to seeing you then."

5. **Not having repercussions for missing the appointment**. *We teach people how to treat us.* If a patient can miss their appointment, and get another similar appointment whenever they want, without any negative consequences, then why shouldn't a patient not show or reschedule when they don't want to come to an appointment for any reason?

   There must be repercussions: they won't be able to reschedule when they want, or they will be charged for a missed appointment without adequate notice, or they won't be rescheduled at all.

If a scheduled patient should call to cancel or reschedule, the way the office representative responds is critical to controlling cancellations and failures. Without a doubt my biggest aggravation of all time has been walking by my business office and hearing my team member taking a cancellation call and saying, "Would you like to reschedule?" Nothing *says your appointment wasn't important anyway, or we're okay whether or not you re-schedule* than that question. In fact, the exact opposite of that should happen.

The conversation should go as follows:

- Start with "Oh dear, are you quite sure you can't make this appointment?" while pulling up the patient's records.
- If canceling or rescheduling forty-eight hours or less before the appointment: "As you know, we require forty-eight-hours' notice to change an appointment."
- If rescheduling more than forty-eight hours before the appointment: "Waiting longer to address _______________ (referring to the patient's record) can result in more problems."
- If canceling without rescheduling more than forty-eight hours before the appointment: "This is an important appointment (referring to the patient's record) for the following reason - ________________," and "I know that _______________ (name of provider – doctor or hygienist) will be sorry to hear you canceled your appointment."

As you can see, the office representative needs to be knowledgeable about dental care and the negative impact of not having it performed as originally scheduled.

If the patient insists on rescheduling the appointment, they should not be given another appointment within the next two weeks. In fact, the longer the patient must wait for the rescheduled appointment, the better, even if one is available before then. The office can always call the patient back later if an appointment is available sooner.

The key is to send a message that rescheduling except for understandably good reasons is unacceptable. If they cancel without rescheduling, a reminder should be made to call them within two weeks if they do not call back and reschedule. Whether they reschedule or cancel, an entry in their patient record regarding the circumstances around the event should be made.

If the communication occurs electronically, via text or email, then the response from the practice is the same, except the office should respond by phone whenever possible. Texts and emails are poorer methods of communication and can send an unintended message. However, if this is the only way of communicating, then it is better than no response at all.

The decision to charge the patient a fee for canceling or rescheduling an appointment without forty-eight hours' notice, or when the patient fails their appointment, depends on several factors. One may be supply and demand. If a practice has minimal competition from other dental offices, is at or near capacity, and has high demand, then notifying the patient in the beginning of the relationship that there is a fee for missed appointments makes good sense. Any ill will is offset by the added leverage the office has in these circumstances.

Many offices do not have the benefit of supply and demand on their side, therefore the charge for missed appointments is used selectively. For example, long procedures (that are not prepaid in advance) that last two or more hours are examples of appointments that would incur a missed appointment charge if the patient failed to notify the practice with reasonable notice. Another example is a patient who has become a repeat offender.

Many offices are hesitant to charge a patient for not showing up for their appointment, fearing the resulting ill will to be greater than the cost of the missed appointment. After all, the barber or the nail salon doesn't charge for a missed appointment. While that may be true, the airline docs, and more and more healthcare professionals are, as well. Seldom is the charge the actual amount of loss the business incurs, and often the charge isn't even collected. The purpose of the charge is more about enforcing the rules of the working relationship and establishing a mindset on the part of the patient that keeping appointments is not just preferred, appreciated, or expected, but required.

The amount of the charge can range from a set amount per unit time (most often) to the entire cost of the appointment (seldom and on a selected case basis). It is not uncommon for a patient to refuse to pay for a missed appointment charge, and it is usually a good idea to not pursue an overdue amount for this charge, but to write it off as "bad debt." When this is done, an entry should be made in the patient's record, and the account flagged as one in which special financial accommodations must be met for all future scheduled appointments, should the practice decide to maintain the patient in the practice.

6. **Allowing repeat offenders to repeat**. As mentioned previously, we teach people how to treat us. If you have informed people in advance of your cancellation/failure policy, and they violate it, then they should be reminded. If they violate it a second time, then they should get another chance with a different policy – appointments are only scheduled if paid for in advance. If they violate it a third time, then they can no longer be a part of the practice. To those who feel this policy is too severe, I would suggest that you very likely have several patients who are repeat offenders, yet you continue to lament the fact that you have a cancellation/failure problem.

At the core of any successful relationship is trust. My father taught me at a young age the value of keeping your word. It was in the context of being on time. He said,

"Son, don't put your trust in someone who is late for an appointment. They've already lied to you once."

The same applies to patients who habitually run late or, worse, cancel at the last minute or fail to show. They've broken trust. That's not to say that they can't earn back trust over time, but for the time being, you have learned something about them. Not learning the lesson is on you. Fool me once, shame on you; fool me twice, shame on me.

MONITORS FOR SCHEDULE EFFICIENCY

- Production
- Collections
- Overhead %
- Practice profitability

Production System #6 – Facility

The physical space must not be an obstacle to production potential. How much dentistry can be produced is largely dependent upon how much physical capacity exists, especially the number of treatment rooms. Likewise, the number of treatment rooms determines to a large extent how many new patients a practice can accept.

If proper staffing and demand are in place, the best investment a practice can make in tapping its future production potential is adding more treatment rooms.

This is where the concept of demand and capacity come into play. They are connected: More demand requires expanding capacity to meet that demand. More capacity requires increasing demand to meet that capacity.

What I see in many dental practices is that capacity limits demand, slowing down or halting growth and preventing the practice from becoming more. Highly productive practices increase capacity as demand warrants it. The most productive practices increase capacity *before* demand warrants it.

I realize that just adding more treatment rooms will not by itself increase production. You will need a plan for additional staffing, as well as filling those rooms with additional productive treatment. However, if you do, this is almost always the best investment a dental practice owner can make in his/her business. This applies to both expanding an existing facility or acquiring a new one.

MONITORS FOR FACILITY

- Production
- Collections
- New patients
- Overhead %
- Practice profitability

Production system #7 – Treatment Mix

The type of procedures scheduled must be as productive as possible. Some procedures are more productive than others. I have already touched on treatment mix as a means to a more productive schedule in the section on the Quality New Patient and Scheduling Efficiency.

Most dentists, if asked to describe their ideal day, would not describe a busy day, as busy days are often full of low- or non-productive procedures. A busy practice does not necessarily translate into a productive practice. The ideal day is one filled with productive procedures.

On the Production Wheel, arranging the schedule to perform more productive procedures per unit of time has the biggest impact on practice production vs. effort expended.

A highly productive procedure is one in which 40% or more of a provider's daily production goal can be accomplished in a single appointment. Adding these procedures through continuing education, learning how to present and gain acceptance for these treatments, and marketing targeted to attract the patients who need and want these services, are all necessary to produce more dentistry per unit of time.

Procedures such as cosmetic dentistry (anterior crowns and porcelain veneers), implant dentistry (placement and prosthetics), quadrant or full arch crown and bridge, and sedation dentistry where full mouth rehabilitation is performed, are examples of productive appointments.

Keep in mind that providing more productive procedures also requires capacity in the schedule to perform them. This is where the use of expanded duty assistants (when applicable) and associate dentists can play an important role in allowing the schedule to include highly productive procedures.

MONITORS FOR TREATMENT MIX

- Production
- Collections
- Overhead %
- Practice profitability

Production system #8 – Team Quantity

The practice must have enough team members to be productive. Understaffing reduces the capacity to schedule more dentistry. Along with adding treatment rooms, adding additional team members has the most potential to increase capacity, allowing for more productivity.

Years of consulting have revealed two things regarding team quantity: 1. Most practices are understaffed, especially in the business office, and 2. The most successful practices staff for the schedule they want, not the one they have.

Some of the telltale signs of an understaffed business office are rising accounts receivable, too many statements being sent, decreasing new patients, and an unproductive schedule. Most practice owners, due to their limited exposure and understanding, have no idea what a typical day is like in their business office – incoming and outgoing calls, checking patients in and out, collecting money over the counter, processing payments by mail, handling insurance claims, making accounts receivable calls, confirming appointments, rebuilding the schedule, making financial arrangements, and more.

There isn't any formula for how many business office team members a practice should have, as there are too many variables that affect that number. There should be well-defined roles that address the most important roles the business office accomplishes – scheduling to goal, collecting money, and answering the telephone. If any of these systems is not being performed at a high level, the question of whether that is due to manpower must be addressed and, if applicable, team members must be added. Too often, the decision to add team members comes down to some rule of thumb percentage of staff salaries, when adding more team members will actually reduce the percentage of collections paid to staff salaries, as additional manpower will increase collections.

Regarding clinical staffing, the amount of dentistry that can be performed is often as simple as how many hands are available to perform it. Just as with business office staffing, there isn't a formula for how many clinical team members are optimal for most practices. But if there is an opportunity to add capacity, and there is demand or a viable plan to create it, then more team members make sense when more production is the goal.

What often comes to mind when the practice owner considers adding additional team members is that more team members mean more stress. What they are really saying is more people means more people to manage. That's where raising the leadership game of the owner must happen, a big part of which is developing leadership in others. Practices with multiple members in each area – the business office, the assistant department, and the hygiene department – will benefit from having team leaders who are accountable for the success of their departments, and for managing the members of their teams. This removes much if not all the management burden from the practice owner, who can focus more on leading the practice instead of managing it. Much more information about Department Team Leaders can be found in the Leadership chapter.

MONITORS FOR TEAM QUANTITY

- Production
- Collections
- New patients
- Accounts receivable
- Overhead %
- Practice profitability

Production System #9 – Team Quality

The team must be doing the right things the right way to be productive. Your success depends more on the people you surround yourself with than you.

Most dentists would rather invest in honing their clinical skills, or adding technology, or working harder, when investing in the quality of their team would bring a greater return than any of those things.

In my coaching of dental practice owners, I spend most of my time addressing team member issues. At least half of those issues have more to do with the leadership of the practice owner than the team member. But when it is the team member, the practice owner has likely chosen the wrong person, and it is unlikely that the wrong person can ever become the right person.

Early in my working relationship with dental practice owners I ask them to name the most important qualities of an ideal team member. Most of the time the answers can be narrowed down to three things: skills, experience, and attitude. I call these the "Three A's" – Ability, Aptitude, and Attitude. These qualities were defined and explained in the Team chapter.

I then ask the owner to rate each one of their present team members in these three categories on a scale of 1-10, where 1 is awful and 10 is the very best.

Once they're finished, I ask them two more questions: 1. On a scale of 1-10, what kind of practice do you want? They always say "10." (Quite frankly, if they said anything other than "10," our working relationship would be over.)

Then I ask them the second question – How are you going to have a "10" practice with team members who are fives, or sixes, or sevens? Only if those team members rate low in aptitude do you have a chance of raising their number.

I realize that "10" quality individuals aren't common, which has a lot to do with why "10" quality dental practices are not common, either.

I also realize that the "10" team member comes at a high price.

The great thing about high-quality team members is this: it's nearly impossible to overpay them. If they want more, they will become more. However long it takes, whatever you must do, don't compromise on the quality of your team.

MONITORS FOR TEAM QUALITY

- Production
- Collections
- Collection rate
- Accounts receivable
- New patients
- Practice expenses
- Overhead %
- Practice profitability

Production System #10 – Fees

The practice must charge the patient appropriately for its services. Raising fees periodically to account for rising costs, and to reflect higher levels of care, makes sense.

Dental practice owners have invested much in their training, technology, team, and facility, among other costs, to provide high-level care. It is more expensive to be educated in and practice dentistry than any other healthcare profession. Factors such as student debt, a proliferation of dental service organizations, an oversupply of dentists, and discounted fee plans make the average salary of a dentist not representative of the value of the service they provide.

It's a good thing you aren't average. Another good thing is that dentists can make choices that allow them to become more, and, as a result, make more. One of these choices is what they charge for the services they provide. Certainly, those fees should be within the realm of fees charged in the marketplace in which they practice. Dentists should decide what percentile of that group represents the value of services they provide.

The highly productive dental practice should be charging at the 80th percentile or higher for their area.

Reports on what dentists are charging for dental procedures for a zip code are easily obtained. Correcting a fee schedule deficiency makes for increased production without working more or harder, or incurring any additional expenses.

It is better to raise fees a modest amount every year than to raise them a large amount every few years. Raising fees is usually not giving the practice a raise, but rather keeping pace with dental inflation, the average annual increase in the cost of providing dental services. On average, this increase amounts to four percent annualized, but will be more during periods of higher than average inflation.

MONITORS FOR FEES

- Production
- Collections
- Overhead %
- Practice profitability

Production System #11 – Quantity of Days Worked

You must be present enough to produce enough. Even if the days worked by the practice are productive, if not enough days are worked to meet monthly practice goals, the practice is unproductive relative to its needs. Therefore, practices must have enough provider days in order to accomplish financial objectives. Part of creating a practice budget is planning how many provider days the practice needs to meet these objectives.

The good news is that the owner dentist doesn't have to be present for the practice to be productive. Adding providers - hygienists and associates - increases the quantity of days worked without the practice owner working more days. This is the concept of leverage.

As a dental practice owner transitions their practice into one that has more cash flow and equity value, adding associate dentists that may become partners allows the practice owner to retain ownership, while maintaining control over business decisions and work schedule.

MONITORS FOR QUANTITY OF DAYS

- Production
- Collections
- New patients
- Overhead %
- Practice profitability

Production System #12 – Clinical Speed

You must work efficiently to reach your production potential. If more dentistry can be produced in a shorter unit of time, then more dentistry can be scheduled per day, increasing capacity and the potential to consistently schedule to goal.

Producing more dentistry per unit of time is sometimes simply a factor of efficiency.

Being organized, properly equipped and supplied, focusing on more efficient delivery, and delegating as much as possible – all have a positive impact on making the most of the available time scheduled each day.

Efficiency in this sense refers to making better use of time, so we are not necessarily referring to working faster, although there is often room for dentists to do that. The standing joke about how fast a dentist works goes like this:

Question to dentist – "How long does it take you to do <insert any dental procedure>?"

Answer – "How long do I have?"

If you desire to make more, keep more, and enjoy more, you must understand the concept that dentists in private practice don't make more by providing great dental care, they make more by providing great dental care faster.

Dental practice owners should analyze the time they and other providers in the practice use for dental procedures and establish consistent standards and plans for maximizing clinical speed.

MONITORS FOR CLINICAL SPEED

- Production
- Collections
- New patients
- Overhead %
- Practice profitability

FINANCIAL SYSTEMS

While there are several business office systems critical to building the prosperous dental practice, the three most important are: scheduling to each provider's production goal, collecting money, and answering the telephone. In order to use these systems effectively, the business office must be organized appropriately. While well-defined roles are essential, all business office team members should be cross-trained and able to perform the duties of others in the event of an absence so that no area falls behind or suffers.

The Business Office Structure

As in other areas of the practice, the business office must be organized with updated job descriptions for each member of its team. Here, especially, the Key Concept of Accountability Versus Responsibility is especially important for the overall effectiveness of business office operations.

Every member of the team, whether they play their major role in the business office or not, is responsible for financial systems. The three most important systems (scheduling to goal, collecting money, and answering the telephone) require accountability for the three key business office roles – the Scheduling Coordinator for scheduling to goal, the Financial Coordinator for collections, and the Receptionist for answering the telephone and greeting patients. Job titles are important in identifying individual accountability. The Scheduling Coordinator and Receptionist positions have been described in the Production Systems section. Job descriptions for each are included in the Glossary.

The Financial Coordinator

The Financial Coordinator is accountable for all financial systems performed by the business office. This person needs to be completely committed to the financial goals of the business and the concept that the practice deserves to be compensated for the dentistry it performs. With this commitment, they can ask for payment with a confident attitude that leaves little to no room for any other response than payment in full. They take immense pride in collecting as much money as possible in advance or at the time of treatment, and delight in attaining the lowest accounts receivable amount possible. Each delinquent account collection is a victory for this individual. While the receptionist in the DISC personality profile is "S-oriented," and the scheduling coordinator is "D-C-I (in that order) oriented," the financial coordinator should be "C-D-I oriented." This person needs to be analytically inclined, but also have a sense of urgency and influential approach to the financial matters of the practice.

Collection Rate

Ideally, the dental practice should collect the same amount of money as the fee charged for the dentistry it produces. This ratio, called the Collection Rate, in the ideal scenario is 100%. It is the net collections divided by gross production. Collection Rate is one of the three components of *The Profitability Formula* covered earlier. The prosperous dental practice strives to attain the highest collection rate possible.

THE SIX FACTORS THAT HAVE THE GREATEST IMPACT ON COLLECTION RATE

1. Practice Financial Policy
2. Signed Financial Arrangements
3. Participation in Discounted Fee Plans
4. Insurance Management
5. Accounts Receivable Management
6. Adjustments Management

Collection Rate Factor #1 – Practice Financial Policy

The practice needs to fully implement a financial policy that reflects the vision and core values of the practice owner, and one that the team believes in and is committed to upholding.

All new patients should read and sign that they have read and will abide by the financial policy.

The key points to any practice financial policy are payment options; when payment is expected; penalties for delinquent payments; the relationship between the insurance carrier, the patient, and the office; penalties for late cancellations and failed appointments; and a signed statement that the patient has read, understands, and agrees to abide by the office policy. Here is an example of such a financial policy:

<NAME OF PRACTICE> FINANCIAL POLICY

Thank you for choosing <Name of Practice>. Our primary mission is to deliver the best and most comprehensive dental care available. An important part of our mission is making the cost of optimal care as easy and manageable as possible for our patients by offering several payment options.

PAYMENT OPTIONS:

Cash, Check, VISA, MasterCard, Discover, or American Express.

- We offer a 5% courtesy accounting adjustment to patients who pay for their treatment with cash or check in full, prior to the day of the appointment.
- Monthly payment options are available from CareCredit Healthcare Credit Card or The Lending Club. (Allows you to pay over time, with no annual fees or prepayment penalties. Subject to credit approval.)

PLEASE NOTE:

- We require payment prior to or at the time of your treatment. If you choose to discontinue care before treatment is complete, your refund will be determined upon review of your case.
- For procedures requiring more than 2 appointments, alternative arrangements may be provided. (Sedation appointments are not eligible for alternative arrangements.)
- For patients with dental insurance, we are happy to work with your insurance carrier to maximize your benefit and directly bill them for reimbursement for your treatment. However, if we do not receive payment from your insurance carrier within 45 days, you will be responsible for payment of your treatment fees and collection of your benefits directly from your insurance carrier.
- Any estimate of insurance benefits provided is an estimate only. We cannot guarantee payment from your insurance carrier.
- All fees and estimates given are valid for 60 days. Treatment and fees depend entirely on the condition of the mouth at the time services are rendered.
- Any balance that remains on your account for 60 days or more will be charged a finance charge of 1.5% per month, or 18% per annum of the balance, or $5.00, whichever is greater. The finance charge will accrue monthly until the balance has been paid or until the account has been forwarded to an outside collection agency.
- A fee of $80.00/hour is charged for patients who miss or cancel their appointment more than one time in a calendar year without a full 2 business days' notice.
- Patients scheduled for sedation must provide a full 3 business days' notice of cancellation, with a cancellation or missed appointment fee of $410.00.
- Patients scheduled for sedation are required to pay for their sedation appointment in full at least 2 weeks prior to their scheduled appointment date.
- We charge $25.00 for returned checks.

If you have any questions, please do not hesitate to ask. We are here to help you get the dentistry you want or need. By signing below, you confirm that you understand that you are financially responsible for any treatment completed by <Name of Practice>. You confirm that you understand the policies listed on this form and the information contained herein.

Signature: ______________________________ Date: ________________

Collection Rate Factor #2 – Signed Financial Arrangements

The objective is to collect as much as possible of the full fee for the dentistry planned prior to or at the time of treatment. It is essential that the patient is informed of the costs involved prior to treatment, that an arrangement for payment is made with the patient, and that the patient commits to that arrangement by signature. That arrangement should be payment in full, minus any estimated insurance reimbursement or adjustments, if the practice chooses to accept assignment of insurance benefits.

Every procedure other than hygiene re-care and appointments where there is no charge should have signed financial arrangements. All clinical personnel should be capable of and responsible for presenting financial arrangements using the correct language, but the financial coordinator is accountable.

.: TREATMENT CASE

#4 Veneer

VISIT	TOOTH	SURF	CODE	PROV	DESCRIPTION
1	4		D2962	DMD1	Labial veneer (porceln lam)-lab
2	4		D102	DMD1	Seat Veneer

:: INSURANCE PROVIDER(S) ::

Primary	Secondary
Delta Dental of KY	

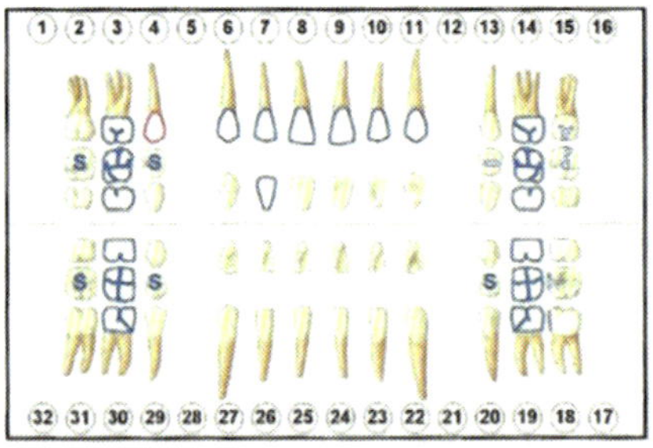

:: FINANCIAL SUMMARY ::

Treatment Plan Total	1438.00

Alternate Cases:

Case notes:

INSURANCE PAYMENT:

Ins. Estimate: $ Ø

Ins. Adjustment : $ Ø

Patient Estimate: $ 1438.00

PAYMENT OPTIONS:

1. We offer a 5% discount with cash or check if paid in full.
   5% discount: (-$ 71.90) = $ 1366.10

2. Carecredit: 12 months interest free option.
   $ 120.00 monthly estimate payment.

3. 2 payments of: $ 719.00

Collections in Advance

COLLECTING PAYMENT IN ADVANCE OF A SCHEDULED PROCEDURE HAS THREE DISTINCT ADVANTAGES:

1. That income begins to work financially for the practice in terms of interest accrued.
2. There are no further costs associated with collecting that money.
3. That patient is highly committed to continuing treatment to completion.

Because of this, offering a percentage discount of five percent when payment is collected in advance is justifiable as an incentive. Therefore, every financial arrangement over a certain amount of money (for example, $1,000) should offer payment in advance with a prearranged percentage discount.

Collections at Time of Treatment

All payment due for treatment performed, minus any payment collected in advance, should be collected in full at the time of treatment. An exception is if the practice accepts insurance assignment, in which case the estimated portion after insurance payment is collected at time of treatment. If the practice participates in a discounted fee plan, then only the amount allowed by that plan's fee schedule is allowed to be collected.

Another exception is if the practice allows patients to pay over the number of appointments to complete a procedure. For example, a crown may take two appointments to complete if the practice uses an external lab for fabrication. The patient could be offered three total options for payment: pay their portion in two payments, pay in full in advance and receive a 5% discount, or finance with a finance company. When paying over the course of treatment, the patient doesn't feel they are paying for something that hasn't been completed, and it is less money out of their pocket at one time. While this option may be favored by the patient, it must be clear to the patient when the additional payment is due to avoid any misunderstandings. There is additional risk to the practice should the patient not complete the treatment for financial reasons, although the practice has already paid for the majority of the cost involved in providing the completed treatment.

Collection Rate Factor #3 – Participation in Discounted Fee Plans

Preferred Provider Organization (PPO)

A preferred provider organization is a discounted fee schedule plan that a dental practice may elect to participate in. These plans have fee allowances that typically range anywhere from 30 to 80 percent of the practice's regular fees. Allowances can be negotiated with some plans, but most plans base allowances on the area or region of the practice location. Of course, the number one determinant of the plan fees is the desired profitability of the company administering the plan.

Obviously, participating in a PPO plan will have a significant impact on the practice collection rate, which begs the question, why would *any* practice consider participating in such an arrangement?

To answer this question, we must clarify what the PPO arrangement is to each of the participants involved.

To the patient, the arrangement means a savings for the cost of receiving care. This along with convenience are the primary considerations, as many, if not most, patients perceive that the care they receive will be performed to at least the standard of quality of care.

To the PPO administrator, the motivation is profit. This is accomplished by making the plan as attractive as possible to the employer, their employees and other subscribers, with the selling points being cost and convenience.

To the participating dentist, who will absorb the discounted cost, the motivation is increased profits from the anticipated increase in volume of PPO participating patients to the practice. Another motivating factor is fear. Dentists fear that if they don't participate, they will lose and/or not acquire the patients they need to succeed in their businesses.

Whenever possible, dental practice owners should NOT participate in a PPO plan if they can avoid it. It makes more sense for the provider to be paid their established fee for the care they provide.

However, there are circumstances that justify participation. This is substantiated by the success of many the dentists I have worked with over the years who are heavily involved with discounted fee plans, while still being highly profitable.

How is it possible to be highly profitable while participating in discounted fee plans? By outproducing the discount, while keeping overhead low.

Remember the Profitability Formula: Profit = Production X Collection Rate - Overhead. When participation in a discounted fee plan is strong, the collection rate will be low. However, this can be overcome by adjusting the two other parts of the formula – increasing production and decreasing overhead.

Consider the following scenario in Practice One and Practice Two. They do the same kind of dentistry, and both practices participate in the same PPO plan that has an average discount relative to the practices' regular fee schedule of forty percent.

Here's where the practices are different: Practice One produces one million dollars annually on those PPO patients with an overhead of sixty percent, while Practice Two produces four million dollars annually on those PPO patients with an overhead of fifty percent. (Increasing production typically lowers overhead as fixed expenses remain the same, and the increase in variable expenses is negated by the increased collections that result from increased production.).

EXAMPLE OF PRODUCTIVITY'S IMPACT ON PROFITABILITY WHEN PARTICIPATING IN A DISCOUNTED FEE PLAN

Practice One and Practice Two

Both Practice One and Practice Two participate in the same average 40% discounted fee plan. Practice Two produces four times as much as Practice One and has a lower overhead percentage resulting from its higher production.

Practice One

Gross Production of $1,000,000 X Discounted Rate of 40% = Net Production of $600,000
$1,000,000 X 60% Overhead (cost to provide $1,000,000 of care) = $600,000
Practice One Profit = $600,000 (production charged for and collected) - $600,000 (cost to provide that production) = $0 Profit

Practice Two

Gross Production of $4,000,000 X Discounted Rate of 40% = Net Production of $2,400,000
$4,000,000 X 50% Overhead (cost to provide $4,000,000 of care) = $2,000,000
Practice Two Profit = $2,400,000 (production charged for and collected) - $2,000,000 (cost to provide that production) = $400,000 Profit

Given the above scenario, the dental practice owner desiring to be a prosperous dental practice must have a high degree of capacity (the facility as well as the number of providers), and a profit margin (100% minus Overhead %), that is greater than the PPO fee discount. Even then, the prosperous dental practice owner should only consider participating in a PPO plan for one of the three following reasons:

THREE REASONS TO CONSIDER PARTICIPATING IN A PREFERRED PROVIDER ORGANIZATION PLAN

1. The practice is located in a market where PPO plans are heavily used. There are locations where the region may have a major employer or employees make up a high percentage of the population that have a PPO dental plan as part of their employee benefit package.
2. The practice is located in a market where there is a high dentist/population ratio and marketing for fee-for-service patients is highly competitive. Practice owners who profit through participation in PPO plans recognize PPO plans for what they are – marketing plans. The arrangement between the PPO plan and the participating dentist is that the dentist agrees to provide dental care at an agreed-upon price point, and the PPO plan agrees to send patients to that dentist. If that dental practice has low overhead, enough capacity (facility, team, and providers) to provide more care, and the new PPO patient can enter the practice within ten days of calling to make an appointment, then PPO plans (those with lower discounted fee schedules) are one of the best forms of marketing sources that exist for a dental practice when it comes to potential volume from a source.
3. The practice is a start-from-scratch practice and desires to grow its patient base as quickly as possible. Given the potential patient volume from using a PPO plan as a marketing method, then a scratch practice with an abundance of capacity can fill a schedule quickly. While the percentage of PPO patients in the new practice will be high, developing these PPO patients as referral sources for other patients, some of whom will be fee-for-service patients, can be an effective technique for growing a patient base quickly. The practice can then gradually phase out the PPO plans over time.

There are other methods (we've already discussed increasing production and lowering overhead) to reduce the impact of a discounted fee schedule plan. These methods involve treating the PPO patient differently than the fee-for-service patient. The contractual arrangement the dental practice owner has with the PPO plan may dictate whether any of these methods can be utilized. It is the responsibility of the practice owner to determine this before implementing any such methods.

Many dentists have trouble reconciling the concept of treating some patients differently than others based on whether they are part of a discounted fee plan or not. Others operate on the belief that patients who pay more should get more. It is clear that the fee-for-service (FFS) patient is paying more to the practice for their care, and whenever the practice raises its fees, more of the relative burden of the increased fees is placed on the FFS patient than on the PPO patient whose fees are not affected. In other words, the FFS patient subsidizes a portion of the cost of providing dental care to the PPO patient.

Other methods to reduce the financial impact of participating in a PPO plan include the following:

1. **Controlling the percentage of PPO patients in the practice**. Regardless of the amount of production, the overhead percentage, and the discounted fee schedule percentage, the goal of a prosperous dental practice should be to collect as much as possible of the dentistry it produces. Therefore, if PPO participation is to be undertaken, the goal is to keep the ratio of FFS to PPO patients as high as possible. This ratio can be controlled by measuring it periodically and, when necessary, controlling the number of PPO patients that are allowed on the schedule. This can be accomplished by reserving spaces in the schedule for FFS patients (see below) or limiting the number of PPO plan patients your practice accepts at any given time. Just because a practice has a PPO agreement doesn't necessarily mean that they have to accept every new patient that calls the office from that plan. The dental practice owner considering participation in a PPO plan should know in advance the viability of controlling the number of patients from the PPO plan that enter the practice.
2. **Controlling the percentage of PPO patients in the schedule**. One of the most important factors determining the quantity as well as the quality (net production potential to the practice) of a new patient is the availability to schedule them within ten days for a non-emergency, and within one day for emergency needs. If the practice schedule's allotment of time for new patients is filled mostly with PPO new patients, there will be less availability for FFS patients to enter the practice, negatively impacting the FFS/PPO patient ratio. When a new patient contacts the office to set up an appointment, their FFS or PPO status can be determined and placed in the schedule so that availability for FFS new patients is protected. The same concept can be applied to existing patients who schedule treatment. PPO patients can be flagged and given access only to pre-designated amounts of time each day. If there is a concern about having holes in the schedule, utilizing an "As Soon As Possible" (ASAP) call list the day before or two days before will allow these available times to be filled with production.
3. **Reducing the overhead of PPO patient production**. Earlier I noted how important the practice overhead is to the profitability of participating in a PPO plan. If the overhead for

the PPO portion of the practice can be reduced, then profitability increases. This can be accomplished by using a different dental laboratory, different materials, or even different providers. Keep in mind I am not recommending different standards of quality care, only different methods of controlling expenses. This is a widely accepted practice in the business world – when people pay more, they get more. When you fly on a commercial airplane, the airline spends more on the people who pay more. The same thing applies to hotel rooms and healthcare. The prosperous dental practice owner should be constantly cognizant of the both the purposes of the practice as well as the business.

4. **"Unbundling" charges for PPO production**. The fees that dentists charge for treatment include not only the title of that fee (example: Molar Endodontic Treatment), but all the things that are included, or bundled in, with that treatment, such as disinfection, oral hygiene instructions, nutrition counseling, pulp capping, and others. Because many PPO plan fee schedules allow charges for these services, the normally bundled procedures can be unbundled and charged separately.
5. **Negotiating the fee schedule with the PPO plan**. It is no secret that PPO plans have different fee schedules for different dentist subscribers. Dental Service Organizations (DSOs), buying clubs (for example, Smile Source ®), and large group practices negotiate more favorable fee schedules. Smaller, independently owned private practices can do the same thing. It helps if they have many of the PPO plan's subscribers as patients. It also may help to hire the services of a PPO plan negotiator. These individuals work for a percentage of savings or have a set fee per plan they negotiate favorably.

Which PPO Plans to Participate In?

In deciding which plans to participate in, there are three factors the dental practice owner should consider, in order of importance:

1. **The discounted plan fee schedule**. The average discount percentage of the PPO fee plan should be less than the profit margin of the practice (where profit margin is defined as one hundred percent minus the overhead percentage). More specifically, the allowable fees of the discount plan can be compared to the regular practice fees of commonly performed procedures to get a good feel for the average discount percentage of the PPO plan. The PPO Analysis Spreadsheet compares these numbers and provides an analytical as well as visual picture of how viable it is for the practice owner to participate in the PPO plan(s) in question. An example of the PPO Analysis Spreadsheet can be found in the Glossary.
2. **The potential number of patients from the plan**. Depending on the needs of the practice, it may make more sense to participate with a plan that has fewer (if you desire to control the PPO impact on the practice) or more (if you desire to increase demand as much as possible) participants. This information can often be collected from the plan itself.

   It may also be apparent from the employers in the community who provide that plan, as well as from patients who contact the office regarding a particular plan. It is important to remember that, when considering participation in PPO plans, employers often change their benefit packages year to year. It is crucial to do an analysis and consider that information versus the number of patients who may enter the practice with that PPO plan.

3. **The terms of the arrangement**. While most PPO plan contracts are similar, there may be important differences in participation requirements such as reporting, whether non-covered procedures can be charged for, and terms of suspending or terminating the agreement.

How to Terminate the PPO Relationship

There may come a time when the practice owner decides to end affiliation with a PPO plan. Careful consideration of whether to participate in the first place should be given as the termination process involves time, effort, and – even when done well – some pain in the form of lost patients and ill will. The patient often has difficulty separating themselves, their plan, and your practice in their mind. In other words, they see your decision to no longer accept their plan as a decision to no longer accept them as a patient. If the practice is to separate from the PPO plan, careful analysis, planning, and implementation must be undertaken to keep the pain to a minimum.

Analysis

The practice must determine which plan(s) should be canceled. The PPO Analysis Spreadsheet will be helpful in determining which plans are the least profitable, but the practice also needs to know how many practice patients use a plan. This is essential because any good plan to terminate a PPO relationship should assume that all the patients who have that plan will leave the practice. Not all the patients will leave, of course, but because some will, and since you don't know how many that is, you should safely assume that all will leave. Therefore, unless the practice plans to shrink the patient base, the practice should know the number of FFS patients that will be required to replace the terminated PPO plan patients, so that an appropriate marketing plan can be developed.

The following grid is a useful visual to help determine the optimal order in which plans should be dropped. If a plan has a large relative discount and there are a small number of those patients in the practice, then that plan can be dropped quickly without much potential harm to the practice. If, however, a plan with a large discount involves a large number of patients, then that plan should be dropped slowly, allowing for measures to keep as many of those patients to be implemented, as well as time for marketing to replace those patients with fee for service (FFS) patients.

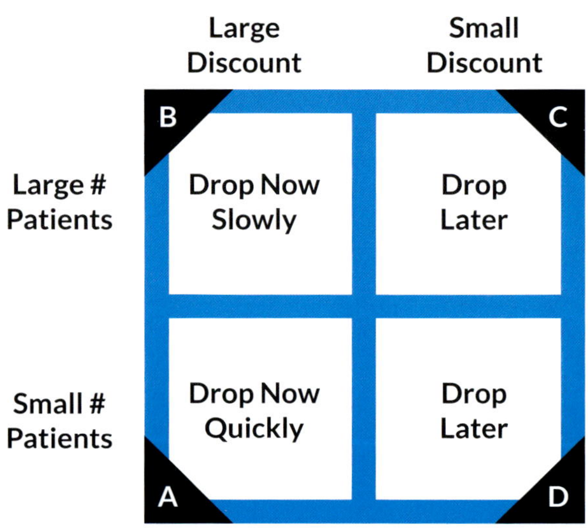

If a plan being dropped involves a small discount, regardless of the number of patients, then there is no rush to drop that plan. It can be dropped later, once marketing to attract more FFS patients has had time to work.

Developing a plan

Once the decision has been made to drop a plan, and you understand its impact, you must develop a timeline so that the process is as efficient and effective as possible.

First, let's start with the wrong way to drop a PPO plan that involves a significant percentage of the practice: Terminate the agreement as soon as the agreement allows (usually 30-60 days), and send a notification out (letter, email, text, or phone) to all patients who use that plan in your practice. This is a sure way to create a lot of stress for you and your team (especially the business office). This is also a sure way to disappoint and antagonize those affected patients, create ill will, and force them out of your practice.

Your goal should be to drop the plan and keep as many patients as possible. The right way of accomplishing that should be to establish a timeline for phasing out the PPO plan and communicating that information clearly to the patient.

The message to the patient is critical. It needs to communicate that the plan prevents you from providing the high standard of care you have been providing and are committed to providing in the future. It needs to communicate that the fee schedule of the plan has not kept up with the rising costs of providing that quality dental care, and now it costs you more to provide that care than the fee schedule allows.

The message communicates that you are about quality, while the plan is about preventing you from providing that quality. Also important to the message is how difficult the decision was to make, because you value the professional relationship you have with your patients, and you want to continue that relationship.

As critical as the content of the message is the method by which it is communicated. Despite how carefully you word the message, the patient still is left with the conclusion that they may have to look for a new dentist.

The best form of communication is face-to-face from a trusted person, such as the dentist, but it can come from any member of the practice team. A distant second is over-the-phone communication, and a distant third is written communication. The prosperous dental practice should plan to speak face-to-face, in the office, to every patient who participates in the PPO plan being dropped at a recare or other scheduled treatment appointment. The message should be communicated by the individual or individuals who do that best, whether that's the doctor or another member of the team. Everyone on the team needs to know the message, how to communicate it, and how to address questions and concerns. This means that it will take at least six months to drop the PPO plan.

The termination terms of the contract with the PPO plan are determined so that the proper notification method and length of notice are followed.

A marketing plan is developed to replace the patients that are lost from the PPO plan. Marketing plans will be covered in detail in the section on Growth Systems.

Implementation

Prior to communicating the message to the patient, the team must buy in to the reason behind the decision to drop the PPO(s) in question. Otherwise, the message will not be delivered with sincerity and belief, and it will fail in its purpose. This can be a challenge, because team members often feel more aligned with the patient in these instances as they themselves may be part of a discounted fee plan for healthcare.

This is where sharing information about the business is useful, giving team members a quantitative accounting of the numbers as they relate to profitability. It isn't difficult to communicate that the practice cannot provide dental care at a loss. The challenge may be in convincing the team member that the profit margin of the practice is less than the discounted fee schedule of the PPO. I recommend sharing overhead numbers with the team for this reason as well as others. Otherwise, the team will have to rely only on the word of the practice owner.

Next, the plan and timeline for the PPO elimination should be presented to the team. Before the timeline begins, the team must understand that the message will be communicated to each member of the plan face-to-face. Each team member should role-play the conversation in a team meeting designed for that purpose. An example script should be provided, but team members are encouraged to use their own vernacular to make the delivery of the message more comfortable for them. The owner and/or team leader gives final approval to the team members' presentations.

First, identify what *shouldn't be said* - *"We will no longer be a provider for your insurance"* or *"We cannot afford to continue to accept your insurance."* This sends the message that we don't value the patient, or we are just plain greedy, or both. It concentrates on the negative – what we *won't* do anymore. Patients view their dental benefits as part of their compensation package. When we say we no longer accept it, it's like saying their money isn't good here anymore. Although it is a true statement that we are no longer a provider, it is also the truth when we phrase it in a more positive way to stress what we *will* be doing.

DROPPING A PPO - WHAT TO SAY TO PATIENTS

"The next time you come in, you will notice a change in what you pay for the services we provide for you.

We are ending our relationship with ___ PPO because their allowances for what we can charge for our services do not cover our cost of providing those services. We simply cannot operate our practice at a loss.

While some practices choose to reduce the quality of their care so they can afford to participate in a PPO with low fee allowances, we've decided to provide the best care we can for all our patients.

We'd love to continue to provide care for you and are committed to continue providing that care at the highest possible level. Does that make sense? Do you have any questions?"

This would be a perfect time to offer your in-house plan, which is covered later in this section.

The dates for the start of implementation are determined, as well as the date for notifying the PPO plan. A list of patients in the plan should be checked against the appointments on the schedule, and as they are communicated with, they should be marked off the list. If, at the five-month mark on the timeline, any patient cannot be contacted face-to-face, a phone call can be made communicating the message. If a patient cannot be reached by phone, then a letter or email can be sent.

AN IMPORTANT MESSAGE TO OUR PATIENTS WITH (PPO, Insurance) COVERAGE
Effective <Date>, there will be some changes to how your (insurance coverage, dental benefit plan) is handled with our office. First of all, most things will stay the same. You will continue to receive the same excellent care you deserve and have come to expect. We use the best labs, the finest materials, the most up to date techniques, and have the finest dental personnel in the region. In order to continue to provide you this level of care, the following changes will go into effect on <Date>: 1. You will receive your care as always and can pay for that care by one of six different methods we offer to make dentistry as convenient and affordable as possible. 2. We will file your insurance claim promptly for you, and you will receive payment directly from the insurance company. 3. Oftentimes, you will receive your reimbursement faster than we do, and sometimes at a higher level. 4. We will work hard to maximize your benefits so that you receive the most from your dental benefits. We will also write any letters or support you in any dispute with your insurance company over payment to the maximum of our ability. Please call our office with any questions or concerns about this policy. We will be happy to address anything that may remain unclear to you. Finally, we want to assure you that our goal is to care for you and your family in a way consistent with providing the best that dentistry has to offer. Be assured that we will continue to be your home for dental excellence. The Team at <Name of Practice>

The In-Office Plan

If a practice with a significant portion of PPO involvement (40% or more) is to properly implement the plan outlined above, it is helpful to have an alternative to offer the patient who is losing their PPO plan benefits with the office. That alternative is another plan, but one administered in part or in full by the practice, with terms that are affordable to both the patient *and the practice.*

Today's consumer mindset is that in order to receive healthcare, they need to be part of a plan that offers favorable discounts off standard fees, as well as other preferred treatment (whether real or not). The practice can offer an in-house plan that goes by various labels, whereby the practice offers individual and family plans with monthly fees that allow the participant access to complimentary as well as preferred pricing services with the practice.

The practice may market and administer the in-house plan or pay an outside service to do some or all of that.

There are both advantages and disadvantages to creating an in-house membership plan.

ADVANTAGES OF AN IN-HOUSE PATIENT MEMBERSHIP PLAN

1. The practice keeps many of its existing patients who may otherwise leave because of their existing plan.
2. The practice attracts new patients because of the plan (a unique selling point).
3. The practice gains an additional income source in membership fees.
4. The practice sets the discounted fees at a level that it can afford.

For instance, if a practice has an overhead of 70%, then offering a discount of 15% still allows a reasonable profit margin, especially compared to a typical PPO discount of 30% or more. Another advantage is that the practice also can tailor its in-office plan to patient needs to give a more personal feel. The practice can market this aspect of the plan so that the patient is getting a personalized plan rather than being just another person in a collective plan offered by a PPO. Having a plan in place allows the practice to offer the patient an alternative to enrolling in their employer-based plan during open enrollment. The patient would be paying their premium to you, someone they can see and easily speak with, rather than a large, impersonal company.

DISADVANTAGES OF AN IN-HOUSE PATIENT MEMBERSHIP PLAN

1. There is a cost to administer the plan, whether that administration is performed within or outside the practice.
2. The practice's fee-for-service patients may now want to participate in the in-house plan.

Offering the in-house plan only to new patients or to patients with a pre-existing PPO plan is discriminatory, so the practice must be willing to accept this disadvantage. This can be minimized by not marketing the plan, and by offering it only under certain circumstances (but making it available to anyone in the practice upon request). Another way to minimize the in-house discount is through sheer volume – to sign up as many patients as possible. It is easier to overcome the lesser discount of the in-house plan through volume than to do so with an outside PPO.

Outside Financing

The case was made earlier for larger treatment plans being an essential part of the Goal-Focused Scheduling System. And in the section on Case Acceptance, addressing the common objection of affordability was highlighted as essential to the patient moving forward. Moving forward is more than dealing with the emotional aspect of the buying decision; it also involves the very real practical aspect – Where is the money going to come from?

The answer is often from an outside source. This could be a family member or a friend, but often it is a financial institution – a bank or other financing service organization.

While banks (especially small ones heavily invested in the local community) are a potential source, they lean heavily on collateral to guarantee loans. They cannot seize dental work in return for a defaulted loan, so they look at other resources of equity. This tends to make access to bank loans for dental treatment less available and more limited.

Lending services that specialize in healthcare provide both the patient and provider with options more suited to the specific needs of dental treatment. These services, unlike that of a bank, require the provider to pay a fee, and usually require the applicant to pay a fee as well. This allows the financier to provide more appealing terms to the applicant, thereby increasing acceptance. The fee that the provider pays is affected by the length of time as well as the amount that the applicant is financing.

There are many such services to choose from, with minimum credit score requirements that range from 550 and upward, terms from 3-180 months, and interest rates from 0 to 36%. Acceptance can be limited and, even when accepted, the patient may not accept the terms. One such company, *CareCredit®*, has a dominant share of the healthcare financing marketplace, and for several reasons is the first choice of many healthcare providers, including dentists, when it comes to dental financing.

With *CareCredit®*, the patient applies for a healthcare credit card that can be used at hundreds of thousands of enrolled provider locations in the U.S. Once accepted, the patient can use the card again and again at any location that accepts *CareCredit®* up to the maximum amount allowed for that individual. Applicants may be eligible for financing at no interest for up to 24 months, as well as up to 60 months for interest rates that range from 14.9-17.9% APR. The application can be made by phone in a relatively short time with a limited amount of information.

For the provider, it means access to financing for patients to increase case acceptance, and payment in full within two business days. *CareCredit®* also provides free training, phone support, and pre-approval for scheduled patients.

Despite these advantages, the dental practice owner should have a business relationship with more than one financing service. This increases the odds that a patient will be accepted for financing, as the rate of acceptance can be impacted by the loan-equity ratio of the lending institution on the day the credit is applied for. Having more than one finance company is also beneficial because while one company may offer interest-free options at one administrative rate to the practice, another may offer a lower interest rate to the patient and a lower administrative fee to the practice for interest-bearing extended payment loans.

Collection Rate Factor #4 – Insurance Management

If the patient has traditional indemnity dental insurance, then a claim can be filed for reimbursement for dental services performed. The policy is tied to a deductible and an annual maximum amount in nearly all cases. This type of policy is not as prevalent as in the past due to the competitive advantages that Preferred Provider Plans (PPO) have for the employer – as well as for the public seeking to purchase a discounted dental plan independent of an employer.

When dental insurance is encountered, whether or not it is a plan that the practice participates in, the practice should fill out and submit the insurance claim on behalf of the patient. This is a straightforward process built into all dental practice software platforms. What the dental practice owner must decide is whether the patient or the practice accepts assignment of insurance payments. Some insurance plans, when the practice is an out-of-network provider, will automatically deny the acceptance of assignment to the provider and will send the payment to the patient. By using this tactic, they are hoping that having to pay the practice in full at the time of treatment will encourage the patient to leave that practice and go to an in-network participating provider.

It is certainly most advantageous for the practice to accept payment in full from the patient before or at time of treatment, and have the patient reimbursed by the insurance carrier. This prevents delay in payment to the provider, as well as the cost of follow-up by office personnel. However, healthcare practices have traditionally accepted insurance assignment resulting in an expectation of this on behalf of the patient.

It is imperative that any payments received after treatment is performed are limited to insurance payments.

In other words, the dental practice should do everything it can to avoid sending statements to a patient after treatment is completed. (The only exception would be prior-made payment plans which should be kept to an absolute minimum). If the practice makes financial arrangements ahead of treatment properly, then for those patients who have dental insurance and the practice accepts insurance assignment, the expected insurance payment is underestimated, so if there is a balance after insurance payment is received by the office, it is a negative balance. Most dental office software allows for the practice to track what different insurance companies pay for services so that these estimates can be properly made. If this is done properly, the only positive accounts receivable balance (owed to the practice) should be outstanding insurance.

The financial coordinator should file all insurance claims on the day the service is provided. Batch filings days or weeks later guarantee that some insurance balances will be overdue. Any unpaid insurance claims should be followed up two weeks after filing to confirm that the claim and any supporting materials were received, and to get an updated status on the processing of the claim. If the claim is not paid two weeks after that, another call should be made to the insurance claims processing department. The speed of claim processing is often impacted favorably by the practice checking in (the squeaky wheel gets the grease).

If the claim is not paid within 45 days, the patient should be notified. As a reminder, the financial arrangement made with the patient includes a statement that says:

PRACTICE POLICY REGARDING DENTAL INSURANCE

"The practice will accept assignment of benefits for any dental insurance claim filed for services provided. However, your dental insurance is an arrangement between you and your insurance company. In other words, you are their client – not us. We will file a claim on your behalf as a courtesy to you. You agree to pay for the estimated balance after insurance benefits are received at time of treatment. Once your insurance company has paid our office from the filed claim, you will be notified of any remaining balance, which will be your responsibility to pay to our office. If the claim is not paid within 45 days of being filed, the entire remaining balance is your responsibility."

While insurance claims can be filed by posted mail, electronic filing is preferred so that the insurance company receives the claim more promptly. The practice can employ an electronic claims processing platform to simplify and streamline the process. Outside insurance and billing services are also available and becoming increasingly popular, because they manage the process efficiently and cost effectively.

Billing Administration

As previously stated, the number of statements sent to patients should be small if financial arrangements are properly administered and insurance administration is effectively and efficiently managed. If, however, accounts receivable balances remain, these require proper management, including timely (as soon as possible) and accurate execution.

Collection Rate Factor #5 – Accounts Receivable Management

Accounts Receivable – The Main Goal

The goal of every dental practice should be to have no overdue accounts receivable (more than thirty days). As each dental practice should pay its accounts payable (expenses) within thirty days, all the income from dental services provided should be collected within the same time frame.

Since the dental practice owner has paid all the expenses related to providing care within thirty days, any overdue accounts receivable (beyond thirty days) that exist go directly (or should) to the bottom line (the owner's account) because everyone has been paid for those services except the owner.

The sad fact is that many dental practices carry a large delinquent accounts receivable balance, and the money owed in that category is worth less than it was the day the services were provided, due to the costs in collecting that money and the inevitable write-off of old accounts that will never be collected.

Accounts Receivables & The AR/Monthly Production Ratio

If the practice is to have zero accounts receivable, then a completely fee-for-service practice will be required. In other words, the practice provides a service, and the patient pays in full for that service. When a practice accepts insurance assignment or allows payment plans, there will be balances in accounts receivables. Keeping this amount within an acceptable range is important to the financial health of the business. The Accounts Receivable/Monthly Production Ratio defines this acceptable range. This ratio should be 0.4 or less. In other words:

The total amount of accounts receivable should be forty percent or less of the average monthly production.

For example, if the practice averages $200,000/month in production, the total accounts receivable should not be more than $80,000.

Delinquent Accounts Management

Any delinquent account balances (beyond thirty days) should be evaluated and a plan for collecting each one created and implemented. Such a plan may involve contacting an insurance company or a patient to determine how best to pay off the balance of the account as quickly as possible.

The reasons for delinquent account balances and the appropriate actions are:

DELINQUENT ACCOUNTS ACTION FLOWCHART

Reasons for:

1. Team not following office financial policy

When the practice accepts insurance assignment:

2. Team underestimating the patient's portion after insurance
3. Insurance company not paying at all, or not paying in a timely fashion

The following actions should take place to address delinquent accounts:

Time	Action
0 days	Treatment performed. Any payment not collected should be due to insurance assignment. At two and four weeks, insurance company contacted. Account status is current.
30 days	Patient is contacted. If unsuccessful, friendly reminder sent by mail, text, or email. Practice owner is notified at Delinquent Accounts Meeting.
45 days	Patient is contacted by phone. If unsuccessful, past due notice sent by mail, text, or email.
60 days	Patient is contacted by phone. If unsuccessful, final notice sent by mail, text, or email. Practice owner is notified at Delinquent Accounts Meeting.
75 days	Account is turned over to collection agency. Practice owner is notified at the next Delinquent Accounts Meeting.

At the 30-day mark, the patient should be called to collect payment. If the patient cannot be reached, a friendly reminder statement should be mailed with a notice that the account is now overdue and prompt payment is appreciated.

A FRIENDLY REMINDER

Date ______________________________

Dear ______________________________

Just a reminder that your balance of $__________ is past due. Please remit payment by __________. Perhaps your check is already in the mail; if so, thank you for your payment. If you have any questions, please feel free to contact our office.

Sincerely,

<Name of Practice>
<Phone Number>
<Street Address>
<City, State, and Zip Code>

At 45 days, if the patient has not responded to the first statement, then the patient should be contacted by phone notifying the patient that this is the second delinquent account notice, and that payment of the balance must be taken care of as soon as possible. If the patient cannot be reached by phone, then a second delinquent notice should be mailed with the same message, including the option to contact the office to make other arrangements for payment. If the balance is not paid due to insurance, the statement should state that the patient's insurance has not paid the practice and that the balance is now due. This usually prompts a call from the patient and the patient's help is elicited in contacting the insurance company to address the unpaid claim.

PAST DUE NOTICE

*Date:*______________________________

Dear <Name of Patient> ______________________________

*This is a reminder that your balance of $*____________ *is now 45 days past due. A request for payment has been sent to you (or your insurance company if applicable) without any response. Perhaps there is a reason for your non-payment or perhaps it has been an oversight. Please remit payment immediately or contact us to make other arrangements. If you have any questions, please contact our office.*

Sincerely,

<Name of Practice>
<Phone Number>
<Street Address>
<City, State, and Zip Code>

At 60 days, if the patient has not responded to the first two phone calls or statements, then the patient should be contacted directly by phone and informed that if the account balance is not taken care of within the next month, the account will be forwarded to a collection service. If the patient cannot be reached by phone, then a third delinquent account statement should be mailed to the patient by certified mail, return receipt requested.

FINAL NOTICE

*Date:*______________________________

Dear <Name of Patient> ______________________________

*Your balance of $*__________ *is seriously past due. If your account is not paid in full by* ____________*, it will be forwarded to <Name of Collection Agency> for collection.*

Your prompt attention in this matter will be greatly appreciated.

Sincerely,

<Name of Practice>
<Street Address>
<City, State, and Zip Code>

At 75 days, if the patient has not responded to the sixty-day call, or the final notice, the account should be forwarded to a collection service.

Specific limitations and conditions of a patient's insurance plan should be discussed before treatment is begun. A balance may be left on an account by insurance if, for example, the insurance pays for a crown on the seat date instead of the preparation date. If the patient has not returned to have the restoration seated, the patient should be reminded of this in the delinquent account statements. The statement should emphasize the importance of having the permanent restoration seated in a timely manner and note that, if the crown is not placed, insurance will not consider coverage for the service, will not remit payment, and thus the entire balance will be the full responsibility of the patient.

Sending a patient's account to a collection service is something that many dental practice owners as well as team members have a hard time coming to terms with, especially when there is a long-standing relationship with the patient.

Let's revisit how we arrived at this place. We arranged with a patient to provide a service. They signed financial arrangements clearly describing each party's responsibility. The practice fulfilled its part, and in the process incurred expenses that were paid at least forty-five days ago. The delinquent account patient was notified on at least three occasions of the status of their account and given the opportunity to contact the office to communicate extenuating circumstances and make arrangements.

Yes, this will probably mean the loss of a patient, and likely some ill will.

The practice needs to decide what kind of patients it wants to treat – those who will appreciate and pay for their services, or those who will not.

If the practice owner wants to provide charitable work for those they choose, then that is great. But he/she should know ahead of time who those patients are. Most of these uncomfortable encounters can be avoided by implementing sound financial systems.

Using a collection service has a cost. Most will keep 50% of any money collected. Then there's the ill will between a collection service and the former patient that is extended to the practice. On the flip side, having practice personnel trying to collect a balance that is 75-plus days overdue is costly as well, and not a good use of their time. At the point where the practice has exhausted all its efforts to collect the overdue amount, the option to send the account to a collection service may be exercised. The practice owner should evaluate each of these accounts on a case-by-case basis. If the collections service is not used, then the practice owner can choose to write off the debt as a bad-debt.

Whenever a patient account is sent to a collection service or their debt is written off, that patient is inactivated, and their account flagged in the practice software as "do not schedule without permission of the practice owner. If the practice owner opts to see the patient, the past debt must be paid, and all future dental care must be paid for with cash at time of treatment.

Let's reiterate: delinquent accounts are almost 100% preventable. Allowing a large portion of accounts receivable to become delinquent can happen relatively quickly. Restoring accounts receivable to a healthy status takes time and is costly. Signed financial arrangements plus adhering to the collection systems outlined here will keep accounts current and prevent the time-consuming, costly process of cleaning up delinquent accounts.

To implement these financial systems the practice must be properly staffed in the business office, and everyone in the practice must be committed to following the systems. One of the ways the practice owner can hold the practice, and specifically the team member accountable for keeping accounts receivable current, the financial coordinator, is to hold a Delinquent Accounts Meeting once a month.

The Delinquent Accounts Meeting

The purpose of the Delinquent Accounts Meeting is to inform the practice owner of the status of all delinquent accounts, to make a plan to resolve these balances, and to hold the financial coordinator accountable for that resolution. Present at these meetings should be the financial coordinator, the business office team leader (if different than the financial coordinator), the office manager/COO if applicable, and the practice owner(s).

The financial coordinator should prepare an accounts receivable report of all accounts that are 31 days or older, with the report ordered from largest balance to smallest balance. The financial coordinator should provide an update on the status and plan to resolve each balance. The practice owner may be asked about any accounts that are due to be sent to the collection service. More information regarding the Delinquent Accounts Meeting can be found in the Leadership chapter.

Collection Rate Factor #6 – Adjustments Management

Adjustments

Adjustments to production and collections are deviations from the normal fees charged to and collected by the practice. These come in many forms and can be either positive (beyond the normal amount that is collectible) or negative (reducing the normal amount that is collectible and including write-offs). Some negative adjustments are desirable in that they have an indirect or direct positive influence on profitability.

Positive adjustments may involve procedures that will take more time and/or involve more expenses. Negative adjustments usually fall in to one of two categories - Discounts or Uncollectible Accounts. Negative adjustments, and how they affect profitability, will be covered in more detail in the Profitability section. The write-offs that will be covered here are Bad Debts, Refund Overpayments, Pay In Advance Adjustments, and Outside Financing Adjustments.

Bad Debts

These write-offs have been described in the previous section on delinquent accounts receivables. Obviously, this is an undesirable adjustment that eliminates some or all of the profitability from providing the dental care associated with that account.

Refund Overpayments

As mentioned previously on insurance management, a positive balance may result after an insurance claim is paid due to underestimation of insurance benefits on the part of the practice.

These balances are usually small. The practice can contact the patient and ask them if they want a refund check mailed to them or the balance left on their account for future transactions. This is a desirable adjustment.

Pay-In-Advance Adjustments

Every financial arrangement over a predetermined amount should include the option to pay in advance of the appointment day and receive a five percent courtesy allowance. Sometimes referred to as a "bookkeeper's allowance," the five percent is not only an incentive to pay in advance, but it can also be justified as a way to guarantee that the account will be paid and ensure that the appointment will be kept.

When presented, the five percent courtesy allowance should be calculated in dollar amounts, as five percent may not sound like much until the actual numerical savings are mentioned. Obviously, the larger the account, the bigger the discounted amount. The five percent courtesy can be used with patients who have insurance as long as the insurance claim also reflects the discounted fee, and can only be paid by cash or check, as credit card adjustments would increase the five to seven percent or more. This is a desirable adjustment.

Outside Financing Adjustments

Outside financing has already been covered as a method to help make dental care more affordable and increase case acceptance. The adjustment that the practice would make is the discount paid to the outside financing service by the practice. Since this adjustment leads to higher case acceptance, it is considered a desirable adjustment.

Monthly Financial Review by Practice Owner

It is imperative that the practice owner reviews financial data on a regular basis, at least once a month. The critical financial systems that have the greatest impact on profitability need to be monitored, allowing the practice owner to determine if those systems are working in the manner they were intended.

In the *Production Systems* section, each of the twelve production systems had monitors to measure their performance. To determine how the *Financial Systems* are performing, the following monitors need to be examined each month:

MONITORS FOR FINANCIAL SYSTEMS

- Practice Production (before and after adjustments)
- Practice Collections (before and after adjustments)
- Collections Compared to Goal
- Practice Collections Compared to Historical Collections
- Net Collections as a Percentage of Gross Production (Collection Rate)
- Total Accounts Receivable Balances Aged
- Accounts Receivable Trend
- Over-The-Counter Versus In-The-Mail Collections
- Accounts Receivable/Monthly Production Ratio
- Practice Adjustments (Write-Offs)
- Practice Profitability

Unaccounted-for Money

In addition to the above financial system monitors, I've created a very simple and quick spreadsheet to verify that the difference between production and collections for a designated time period can be accounted for by a legitimate explanation, called the *Verification of Practice Financials Spreadsheet.*

The purpose of the spreadsheet is to calculate the designated time period's (usually a month) *Unaccounted-for Money*. The owner enters the following data into the spreadsheet for the time period being evaluated:

- Practice Production
- Practice Collections
- Beginning and Ending Accounts Receivable Balances
- Adjustments (write-offs)

All these practice metrics are shaded in yellow in the spreadsheet.

The spreadsheet automatically calculates the difference between Production and Collections, the difference between this time period's Beginning and Ending Accounts Receivable Balances, and the time period's Unaccounted-for Money. All these calculations are shaded in green.

Ideally, the difference between Production and Collections should equal the sum of the difference between Beginning and Ending Accounts Receivable and the Adjustments for the time period being measured. In other words, there are only two legitimate explanations for why there is a difference between production and collections – the money either went into the AR, or it was adjusted off.

If the equation doesn't balance, then the most likely reason is that some treatment produced during the time period being measured was paid for in advance of that time period. The practice owner should confirm that this is the case, because another possible reason for unaccounted-for money is embezzlement.

According to the *National White Collar Crime Center*, it is estimated that employee theft and embezzlement cost businesses and organizations $400 billion per year. The *FBI Financial Crimes Report to the Public* estimates that financial crimes account for approximately thirty to fifty percent of all business failures. Dental practices are certainly not immune to employee theft, with studies reporting a thirty-five to fifty percent likelihood that dental practice owners will experience embezzlement.

Not only is this an important topic, but a wide-ranging one as well, with enough information to fill a book by itself. *The dental practice owner* should have a financial audit of practice financial and office protection systems performed by an industry embezzlement service every five years, and more often if those protection systems point to potential inappropriate activity.

In some cases, a forensic investigation will need to be performed.

THE KEY CONCEPT

The Key Concept of Trust But Verify – The business owner must trust that everyone in their employment will conduct themselves in a moral, ethical, and legal manner. This is critical given that team members will be delegated important responsibilities involving the organization's success. A lack of trust with any individual must be resolved to the business owner's satisfaction as soon as possible. Even in the presence of this trust, the business owner must perform due diligence to confirm that trust is well-placed.

Verifcation of Practice Financials		**Practice Name**	**Prosperous Dental Care**
A. Production	$ 257,826.00	**Time Period**	
B. Collections	$ 190,026.00		
C. (A - B)*	$ 67,800.00	*C can only be accounted for by an increase in AR (F), or through adjustments (G), or both	
D. This Month's AR Balance	$ 179,165.00	At end of time period being measured	
E. Last Month's AR Balance	$ 168,163.00	At beginning of time period being measured	
F. (D - E)	$ 11,002.00		
G. This Month's Adjustments	$ 44,549.00		
H. $ Unaccounted For (C - F - G)**	$ 12,249.00	**H can be accounted for by payments made for this time period's production (A) in advance of this time period. The practice owner should confirm.	

GROWTH SYSTEMS

"Growth" in this context refers to increase of the practice patient base. New patients are the lifeblood of any dental practice. Not only do they replace patients lost from natural attrition, but the lion's share of practice production comes from the new patient's first nine months in the practice. A healthy new patient flow allows for expansion of the practice with an accompanying increase in productivity, and, when coupled with profitability systems, profitability as well.

For these reasons, just about all dentists I ask say they desire more new patients. When I ask them how many they need, they appear bewildered and usually respond by saying, "as many as possible," or they come up with some number that is more than they currently have. Like all systems of the prosperous dental practice, Growth Systems are defined by quantitative, objective goals. If the goal of a practice is to simply attract as many new patients as possible, then it may spend more than it needs to in marketing costs, and/or it may exceed its capacity for new patients, which can have a negative impact on production, quality of care, and ultimately on the number of new patients.

How to Determine How Many New Patients You Need

Accepting that most of the production comes from the needs of new patients, the practice can determine the number of new patients needed by dividing the Production Needed from New Patients to reach the Practice Production Goal by the Practice Value of a New Patient. This calculation can be arrived at by using the *New Patient Goal Worksheet.*

NEW PATIENT GOAL WORKSHEET

Name of Practice

Experience indicates that the lion's share of a practice's production comes from new patients, and occurs typically within the first nine months after the new patient enters the practice. Therefore, if you know the average value of a new patient, and you know this "lion's share" percentage of production expected from new patients, then you can work backwards from your practice production goal to determine the number of new patients needed.

Historical # of New Patients Averaged Per Month (use last 12 months average value)	40	A
Practice Value of a New Patient (Doctor & Hygiene)	$ 2,417.00	B
Total Average Historical Monthly Production (use average of last 12 months)	$ 159,000.00	C
New Total Monthly Practice Production Goal	$ 250,000.00	D
A x B = Historical Monthly Production from New Patients	$ 96,680.00	E
E/C = Percentage of Historical Monthly Production from New Patients	61%	F
F x D = Production Needed from New Patients	$ 152,012.58	G
G/B = Number of New Patients to Satisfy New Practice Goal	62.89	H

In order to make this calculation, the following numbers are needed:

- Historical number of new patients averaged per month (use average of last 12 months). This is the "A" in the New Patient Goal Worksheet.
- Practice value of a new patient (doctor & hygiene). This is the "B" in the New Patient Goal Worksheet.
- Total average historical monthly production (use average of last 12 months). This is the "C" in the New Patient Goal Worksheet.
- Latest total monthly practice production goal (determine by practice budget). This is the "D" in the New Patient Goal Worksheet.

The Average Value of a New Patient

The standard for determining the average value of a new patient (VNP) is the amount of production (both dental and hygiene) from a new patient in the practice for the first nine months after their initial comprehensive exam. This is arrived at by looking back on the practice schedule nine months ago and listing the last thirty new patients that had comprehensive exams prior to that date and adding up the amount of treatment they have had performed in the subsequent nine month period.

The total production from those patients is added up and divided by thirty to determine the average value of a new patient in the practice. The practice may choose to use more than thirty patients for this calculation to dial the number in even more specifically. There may be some patients with zero production. These should be used as well in order to determine an average.

The VNP, in addition to being part of the New Patient Goal calculation, can serve as an indicator as to how certain production systems are performing. For example, Diagnosis & Treatment Planning, Case Acceptance, and Quality of a New Patient can all impact the VNP. If the VNP is low in hygiene compared to total production (<30%), this could be an indication that hygiene production systems are not being implemented correctly.

Value of a New Patient Calculation Form

SUNRISE DENTAL SOLUTIONS

make more, keep more, enjoy more

Value of New Patients Data Form

Practice Name: ______________________

Provider: ______________________

Month: ______________________

Year: ______________________

New Patients

	Patient Name	Dental Production	Hygiene
1)	Patient Name		
2)	Patient Name		
3)	Patient Name		
4)	Patient Name		
5)	Patient Name		
6)	Patient Name		
7)	Patient Name		
8)	Patient Name		
9)	Patient Name		
10)	Patient Name		
11)	Patient Name		
12)	Patient Name		
13)	Patient Name		
14)	Patient Name		
15)	Patient Name		
16)	Patient Name		
17)	Patient Name		
18)	Patient Name		
19)	Patient Name		
20)	Patient Name		
21)	Patient Name		
22)	Patient Name		
23)	Patient Name		
24)	Patient Name		
25)	Patient Name		
26)	Patient Name		
27)	Patient Name		
28)	Patient Name		
29)	Patient Name		
30)	Patient Name		
	total	$ -	$ -
	average	#DIV/0!	#DIV/0!

The Seven Necessary Ingredients Needed to Grow the Prosperous Dental Practice

If a practice is to experience significant growth, certain ingredients must exist.

1. Good Dentistry

The first four ingredients all have something to do with reputation. It is difficult to overcome a reputation for poor dental work. Conversely, having a reputation for being a good dentist will overcome an inconvenient location and schedule, as well as cost. David Ogilvy once said: "Great marketing only makes a bad product fail faster." Practicing dentistry at or above the standard of care is an essential ingredient to growth.

2. Friendly, Caring Team

The team is more important to a practice owner's success than the practice owner is to his or her own success. Team members will have more exposure to patients and often have more influence on the patient's relationship with the practice. It is not uncommon for an existing patient to refer a new prospective patient to a practice because of a hygienist or an assistant. Conversely, a hygienist who handles a patient roughly, or an assistant who appears incompetent, is an indirect reflection on the dentist and the practice. Making patients feel special and valued through friendly, caring exchanges goes a long way in creating disciples for the practice who, when prompted, will go out of their way to refer a patient.

Patients also like to see consistency in the team. Frequent turnover implies that people are not being treated well or that the environment of the office is not conducive to team stability. Patients don't want to break in a new hygienist or assistant every time they visit the practice, and they appreciate a familiar voice and face each time they return.

3. Well-Run Business

Just as the dental work and the team are important to the patient's overall impression of the practice, so is the way the practice is administered. Today's consumer notices when the practice appears efficient, competent, organized, and prepared. Conversely, if the practice frequently reschedules appointments, consistently runs late, makes billing mistakes, and appears frazzled and disorganized, the patient's perception of the practice will suffer.

4. Modern, Clean, and Comfortable Atmosphere

The environment where patients receive their care is as important as the care itself. I suggest that dental practice owners see their practice through the eyes of the patient. This can be done through a survey. It can also be done through sitting in the reception area or the operatory, and seeing, hearing, and feeling the atmosphere of the office. Practice owners are often surprised to see untidiness, dust, worn furniture or equipment. They might hear sounds or conversations that are inappropriate. They are often insensitive to the odors of a dental office, but if they ask those who aren't, they might hear that there is an unpleasant smell. There may be outdated decorating or equipment that appears to be in disrepair. Patients take all of this in and form an impression about the practice, and that impression affects their perception of the quality of care provided.

5. Good Location

Today's consumers are convenience oriented. They need a compelling reason to drive past other dental practices that are closer to where they work or live. They want easy access, and they don't want to have to fight heavy traffic. The best location for a dental practice has as many of the following as possible:

- High visibility to drive-by traffic
- Few signage restrictions
- Easily recognizable area
- Growing area with high population of the type of patients desired by the practice
- Ample parking
- Low dentist-to-population ratio

6. Adequate Capacity

A practice can only grow as much as the capacity of the practice allows. Many years ago, I served on the financial committee of a church expansion campaign. In researching how best to expand the church building for a growing congregation, we interviewed consultants in the industry. What we heard consistently was that the size of the congregation was directly proportional to the size of the parking lot and the auditorium. Once either of those two things reached capacity, the growth of the congregation would slow down or stop. I've seen the same thing happen to dental practices. If a new patient cannot be seen for a month, then they are more likely not to schedule an appointment, or not keep one they scheduled. If an existing patient has trouble getting an appointment when they want one, or they see a practice that is busy and running behind, they are less likely to refer others.

Capacity in dentistry refers to treatment rooms and providers and staffing for those rooms.

Throughout my experience in coaching dentists who want to grow, it has become apparent that the very best investment they can make is to add operatories.

An analogy I often use is the pizza restaurant. Pizza restaurant owners make money selling pizzas. The more pizzas they bake, the more they can sell. How many pizzas they can bake is limited by how many pizza ovens they have. Dental operatories are like pizza ovens. The more you have, the more dentistry you can do. Also, the more operatories you have, the more patients you can see.

I've seen two types of dental practice owners. The first type is by far the most common. This owner increases capacity when the demand warrants it. In other words, when the schedule is consistently fully booked for four or more weeks, they consider adding capacity. The second owner increases capacity *before* the demand warrants it. They believe that adding capacity will stimulate growth. *They staff not for the practice they have, but the practice they want.* In my experience, the second owner grows not only faster, but bigger.

THE KEY CONCEPT

The Key Concept of Build It and They Will Come We attribute this famous quote to the film "Field of Dreams," referring to building a baseball diamond in a cornfield where players of past eras would return. In the business world, it refers to creating capacity for growth. Savvy business owners don't just respond to demand, they create demand, and remove all obstacles to the flow of new business.

7. Good Marketing Systems

Every practice markets, whether they intend to or not. Every impression that is made sends a message to someone about the practice good, bad, or somewhere in the middle. The good impressions have potential to grow the practice. These impressions can either happen on their own, or the practice can employ systems to make them happen more often and with more effect.

Marketing Systems

Systems to grow the practice are designed to grow the patient base. They may target certain types of patients, they may be internal (based within the practice), or they may be external (reaching outside the practice). Regardless of the intent or the method, *effective marketing* must exploit all the components of "The Marketing Formula."

The Marketing Formula

The Right Message, to The Right People, The Right Number of Times

Component #1: The Right Message (Unique Selling Point)

The most effective marketing message is one that addresses what makes you different. I recall the best marketing message I've ever seen while driving one day and looking up at a billboard. The advertisement was for a funeral home, but it could have been an advertisement for any business, including a dental practice, because of the power of its message. The message was very simple, but effective, and consisted of only two words – "We're Different." Think about that. People probably think most funeral homes are very similar. Guess what? They probably think the same about dental offices.

"We're Different" should be your marketing message. It says that your dental practice is not just unique, but that uniqueness is worth any extra inconvenience and cost.

Of course, you need to be able to explain why you're different. The words "We're Different" need to be backed by a compelling explanation of your unique selling point. This is where many dentists get hung up. When it comes down to it, they just don't believe they have a unique selling point (USP). I know that having a USP is worth hundreds, maybe thousands, of new patients each year, and that many new patients means hundreds of thousands of dollars, and often as much as millions. Therefore, I recommend dentists spend introspective time and include their team in answering *"The Million Dollar Question."*

The Million Dollar Question

I recommend that both you and your team (they will have invaluable input, and they are more likely to buy in if they participate) spend an entire team meeting, and more if needed, answering the following question:

"Why would someone drive by a hundred other dental offices to come to our practice and pay more?"

In the book "Blue Ocean Strategy," authors Kim and Mauborgne write extensively about the concept of the unique selling point, using the analogy of two contrasting methods of marketing. One is the Red Ocean, colored red because of the fierce competition (the red of blood) for the same market advertising the same message. The other is the Blue Ocean, not bloodied due to less competition as a result of strategies that separate the marketer from the rest of the marketplace.

I encounter dentists on a regular basis who put more focus on new patient flow than they should (at the expense of patient retention systems), and who don't have a USP. What they want from me, or anyone who has a marketing product to sell them, is just to tell them how much to write the check for.

Until you can answer The Million Dollar Question, you don't have a marketing message. If you don't have a marketing message, you can't effectively market. And if you can't effectively market, you should not pay for marketing because your return on your marketing dollar will be disappointing.

So, what is unique about your practice? Is it a service that you provide that no one else or very few in your marketing area provide? Is it your office hours? Is it your experience? Is it the training and/or accreditation that you have? Is it your team? Is it a combination of the above, or something else?

Perhaps it is something that you don't have yet, but that you know will set you apart. Remember, there's a reason it's called *The Million Dollar Question*. Therefore, whatever it takes you to develop a good answer is well worth the resources you must invest in that answer.

There is one more consideration when developing your marketing message: Who do you want to attract to your practice?

Component #2: The Right People (Reach)

Now that you have the right message, you need to communicate it to the right people. The parable in the Bible regarding sowing seed comes to mind. If the message is the seed, and the audience is the soil, sowing that seed in fertile soil makes for the best potential growth. Determining the right audience, what is often referred to as your target market or "Reach," requires answering four questions:

1. **What kind of patient best matches up with the *type of dental appointments you want* to have on your schedule?** Let's revisit the fact that you own your own business. You have the right and privilege to choose what you do when you go to work each day. Don't discount the importance of doing what you enjoy.

2. **What kind of patient best matches up with the *type of dental appointment you need* on your schedule?** Your business has goals. What type of patient best allows you to reach your goals consistently?

3. **What kind of patient *best matches your Unique Selling Point?*** Referring once more to Blue Ocean Strategy, your audience (the ocean you fish in) must match your message (the hook and bait).

4. **What kind of patient *best matches your marketplace?*** You must acknowledge what your market gives you. If who you want or need is in very short supply in your market, then perhaps you need to focus on the haystack, and not the needle.

The Four Parts of Determining Your Target Audience

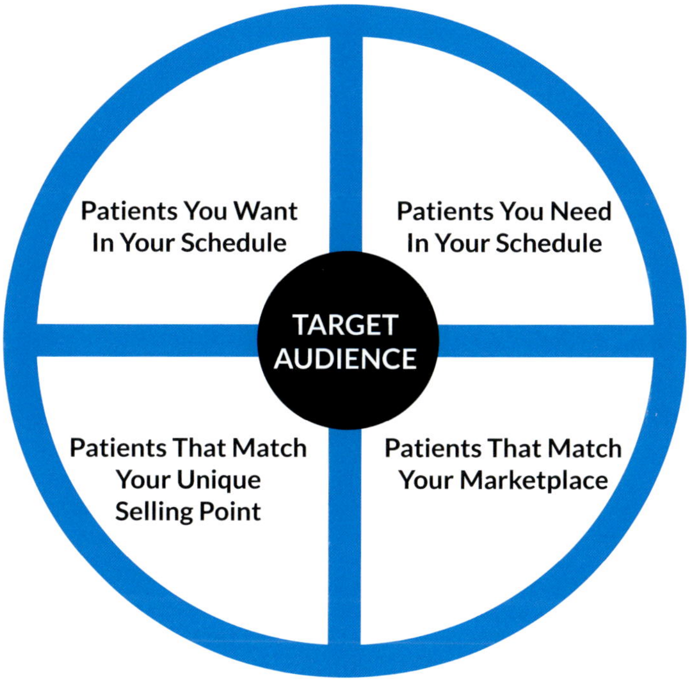
Patients You Want
In Your Schedule
Patients You Need
In Your Schedule
TARGET
AUDIENCE
Patients That Match
Your Unique
Selling Point
Patients That Match
Your Marketplace

The point where all four of these parts intersect is your target audience.

When defining your target, the more specific you can become, the better. Being more specific does not narrow the size of the audience to the point of being impossible to find, as the audience you market to will have some of these characteristics, but not all of them. Examples of specific characteristics include (in order of decreasing importance):

- Need for dental services (for example, replacement of missing teeth, addressing anxiety, etc.)
- Proximity to the office (this will differ depending on how far patients typically travel to the practice – more for rural areas, less for urban; the type of marketing; and the need of the patient)
- Age (reflects the makeup of the marketplace as well as the need of the patient)
- Gender (impacts the type of dentistry being marketed as well as the decision-maker in the family unit)
- Income and price of residence (for example, annual income exceeding $75,000 – often given too much importance, but important nonetheless)
- Education level (limited impact – Dentistry isn't that hard to understand, and the harder we make it, the lower the case acceptance regardless of the degree of education.)

Except for need, all these characteristics are readily available and can be found online in demographics reports for any designated area.

Still, even when the right message finds the right people, it's often not enough to cause action unless you make more than a fleeting impression.

Component #3: The Right Number of Times (Frequency)

The goal of the marketing message is to cause the right person to take the desired action – contact the office for an appointment. The gap between making a favorable impression with the message and taking the action to contact the office is significantly impacted by the number of times the prospective patients has heard, read, or seen the message and their sense of urgency regarding acting on the impression.

THE KEY CONCEPT

The Key Concept of 15X – In general, consumers need to experience a marketing message at least fifteen times before making a decision to act on that message.

Effective marketing requires repetition and time. You cannot afford to take a day off. One of the main reasons marketing of any kind does not work is that not enough time, effort, and resources are committed to making it work. In following through with our analogy of the seed (the right message) and the fertile soil (the right person), frequency is the rain, and it needs to rain consistently for the marketing seed to grow.

The Role of the Team in Marketing Success (the Marketing Committee/ Department)

Marketing, like most things that make up the prosperous dental practice, is team-driven.

Dental practice owners tend to place more emphasis on outside marketing companies and marketing systems, but it's the practice team that makes or breaks any marketing strategy or system.

First, the team must buy in to the importance of successful marketing. This is best accomplished through practice leadership laying out the vision for both the practice and the role that new patient flow plays in that vision.

Next, the team must see how their individual roles in implementation of that marketing all matter. One weak link impacts results. In fact, if marketing is to work, the team must be given significant responsibilities, as well as accountability through the *Marketing Committee.*

The Marketing Committee is a team within a team, made up of those team members who express an interest in playing leadership roles for specific parts of the marketing campaign. This concept was new to me when I decided to give it a try several years ago. After all, the team leader concept was a proven method of making each department perform better. Why not departmentalize and leverage practice marketing?

I laid out the platform for the committee: one team member would be primarily accountable for each part of the marketing campaign at the time – internal, website (content and SEO) radio, television, and direct mail. (Today, it would also contain social media and Google Adwords.) Committee members were solicited from volunteers and were given freedom to interact with outside marketing agents to develop plans that, when approved by the practice owner, were accountable for implementation of those plans.

Marketing team meetings are held outside normal business hours at a private room in a local restaurant (regular pay and dinner provided), where each member makes a presentation describing their responsibilities, assignments, and creative plans. Those present vote on the best presentation for a $100 gift card. The Marketing Committee has proven to be a great example of how The *Key Concept of Leverage* can help the prosperous dental practice reach the potential of its marketing campaign.

Internal Marketing

Internal marketing is marketing through existing patients or office personnel. As such, every office markets internally. Performing internal marketing at a high level is required *before* attempting external marketing, because internal marketing is the foundation of effective external marketing. Generally speaking, internal marketing brings the best return on investment due to its relatively low cost to implement, its higher response rate, and the higher quality of patient compared to external marketing. Because of this, the practice should strive to receive all the new patients it needs to meet its production goals from internal marketing alone.

The Three Components of Effective Internal Marketing:

Component #1: Answering the Telephone Effectively

I'm convinced that the telephone is the most important piece of equipment in a dental practice – more important than the digital scanner, the milling machine, the cone beam machine, or any other high-tech equipment that costs hundreds or even thousands of times more than a telephone system. This simple but vitally important system is often overlooked, primarily because its value isn't properly appreciated, and the owner of the practice seldom knows how it's being handled. If they knew, a high percentage of dental practice owners would be appalled.

In my years of consulting, my staff and I have played the role of the prospective patient in calling the offices of our clients and heard every conceivable way to handle the incoming phone call the wrong way, resulting in countless lost new patient opportunities. The poor handling of the phone call is seldom the result of office personnel intentionally performing poorly. More often, they are not properly trained, including being held accountable and receiving constructive feedback.

I can recount bad examples too numerous to mention here, but one such call that I vividly recall occurred when one of our mystery shoppers contacted a client's office to inquire about setting up a new patient appointment. During the call, we asked the individual from the office about dental implants, acting as if we were interested and wanted to know more about them. To our shock the person proceeded to tell us that a dental implant was "like a bullet that we put in your jaw." Our dentist client didn't believe us when we told him, until we shared the recorded conversation.

While the example given here is extreme, I know from experience that this incredible opportunity to make a great first impression and procure a patient is all too often lost at the front desk.

How To Effectively Handle the Incoming Call

Let's start with the purpose of any incoming call to the practice – a positive outcome. That outcome can take many forms, but all forms have this in common: giving the patient or prospective patient what they want. That may have to do with scheduling, or finances, or information about treatment, among others. What the practice gets in return is goodwill in the form of a good impression and, whenever possible, a scheduled appointment. Among the most frustrating incoming calls I have witnessed is a surprisingly large number of time-consuming calls from a prospective patient in which office personnel *never asked if they could schedule an appointment.*

Effectively handling the incoming phone call consists of three things:

1. The call is answered within three rings, handled by a real person, and the caller is not put on hold. Nothing says "We're too busy to handle your call" like having to wait for minutes to have your call addressed, and nothing is as impersonal as an answering machine or an automated voice giving you several options.
2. The call is answered with a smile, and handled in a non-rushed, friendly, and professional manner. The business office in a dental practice can be a busy place. But when the phone rings, that's an opportunity to grow the practice, so the business office team member should take a deep breath, smile, give the caller their full attention, and make a good impression. I recommend answering the phone with, "It's a great day at <Your Practice Name>, this is <Your Name>, I can help you!" This is a positive, friendly beginning that sets a favorable tone for the call.
3. The call is not terminated until a positive outcome is accomplished. Whenever appropriate, that means scheduling an appointment. The caller should be thanked for their call and allowed to hang up first.

Component #2: The Over-the-Top Experience

The goal is that every patient visit to the practice exceeds the patient's expectations so that the patient will mention it to others. Today's consumer is accustomed to a good experience, so the bar is higher than ever before (that also means an experience below that higher bar will cause the opposite and undesired review). The practice owner should involve the team in a mastermind session to creatively search for ways to exceed the bar. Suggestions could include:

1. Extra effort and time spent recognizing the patient's name, something personal about them (for example, their birthday), or something they requested from a previous appointment (such as a pillow)
2. Recognizing a patient as "The Patient of The Day" and providing them with a bouquet and/or gift bag
3. Providing the patient with a masseuse and a hand massage, or a manicure
4. Providing a complimentary service (e.g., free bleaching when they have other cosmetic treatment, a free mouth guard for children who participate in youth sports, or a free electric toothbrush after a big case)
5. Offering refreshments and a worktable with charging stations in the reception room
6. Posting a picture of the patient on practice social media with a caption recognizing something the practice appreciates about the patient (with permission, of course)
7. Providing a gift certificate for coffee, a car wash, or a movie

8. The doctor calling new patients the day before, introducing themselves and asking how they can make the patient's first visit a special experience, and/or calling the patient the evening of a procedure to check on them
9. Providing the patient with access to an entertainment system during treatment
10. Giving exceptional dental care

Component #3: Asking for the Referral

You can't assume that patients make the connection between being impressed with their care and referring a new patient. We must ask (see Key Concept of Asking under Case Acceptance). Many dentists and team members feel uncomfortable asking for a referral, believing it makes them look desperate. Performed correctly, it is the natural result of responding to a compliment. The process begins not with asking for a referral but asking a patient about their experience with the office – "How was your visit today?" or "Are you happy with the care we have been providing you?" or "How is your new crown doing?" or some similar question. When a complimentary response is returned, then a natural reply is "That's great to hear. If you know of anyone else who could benefit from the kind of care we provide, please be sure to tell them about us."

Asking for the referral still requires something else to make it an effective system – a reward for everyone involved in making the system successful, and a vehicle to remind each person involved and identify those to be rewarded.

The Reward

To expect team members to ask the patient for a referral, and for the patient to refer a prospective patient, and for the prospective patient to show up in the office involves three steps – and three places where the system can fail. For this reason, you will want to motivate each of the three people involved with a reward. Each team and market is different, but working with practices all over North America for many years, I have found that the following rewards induce action - $100 off a new patient's first appointment, $50 credit to the referring patient's account, and $50 to the team member who asked for the referral. In order to trace the sequence of events – asking for a referral from an existing patient, the existing patient referring a new patient, and the new patient showing up for the appointment – we need a vehicle – a referral card.

The Referral Card

The referral card has taken many forms over the years. Essentially, it is something that the referring doctor or team member can hand the referring source that will remind them to refer someone, as well as allow the referred patient to be tracked back to the source of referral.

The best version of the referral card is something that implies value, in order to identify and encourage the referring patient and prospective patient to both keep the card and to act. I recommend a referral card that feels and looks like a credit card, including a black strip on the back. The card needs to clearly state the value (for example, $100) as well as mention the words "Gift Card." On the back of the card is space where a permanent marker can be used to write the initials of the referring team member and the name of the referring patient.

Example of Referral Gift Card – Front

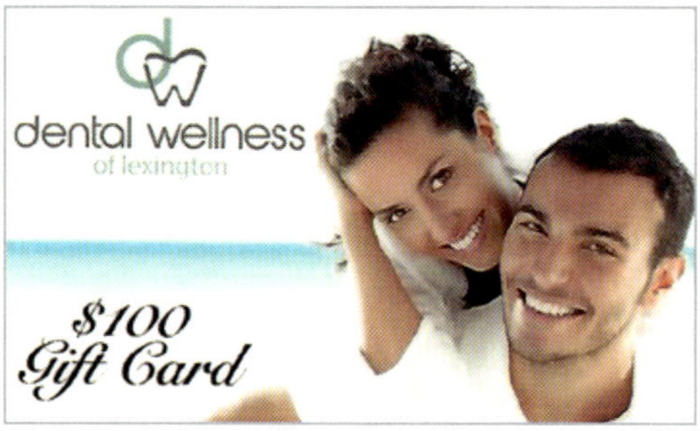

Example of Referral Gift Card – Back

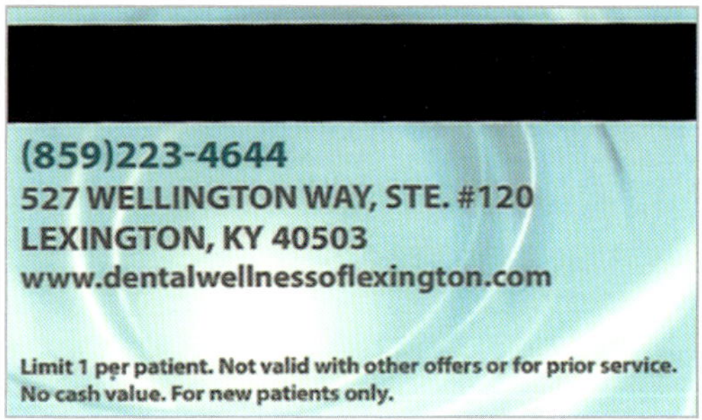

After asking for the referral, the team member can say "Here are some gift certificate cards so that anyone you refer receives $100 off their first visit with us, and for your thoughtfulness for recommending us, we'll credit your account $50 toward any future treatment."

The Gift Certificate Reward Program

Keep in mind that it's a numbers game. The more cards handed out, the more referrals you receive in return. Handing out cards sporadically will yield nothing. Handing out tens or hundreds of cards a day can result in an excellent return on investment.

Team members will need to be reminded each day to hand out referral cards, and they will need to see the practice owner lead by example.

At each month's total team meeting (see Team Communication section in the Leadership chapter), referral card rewards from the previous month should be handed out to team members whose referral cards have returned with their initials on them. The practice owner should make a big deal of these rewards, in order to positively reinforce the behavior. We recommend that the practice owner have a new $50 bill for each referral, and hand the new crisp bill to the appropriate team member by passing it through the rest of the team so that some, if not all, get to feel the money on its way to the recipient. (Be sure to keep track of these payments for accounting purposes.)

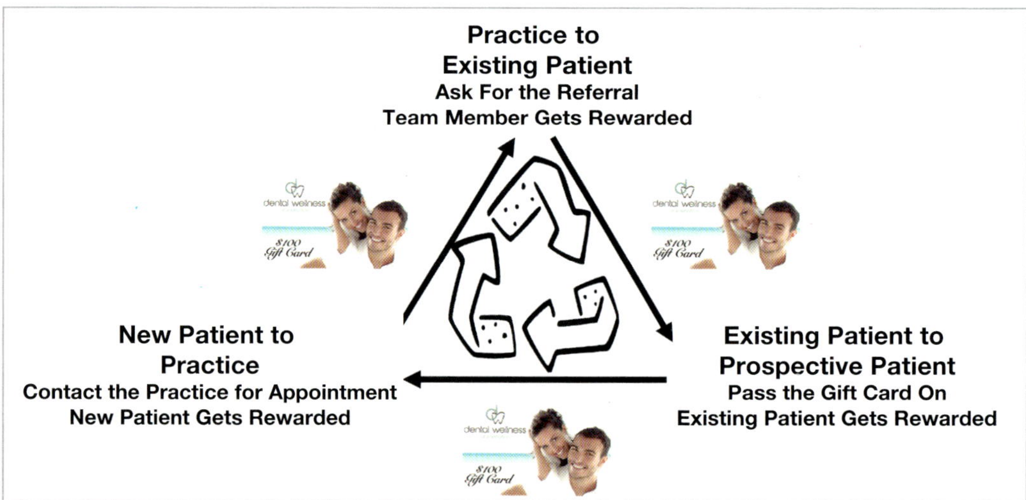

Some offices pool the reward money and divide it evenly among all the team members. The problem with this is that some team members will not ask for referrals, while others do most of the work. Rewarding everyone evenly unfairly rewards those who don't ask and punishes those who do.

The Power of the Testimonial

There is no better marketing than the recommendation of an existing patient. When that recommendation comes from someone a prospective new patient likes, they are more likely to act on the referral due to the heightened degree of believability and trust.

THE KEY CONCEPT

The Key Concept of Believability, Likeability, and Trust (BLT) – Faced with a decision about where to go and who to buy from for any product or service, people rely on trusted sources. They tend to trust those they like, and they often believe those they like. Therefore, if you want to be trusted, first seek to be liked. Then, you are more likely to be believed and trusted.

While not the same as a recommendation from a personal acquaintance, a significant degree of believability, likeability, and trust can be conveyed through a testimonial and recommendation from a patient of the practice. This is most effective when the existing patient tells a compelling story that the prospective patient can relate to, and the storyteller has characteristics in common with the prospective patient.

As with any marketing, the impact of testimonials depends on the message, the audience, and the frequency. Therefore, it is imperative that the practice creates and takes advantage of opportunities to produce and display as many testimonials as possible. Much like asking for a referral, practice personnel can request a testimonial. The difference is that the testimonial is requested from those patients who give the most effusive and emotional feedback, and who are the best match for the desired marketing demographics and treatment.

When this match is achieved it is important to be able to take advantage of the moment while the patient is in the office and the emotion is at its highest level. For this to happen, the practice must be equipped to efficiently capture (audio and video) the testimonial along with any high-quality photos and recording that highlight the testimonial.

The practice should set aside an area (the office photo/recording area) that is equipped with good lighting, a good quality camera, a good background (office logo and/or quote that captures the practice philosophy) and sufficient soundproofing.

Leading questions to prompt an effective testimonial include: "What has your experience been like with our practice?" "How has this treatment impacted your life (ask for an example)?" "What would you say to anyone thinking about having the same kind of treatment you have had?"

It is important that people smile while they are being recorded, and that they tell a story. Be prepared to have the patient do more than one pass so that their testimonial, when edited, conveys the message the practice wants to use for advertising purposes. Editing can be done by an outside source or accomplished by the doctor or team using commonly available video editing applications.

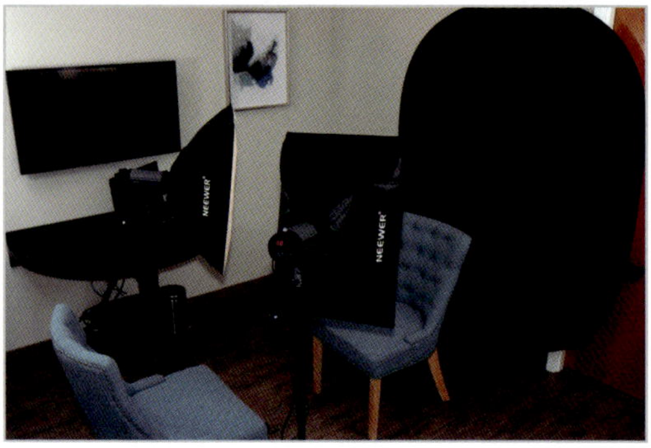

Photo Courtesy of Dr. Christian Yaste

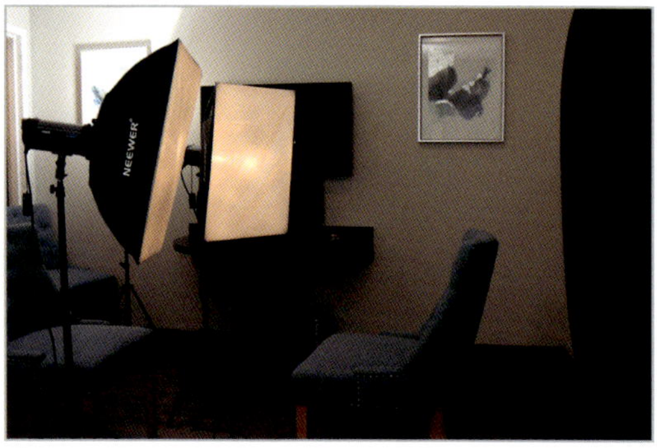

Photo Courtesy of Dr. Christian Yaste

Before the testimonial can be publicly displayed, the patient needs to give written permission to use their testimonial for advertising and educational purposes by signing a media release form. A modified version may be used for team members who participate in advertising and educational productions.

PHOTO, VIDEO, AND TESTIMONIAL RELEASE

I hereby authorize <Name of Practice> and/or any of their assignees to take photographs and videos of my face, jaws, and teeth, and use any written testimonials I may produce for the purposes listed herein.

I understand that the photographs, videos, and testimonials will be used as a record of my care, and may be used for educational purposes in lectures, demonstrations, advertising (including website publication, newspapers, magazines, phone books, television, social media, among others), professional publications (dental magazines and journals), and presentations.

I further understand that if the photographs, videos, and testimonials are used in any publication or as a part of demonstrations, my name (First Name Only) or other identifying information may be used unless stated differently below. I do not expect compensation, financial or otherwise, for the use of these materials.

Please initial:

_______ I do not mind if my first name, face, teeth, and testimonial are used in any of the above stated situations.

Exceptions:

_______ I do not wish to have my first name shown or released.

_______ I do not wish to have my face shown.

_______ I only agree to have my teeth shown without any identifying features.

_______ I do not wish to have my photos used at all.

Name: (Please Print): ____

Name/Guardian Signature: ____

Photographs of any cosmetic treatment the practice wants to use for advertising purposes should be collected on a regular basis. While several team members should be knowledgeable and skilled at taking high-quality photos and video, the practice may want to designate one individual with both artistic and technological aptitude to be primarily accountable for office photography.

Office photos for cosmetic advertising purposes should be full-face, above the hair to below the chin, and should be taken at a consistent distance in order to get the full effect of before-and-after images. Many dentists miss out on the potential impact of before-and-after photos by showing close-up intraoral images. The normal layperson cannot appreciate these images and, worse, may be turned off by them.

On occasion, a high-quality magnified image can have the desired effect for a patient to appreciate the quality of a particular treatment, but the dental team should see any image it takes and displays through the eyes of the intended audience. The question to ask is "If I were a layperson with limited knowledge of dentistry, would this image make the desired impression?"

These images can be displayed in various forms of advertising, including brochures, the practice website, and other internet marketing. Within the office, ***The Office Photo Book***, in either hard copy or electronic form, can be a very effective means of exhibiting dramatic before-and-after images. The more a prospective patient can identify with the before picture, the more compelling the after picture can be in their decision-making process to move forward with treatment.

In addition, after images can be portrayed throughout the practice reception area, consultation room, and hallways for patients to be reminded of what the practice truly accomplishes – the emotional side of cosmetic dentistry – creating confidence, self-esteem, and wellness. Too many offices miss this opportunity, instead choosing to adorn their offices with landscapes or other decor that may be attractive, but don't lend themselves to achieving the goals of the practice and the business.

Reactivated Patients

The definition of an active patient is one who has been seen for a comprehensive examination (in most cases, this examination occurs within or in conjunction with a hygiene appointment) and is scheduled for and/or has a history of having regular, recurring hygiene visits. An inactive patient is one who has only been seen on an emergency basis or has not had a scheduled hygiene visit with the practice for a year or more.

Most dental practice owners don't consider a patient's return to the office, after not being seen in the hygiene department for an extended period of time, as a new patient. Fact is, the returning patient that has or has not received care anywhere else in that period of absence will require a new comprehensive exam and, quite possibly, a new treatment plan. Therefore, any effort to reach out to the patient who has not returned to the office and has not notified the office of their intentions to not return is, in fact, marketing.

All patients, whether their appointment is with the doctor or hygiene department, should have an appointment scheduled before they leave the office. Even if the patient says they will have to "check my calendar and call you back," every effort should be made to make an appointment even if that appointed time has to be rescheduled later. Office personnel can simply respond "even though you aren't sure of your schedule at this time, it's best to make an appointment so we have time reserved for you, and if we need to change that time, it will be easier to move the appointment rather than create a new one." It is more of a challenge to reach a patient by phone to make an appointment than it is to make one face-to-face.

If a patient does not make an appointment before departing the office or fails/cancels their appointment without making another appointment (refer to Cancellations and Failures in the Scheduling Efficiency section), then the patient should be placed on a "Needs Appointment" list. The office software may do this automatically or in part as a "Broken Appointment Report." The scheduling coordinator and other office personnel should contact these patients promptly to reschedule them in accordance with Goal-Focused Scheduling parameters. The longer a patient remains unscheduled the less likely it is that they will ever reschedule.

Office personnel making the outgoing calls should be familiar with the patient's conditions and treatment needs, and be able to competently explain needed treatment and the need for, as well as the consequences of not having the treatment performed. Office personnel should also be trained in case acceptance so as to revisit the patient's chief complaint (SWOT), the emotional basis for moving forward (Dominant Buying Motive), and be able to address patient objections (trust, money, sense of urgency, and fear). When the patient cannot be reached directly, a message may be left to contact the office. Repeated inability to reach the patient directly may require calling after regular business hours.

External Marketing

External marketing involves methods that do not reach prospective patients directly through office personnel or the existing patient base. This is what is commonly referred to as advertising. I have found over the years of consulting that some dentists have negative views about advertising. Admittedly, as a young dental practice owner I viewed those dentists who advertised as unprofessional. After all, if you can't build your patient base on referrals, then you must not be able to do so, and that implies you aren't doing something right – or, worse, that you are doing something wrong. As a result, I also believed that my colleagues would hold me in less regard if I advertised.

It wasn't until I truly appreciated the dual purpose of dental practice ownership – that I owned a business as well as a practice – that I realized the importance of advertising. Effective advertising allowed me to have more control over the quantity as well as the quality of new patient flow, and any old-fashioned and unfounded opinions my colleagues may have had about me were less important than what I thought of me.

I also realized that all the work I was putting in to elevating my skills and making my practice truly unique was unknown to my marketplace.

Stuart Henderson Britt said, "Doing business without advertising is like winking at a girl in the dark. You know what you are doing, but nobody else does."

Truth was, I wasn't just like every other dentist in my area, and the most efficient and effective way to get that message out was through advertising.

Along the way, I learned a lot of lessons about advertising the hard way (trial and error and lots of fails), which was also the expensive way. I'm now confident that I know what it takes and how to gain an excellent return on investment from my marketing dollar. This knowledge has been critical to achieving my vision. Here are the most important things I learned (listed in chronological order of plan implementation):

The Nine Keys to Effective External Marketing

1. Make Sure Internal Marketing is Operating at a High Level

Before you spend a dime on marketing, you must be on top of the three key components to internal marketing mentioned earlier in this chapter – handling the telephone well, an over-the-top experience, and asking for the referral. If you aren't executing here, then you will never realize the true potential of your external marketing.

2. Hire a Marketing Professional

Realize that there are marketing professionals who know more than you about marketing. I wish I had a dollar for every dentist I've encountered who felt like they were best qualified to design their own marketing campaign. Fact is, most dentists are the least qualified to do this because they think like dentists, not like their audience.

I'm not saying that the dental practice owner shouldn't be involved. There's another faction of dentists who don't want to be involved at all. They just want to write someone a check for more new, high quality patients. That's like flushing money down the toilet.

What I am saying is that paying for advice from a marketing professional to assist you in making good objective choices, not influenced by a product that they have to sell you, makes perfectly good sense.

3. Remember the Marketing Formula

As already mentioned, effective marketing must involve the right message, to the right audience, the right number of times. (See previous section.)

4. Have a Goal

As with anything important, you must have a target before you aim and shoot. You will not only likely invest less but get a better return on your investment. This quantitatively-arrived-at goal comes from the New Patient Goal Worksheet directly, and the Practice Budget indirectly.

5. Have a Budget

The dental practice owner should have an approximate amount they are willing to spend on marketing (both internal and external). As a rule of thumb, a practice should not exceed ten percent of collections on marketing. As with any general rule of thumb, this ten percent is neither a hard-and-fast rule for every practice (a scratch practice would likely and appropriately spend more), nor is it as simple as making a certain dollar amount a line in the sand that should not be crossed.

Return on investment must be taken into consideration here, since this percentage is the percentage of practice collections, and more new patients can increase collections. Start with a number that allows the practice to stay well within ten percent of present collections and allows the practice to have diversity in its marketing portfolio. In other words, the practice owner should not spend the entire marketing budget on one form of marketing.

6. Choose the Right Form of Advertising

Of all the keys to success with advertising, this is the most important. It will impact return on investment not only through the number of new patients generated, but also their quality and cost to acquire.

Every market is different. One sure way to know that the wrong person is advising you is when they tell you that one type and form of external marketing works in every market. You should carefully analyze your options with the following five considerations:

1. Who am I trying to reach with my message? As previously stated, your message is dictated by two things – what makes you unique, and what leads you closer to your personal and practice vision. From there, your audience can be defined by the demographic qualities of the individual most likely to be attracted by and be able to respond favorably to your message. These demographic qualities may include age, gender, and income, among others.
2. Where are the most likely places I will find this audience? Do these individuals live or work near my practice? Do they frequent certain localities? Do they read certain publications? Do they listen to or watch certain radio or television stations? How much time do they spend on the internet, and how much are they influenced by internet marketing?
3. What are the options available to me in my market to reach this audience? Among the differences that make a market unique are the advertising options available in that market. There may be numerous opportunities, or in some markets there may be limitations. For example, signage may be restricted in urban and some suburban localities, or there may not be a local television market.
4. What is the competition like for this audience in these areas? Earlier, I referenced the book *Blue Ocean Strategies*. No matter how well a particular marketing medium matches the demographics of your intended audience, or how favorable the costs are, if there is significant competition, you are marketing in a "red ocean," and the cost of acquisition and return on investment will be negatively impacted.
5. What costs are involved and what is the likely cost per acquisition? The costs of marketing must be taken into consideration. However, more important than the top line (the cost) is the bottom line (the return on investment). If the need and potential return is great enough, then there have been times where I have advised dental practice owners to borrow the money to advertise. Case in point would be a start-up practice, but in a few instances it has been in the best interest of turning around a failing business to "bet on the come" (compensation based on future success). In other words, the rewards merited the risk.

Still, when choosing the best marketing options, every effort should be made to shift the risk versus rewards equation toward maximizing rewards and minimizing risk. Two ways to do this are diversification and using historical trends.

In addition to minimizing risk, *diversification of advertising* allows for extending reach and frequency. The dental practice owner must strike a balance between these favorable characteristics and spreading the advertising dollar too thin. A good advertising campaign reaches the potential of as many marketing forms as possible.

The other thing that diversification gives you is potential synergy. In other words, your internet marketing works better because another form of marketing drives the prospective patient to your website. It's as if one form of advertising is the bait, and another sets the hook.

Historical results from previous advertising should carry considerable weight when formulating an advertising campaign. If a particular form of marketing has been successful in the past, or presently is bringing a good return on investment and generating the type of patient the practice is seeking, then consideration should be given to doing more of that form of marketing. In other words, if something has worked or is working, then it makes sense when newer patient flow is needed to do more of that marketing. There is a point where investing more will not bring more, but this point is usually not determined until the additional investment is made. Conversely, if a particular type of marketing was not successful in the past, then it must be determined whether that marketing was incorrectly executed or whether it was wrong for the market.

7. Be Committed

Many advertising campaigns have failed simply because not enough time or other resources were committed to making it successful. Remember the Key Concept of 15X. Even though your marketing message may resonate with prospective patients, they are not likely to act immediately, or even within a short period of time. You must capitalize your marketing campaign for enough frequency for it to gain traction. Many times, I've had new patients enter the practice and say they heard about us from an advertising campaign that I had ended months previously.

Different forms of marketing take longer to gain traction. Signage, direct mail, radio, business to business, and television require greater frequency to be effective, while internet, professional referrals, magazines, and office seminars require less.

8. Be Consistent

Many dental practice owners are penny wise and pound foolish when it comes to their advertising, trying to time the market and looking for ways to save money by cutting corners. Henry Ford said, "Stopping advertising to save money is like stopping your watch to save time." When you start and stop advertising, it's often like starting over each time, losing momentum from the previous campaign.

I've heard practice consultants recommend shutting off external marketing during recessions, Christmas holidays, even election cycles. I've never seen the wisdom in doing this. During the pandemic of 2020 when most offices were closed (ours was wide open to seeing emergencies), we maintained our advertising campaign, just shifting the message to "we're here for your emergency dental needs" and "we place your safety first as we exceed infection control recommendations." Remember, people still see, hear, or read your advertising, and act later when they are ready. Advertising isn't meant to just bring immediate results, but to sow seeds. In addition, when everyone else isn't advertising, that's a prime time to be in front of your market with your message.

9. Track Results

You must establish a method of measuring results to determine if goals are being reached. The increase (or decrease) in number of new patients after a campaign is begun gives the practice owner an idea of how successful the marketing campaign is. However, the total number of new patients is not specific enough for the practice owner to make the best decisions about each specific form of marketing.

I've heard some consultants and many advertising companies with products to sell say that tracking where new patients come from is impossible. Their reasoning is that new patients either don't remember or they come from multiple sources, making specific tracking numbers invalid.

Experience has taught me otherwise. Tracking new patient sources is critical to making good decisions about getting the best results, as well as the best use of ongoing marketing resources. Like any system, if it's performed correctly, a better outcome is assured.

First, your team, especially the business office where new patient intake first occurs, must be committed to obtaining information regarding where the new patient heard, saw, or read about the practice. New patients are the lifeblood of any dental practice, and continued success depends on making good decisions when it comes to marketing choices.

The new patient intake form that the patient fills out must ask specific questions - not the typical open-ended question, "Whom may we thank for referring you to our practice?" or "How did you hear about our office?" Use a multiple-choice question format that allows for multiple answers (because the new patient usually does come from multiple sources).

Ask "How did you hear about our office? Please check all that apply:" and then list all possible sources, including current marketing and advertising, plus "other - please explain," as well as ones you aren't currently using but may use in the future. When the patient selects multiple sources, each source gets some credit, so the total equals one. In other words, if the patient selects two sources, each source gets credit for 0.5, if they select three, each source gets credit for 0.33, and so on. I know that a client is properly tracking new patient sources when their monthly report lists sources in whole numbers *and* fractions.

If the patient does not select a source, then the business office personnel must persist in acquiring this information by directly asking the patient. The category of "unknown" is not an acceptable category for sources of new patients.

THE NINE KEYS TO EFFECTIVE EXTERNAL MARKETING

1. Make Sure Internal Marketing is Operating at a High Level
2. Hire a Marketing Professional
3. Remember the Marketing Formula
4. Have a Goal
5. Have a Budget
6. Choose the Right Form of Advertising
7. Be Committed
8. Be Consistent
9. Track Results

Forms of External Marketing

Signage

There's a good reason why I list signage first. It is hands down the best potential form of external marketing from a long-term return-on-investment perspective. It may be a large one-time investment in the beginning, but it's an investment that brings a return over the life of the signage, which can be decades.

No doubt you've heard the oft-mentioned phrase connected to real estate and other business ventures – "Location, location, location." While this phrase certainly applies to dental practices as well, another phrase is almost as important – "Signage, signage, signage." When I'm consulting with a dentist regarding considering a location for a new practice, or a marketing plan for an existing one, one of the first questions I ask is about the availability of signage.

An external sign not only helps patients who are looking for you find you, but more importantly lets those who aren't looking know you are there. This is signage that plants a seed in the minds of future patients who drive by and see the sign on a regular basis, which they recall when they are considering a new dental practice.

There are two main factors that determine the effectiveness of signage: Visibility and Message.

1. Visibility – Obviously, a sign must be seen to be effective. To be seen it must be placed in the most visible position, so that it is exposed to as much traffic as possible. The higher and the larger the sign, the farther away it can be seen. Internally lit signs show up better during the day as well as at night.

When larger size, position, or illumination is not possible, then the business owner should look for creative ways to get the sign noticed. For example, an American flag, a dental symbol, or a clock, are ways to draw attention to signage. When an internally lit sign is not possible, then external lighting will suffice.

Sometimes, due to local regulations regarding signage, external signage more than a small monument is not possible. In these cases, the glass portion of the office windows and doors can be covered with attractive artwork that doubles as signage.

Electronic signs are excellent forms of signage. They can display images and rotating messages that can easily be changed as often as the business owner wants. In every case I've encountered where an electronic sign was installed, the additional cost was more than justified given the outcome of using this form of signage.

2. Message – The message should leave no doubt in the viewer's mind that this is a dental office. Given the amount of space availability, the most important message is the name of the dental practice and contact information – website address and telephone number (if there isn't room for both, the website address is more important). If additional space is available, and it doesn't decrease the visibility of the practice name and contact information, then a "Doing Business As" name (if applicable), or the name of the practice owner can be added. If an electronic sign is available, additional messaging can highlight services, special offers, and community service announcements.

home page (primarily the owner with other appropriate individuals participating) sharing his/her compelling practice philosophy and unique selling points. Participation in watching this video is optional for visitors, but the click ratio is favorable.

The effective home page includes video patient testimonials and a navigation bar with options that may have drop-down menus with links to About Us, Dental Services, For Patients, (containing information on financing and forms, as well as offers and promotions), Dental Insurance (when applicable), Reviews, Career Opportunities (often overlooked), and Contact Us. These drop-down menus offer separate pages where the visitor can find extensive information about the practice. The more specific the information is to the practice, including video and photos of patients and team members in the practice setting, the better for visitors. Remember, visitors to the practice website have a notoriously short attention span. To retain their interest, the site must be dynamic (action-packed) and interesting (information-packed). Words matter, but images matter more, and videos matter the most.

It is impossible for the website to have all the answers to the visitor's questions, and when a visitor wants answers, it is often after hours, or inconvenient to call the office. That's when a "***Live Chat***" service can be valuable communicating on behalf of the practice in real time with the visitor. Of course, practice owners have legitimate concerns about giving this responsibility to an individual they don't know who is acting as a surrogate team member of the practice. This concern is best addressed by working with a Live Chat company that has experience, demonstrates competence in dentistry, is familiar with the dental practice they are representing and their practices, and is monitored on a regular basis by the dental practice.

The content of the website is much like the advertising copy of any good marketing – it describes what makes the practice unique, including the services they provide, the way they provide them, and the qualifications of the doctor and team. Too many dental practice owners outsource this content, resulting in standardized, impersonal copy. Website content should be reviewed and updated periodically to reflect changes in the practice and fresh information.

If the practice is targeting a particular service (for example, implants), then that service can be highlighted in the practice marketing, including the website, using a "Doing Business As" (DBA) name. A DBA allows a business to use an alternative name to its official name, often for marketing purposes. The DBA is registered with the state and protected from being used by another business. An example is a practice having a DBA of "The Implant Center of Central Alabama." The connotation to the prospective patient interested in implants is that this practice focuses on implant dentistry; that information is likely to be meaningful in their choice of where to have their implant treatment performed. In the website page on implants (or a separate landing page), the DBA could be highlighted in the title – for example, "The Implant Center of Central Alabama, located at Birmingham Dental Care."

Google AdWords is an advertising system through the Google search engine platform and partner sites that places a text or image ad on a page after a user searches for keywords and phrases related to a business and its products or services. This system expands a business's exposure in its market through both reach and frequency when an organic search is made. Google AdWords can be purchased via a vendor (oftentimes the website administrator) for a specified monthly budget. The method by which the AdWords are charged is via a "click" on behalf of the searcher, leading to the system's often-used pseudonym "Pay Per Click." Both the words/phrases and budget play a big role in the effectiveness of the Google AdWord campaign. Whenever an internet marketing campaign needs a boost, *Google AdWords* can bring a good return on investment to the dental practice owner.

Landing Pages are a good way to target patients who want and need a procedure the practice desires to do more frequently. If the patient interested in a specific procedure is directed to the practice website, they may become distracted by all the other information. With a landing page, if a prospective patient searches for "implant dentist near me," and then clicks on the practice advertisement, they will be redirected to content dedicated to the procedure that individual is interested in – in this example, implants.

With the advent of ***Social Media***, the interpersonal communications landscape has changed forever. Now social media users have access to a whole new expanded database of information through interactions with friends, followers, and groups. While in the past consumers acquired their information from a trusted authority (for example, a health care professional they encounter during an office visit), the social media age has transferred much of that trust to members of the group they interact with on their smartphone, tablet, or laptop/desktop.

Therefore, social media is an essential part of any business's marketing plan. When orchestrated correctly, it allows the business owner access to thousands of potential customers with meaningful impressions on a frequent basis for next to nothing in terms of cost. Managing the business social media presence and marketing campaign is often referred to as Social Media Management (SMM), which like any other critical advertising arm of the marketing campaign should start with goals and a plan.

The goal of social media marketing is obvious enough – to increase exposure of the practice-marketing message and establish its brand in the local community. The plan follows the tenets of all effective marketing – reaching the right audience enough times with that message.

To do this, the business must establish a presence in the major social media outlets – Facebook, Instagram, and YouTube, along with an easy-to-remember "handle" (for example, @dentalpracticename). As with other parts of the practice marketing campaign, a team member should be accountable for social media advertising. This individual may enlist the help of other team members who express an interest. Posts and stories should be posted at least weekly and should highlight services, technology, testimonials, team members, and office events.

Managing followers (the audience) is a matter of choosing to follow existing patients and, those they follow, along with searching the "suggested for you" list supplied by the social media platform. Following and accepting followers who have large numbers of followers of their own (influencers), as well as health and appearance-related businesses, give the practice access to those groups. Accepting followers who are potential competitors, such as other dental practices, is counterproductive.

The influencer, an individual who has a dedicated social following and is viewed as an expert within their niche, gives the practice an opportunity to develop economic relationships in return for endorsements. Having an "influencer party" allows the practice the opportunity to host multiple influencers at a time dedicated to developing this part of social media marketing.

Geofence Marketing is a form of location-based internet marketing where a geographic boundary is placed around a point of interest. For a dental practice, this could be a business that high-income or health-and-appearance-conscious people frequent. Or it could be another dental practice competitor. When a mobile device enters this area, the Geofence can trigger an advertisement for the practice.

Business-to-Business Marketing (NEER)

The prosperous dental practice owner should market not only to individuals, but to businesses as well. The idea is for those businesses to promote and/or endorse the dental practice in return for some form of compensation, usually in the form of the dental practice promoting and/or endorsing that business. This form of marketing is often referred to as "Naturally Existing Economic Relationship" marketing or NEER.

Obvious business relationship opportunities with dental practices include those businesses that are within proximity to the practice, or that have customers with interests related to dentistry (cosmetic or health-related for example). The practice owner or representative would contact the business in person with a gift (food or flowers, and multiple gift certificate cards) and request business cards from the business. This gesture may need to be repeated multiple times for the referral relationship to gain traction. It is a numbers game; that is, the more businesses that are approached, the more likely NEER marketing will bring a positive return on investment.

Professional Referrals

Patient referrals from specialists and general dentists to other general dentists are a version of NEER marketing. Specialists see patients who don't have an ongoing relationship with a general dental practice and who request a referral from the specialist. Specialists tend to refer to general dentists who refer to them, or who they want to refer to them. Developing these referral relationships can mean a pipeline of new patients each month.

Developing these relationships is not a passive process, but one in which the general dentist seeks out and negotiates an informal two-way referral arrangement. This is where most general dentists fail, because they assume that, if they refer a patient to a specialist, the specialist will naturally respond in kind with a referral back. Most specialists don't work this way. They feel that their part of the referral relationship ends with taking good care of the referring dentist's patient. And when the specialist has a patient they need to refer to a general dentist, they often will refer to one with whom they have a social relationship. That is not a business relationship. That is a one-sided arrangement that benefits mostly one side – the specialist.

When I address this with general dentist clients, I ask them about the economics of their existing referral relationships with specialists. Most are taken aback by the question as they never considered the relationship to be economic at all, but rather a service that the specialist provides for the referring dentist and their patient. This is because most dentists don't fully appreciate one of the premises this book is based on, that the practice owner not only owns a practice, but they own a business, and nearly everything that happens within a dental practice serves both of those purposes to one degree or another. Most referral relationships serve the practice of the referring dentist, but not the business.

I then ask the general dentist to estimate how much income their referrals have meant to the specialist over the course of a year. The reply is tens of thousands, if not hundreds of thousands, of dollars. My follow-up question is, "How much income do you realize in return referrals?" The answer is almost always somewhere between zero and one-hundredth of the income referred out. Sometimes, the general dentist will follow up that answer with, "But they send me a nice gift every Christmas." One dentist told me how much they look forward every year to getting a cooked turkey from the oral surgeon they refer to. What that dentist didn't understand was they were paying $100,000 a year for a turkey.

The general dentist should buy their own turkey each year, and request referrals instead! I recommend inviting the specialist to lunch, reminding them of how the referral relationship has worked in the past, and how that has helped the specialist's practice. Then, request that the specialist return the favor and refer patients to them. The general dentist doesn't have to say what is implied – that the future of the referral relationship depends on it being more of a two-way street in terms of referrals.

Referrals from general dentists have long been the purview of the specialist dentist. However, general dentists usually overlook this opportunity that has the potential for a large return on investment. As stated earlier, one of the best ways to increase productivity is to perform dental procedures that most other dentists don't do, yet are needed by the general population. Both specialist and general dentists should market to their colleagues any procedure(s) their colleagues might not perform and/or would refer out.

Early in my career I appreciated the need for treating anxious patients, especially for extensive and invasive care. I would refer out these patients to specialists, but for the patients who needed operative or crown and bridge care, nitrous oxide was often not enough to address their anxiety, making for an unpleasant experience for everyone involved (including us). This is what started my journey to learn the art and science of safely sedating my patients with conscious sedation dentistry.

Once I became competent and confident with this modality it quickly became my favorite way of treating patients (and it addressed a major need in our community and surrounding areas). I found that very few of my colleagues wanted to see these highly anxious patients or add sedation dentistry to their repertoire of services. As a result, I developed a brand as a sedation dentist, and a niche in my marketplace that has served and continues to this day to serve both my practice and business objectives extremely well.

Other dentists in my area referred to me the patients they couldn't and didn't want to treat; often they saw these patients as, one referring dentist confided to me, "a 'life's too short' patient." However, when these challenging patients are properly sedated, they suddenly become great patients because they need lots of treatment and they want their treatment completed in as few appointments as possible.

When we realized the positive impact of these referrals to our production, we leveraged our niche market presence by advertising to other dentists. You may question whether another general dentist would refer to a competitor. The key is to alleviate that concern from the beginning. While I am not a specialist, and cannot present myself as one, I act like one in the sense that I tell referring dentists that I am happy to help with "their" patient, and to reinforce their patient returning to them for regular care. Fact is, many of my referring dentists are happy for me to take these patients they cannot treat and for them to become "my" patients.

I advertise my sedation services to other dentists (and nearby physicians) by contacting them personally, visiting them and dropping off breakfast or lunch, plus referral pads. I explain that my practice is happy to help with any of their patients who are too anxious to receive care

dental wellness
of lexington

Referral for Sedation Dentistry

Anthony S. Feck, D.M.D.
Maxie J. Combs, D.M.D.
Carol A. Wilson, D.M.D.

527 Wellington Way, Suite 120
Lexington, KY 40503
(859)223-4644
www.lexingtondental.com

Referring Doctor ____________________

Patient Name ____________________

Appointment Date ____________ **Time** ____________

Comments ____________________

____

____

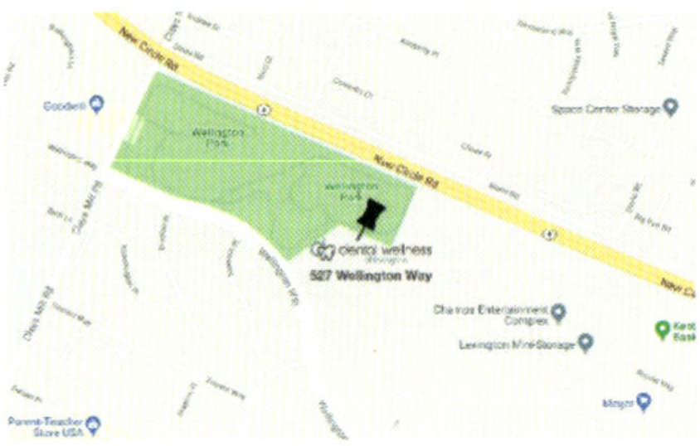

without being sedated. I answer any questions they may have regarding the sedation treatment. Again, I am sure to remind them that the patient will return to them for follow-up care after any sedation treatment in my office.

A modification to the following form can be made for any type of service the practice offers for referring dentists.

For those practices in the region who we are not personally acquainted with, we send a letter addressed to the practice owner, marked "personal and confidential," outlining the same message, with a referral pad. Here is an example of a referral letter:

> Dear Dr. <Personalized Name>,
>
> I hope this finds you well. I am writing to see if I can assist you in the care of any of your patients that may need <name of treatment>.
>
> You may or may not know that we perform <name of specific service> and have been doing so for several years. I have a passion for this particular care and began an educational curriculum many years ago that has allowed me to provide a high level of care for patients who could benefit from this service. I realize it is very possible that others, perhaps even yourself, also share this passion, and have extensive education and background in this field. If you don't and you would like to learn more about pursuing a similar journey in order to provide this care, I would be happy to share my experience.
>
> In case you prefer not to take that path, but believe you have patients who I could serve in the performance of their care by providing this service, I am happy to help here as well. All you have to do is contact me by email, phone, text, or simply have your patient contact our office for a consultation. Please be reassured that I would treat your patient with the highest level of care, and make sure that after they receive this specific care, they return to your practice for the completion of their treatment, and for ongoing preventive and maintenance care. In any situation in which I see your patient, I will be sure to keep you abreast of any interactions, treatment, and the outcome of that treatment.
>
> I have included a referral pad you can distribute to your patient for their use in contacting our office. Should you have any questions, please feel free to reach out to me.
>
> Professionally yours,
>
> <Your name>

When a referring dentist sends a patient, we are sure to communicate with them our findings, treatment plan, treatment, and follow-up post-care. We send a thank-you note and a gift to any referring dentist who sends multiple patients during a year.

Print Advertising

Print advertising refers to printed media in hard copy form, usually brochures, direct mail, magazines, or newspaper. While its impact has lessened as electronic media has exploded on the advertising landscape, there is a place in the marketing campaign for print advertising, especially printed practice brochures.

Practice Brochures may be used for internal or external marketing. In the office, they can be dedicated to specific procedures and distributed to existing patients as educational material. They may also describe office policies as part of a new patient packet.

Brochures for external marketing are designed to communicate the practice's unique selling point, as well as to deliver a call to action – to make an appointment. Every good practice brochure has in common the following five elements:

FIVE ESSENTIAL ELEMENTS OF THE PRACTICE MARKETING BROCHURE

1. High quality paper – Nothing that the practice distributes should look amateurish. Everything about the practice, including its printed advertisements, must reflect a high-quality image.
2. An attention-grabbing image – Pictures speak louder than words. If someone is going to take the time to read the copy, they need to be interested first. This image can be an attractive smile, a before/after image, or a picture of the doctor and team.
3. A compelling message that communicates the unique selling point – The message must describe the brand the practice wants to portray. It can be excellence, patient-centered practice, experienced caring team, a procedure, or a combination of any of the above.
4. A call to action – Now that the prospective patient is sold on your practice, they need a sense of urgency. This can be a special offer for a consult or new patient exam, accompanied by an expiration date.
5. The practice contact information and a locator map – List the practice phone number and website address, along with a locator map to make it as easy as possible to find your office.

Brochures can be distributed to nearby businesses as a part of NEER marketing or mailed as part of a direct mail campaign.

Direct Mail Marketing involves mailing practice brochures or postcards. It has the most potential to succeed when a substantial percentage of patients the practice is trying to attract live or work near the office. There is a direct negative correlation between the distance from the office the patient has to travel and the likelihood they will act on the mailer.

Another consideration with direct mail is the competition within the local dental market. If recipients of direct mail brochures receive multiple mailers from dental offices, the impact of the marketing will be diluted.

Additional considerations to a successful direct mail campaign are initial impression and repetition. The initial impression is critical because no one goes to their mailbox wanting to receive an advertisement from a dentist. In the first few seconds after scanning the brochure, the recipient will decide to throw it away or look at it further. Whether they look at it further or not depends on their interest in the message (the unique selling point and/or the offer), the mailer's images, and, to a lesser extent, the size and weight of the brochure.

Experience shows that a picture of the office staff or a before/after picture of a cosmetic case garners extra attention to the brochure. Both visuals can be used (one on the front, the other on the back) for maximum effectiveness.

Direct mail requires repetition. Recipients may act immediately, but more likely they will not. They might choose to keep a brochure for when they decide to act, or to act after throwing away multiple brochures. The campaign should allow for this.

Zip codes are chosen based on proximity to the office, as well as demographic considerations such as annual income, average age, property values, and education levels.

A typical campaign will choose three mailing areas and rotate these areas on a monthly basis. For example, brochures will be sent to area one in month one, area two in month two, and area three in month three. In month four, the cycle will be repeated. This way recipients receive brochures every three months, or four times each year. Because of the importance of repetition to direct mail marketing, the advertiser should commit to a year-long campaign, evaluating success at three months, six months, nine months, and one year. At each quarter, the response rate should be evaluated for tweaks to the mailing pattern.

Magazine Marketing is not nearly as popular as in the past. Magazines, like much of the print advertising world, have gone online. Still, traditional magazines are distributed and have the potential to reach a target audience of significant size. Cosmetic procedures, especially, have a place in periodicals that cater to health, fitness, and appearance. Placing a full-page advertisement next to an article that the advertiser authors is a good way to get more results.

The advertisement itself must contain the same ingredients as any good print advertisement – attention-grabbing image, compelling message, a call to action, and practice contact information. Magazine advertising, like all print advertising, is subject to the 15X rule. The advertiser would be wise to purchase several copies of the magazine with the advertisement and personally place the magazines (with permission of course) in the reception area of local gyms, hair and nail salons, plastic surgery offices, and high-end businesses.

Newspaper Advertising, like magazine marketing, is a small fraction of its former self. Newspapers have attempted to replace lost circulation through online versions, but newspapers continue to struggle and are no longer considered a primary source of news or other information. Still, there remains a niche market for newspapers, whether it is the traditional paper-based product or the online version.

This market is dominated by the Silent Generation (born 1928-1945) and the Baby Boomers (born 1946-1964). These older patients can have a considerable impact on office production due to their increased likelihood of maintaining their teeth, their need for tooth replacements like crown and bridge, implant-retained solutions, and their ability to afford large sized cases.

Newspaper advertising, like all marketing, works better when it is more visible. Space (full page for example) and position (front page of the first section, front page of a subsequent section, and the back page of any section) make a difference. Here again, the tenets of good print advertising apply.

Where newspaper advertising differs from other forms of print advertising (direct mail and magazines) is its lack of staying power. It is usually a one-shot deal – the recipient acts within a short period of time, or not at all. People do not hold on to newspapers like they do brochures and magazines. Therefore, newspaper advertisements must include a call to action that has a short deadline.

The Office Seminar

Newspaper advertising has been especially beneficial in promoting the office seminar. The office seminar is an event held by the practice to promote special services, such as implants, where the target audience is older (and still likely to read newspapers). The office seminar may reach a small number of potential patients, but the conversion rate can be especially high, and when the case size is large, the return on investment can be quite good.

The seminar is promoted in advance through marketing media such as television, radio, and newspaper. The essential ingredients to print advertising of the office seminar are:

1. A background picture of a smiling person in the age group the marketing is targeting
2. A compelling message such as "Dental Implants Gave Me My Life Back"
3. Bullet points enumerating the advantages of dental implants
4. An offer too good to turn down, such as, "Complimentary Seminar on How Dental Implants Can Change Your Life," "Financial Incentives Available For Those Who Attend," and "Free Refreshments"
5. A call to action such as "Don't Delay - Call Today to Reserve Your Place" or "Seminar Attendance Is Limited And Will Fill Up Fast."
6. Office contact information, including a locator map

Radio promotion of the office seminar would not have an image as with newspaper marketing, but both radio and television advertising would have all of the other elements of print advertising plus a testimonial from a patient.

Seminars are best held on Saturday mornings, at the office. Saturday mornings are best for the older population compared to a late afternoon or early evening time. Hosting the meeting at the office has the advantage of showing the attendee where the office is located, but more importantly allows the team to identify anyone attending who is ready to take advantage of the seminar offer to have a consult with the dentist. The seminar should take no longer than an hour.

Refreshments (for example, coffee and donuts/pastries) are provided, and office literature is distributed. Models of the service(s) being promoted should be available.

The practice dentist-owner makes the presentation, although it can be delegated to a well-trained, capable team member. The presentation consists of five parts, each of which can be portrayed by a slide deck (PowerPoint, Keynote) on a large screen television:

1. A picture of the dentist with either his/her team or his/her family standing in front of the office or office sign. This is where the dentist talks personally about why he/she became a dentist and why they love helping patients improve their lives through dental care, especially the type of care the dentist wants to promote at the seminar.

2. A testimonial or a picture (before/after) of a patient who was treated by the practice and how that patient's life was impacted by the treatment provided, followed by a story about that patient narrated by the presenter
3. A second testimonial from another patient, followed by their story
4. A third testimonial from another patient, followed by their story
5. Question & Answer sessions and "The Offer" (call to action) – *"If anything you've heard this morning speaks to you about your personal dental situation, and how (services listed here) could make a difference in your life, we would love to explore that potential with you. In appreciation for you taking the time to be here this morning, we would like to offer you a complimentary exam, x-rays, CT scan, and consult with the doctor to review your situation and data collected, a $900 value, if you have that done today and schedule a follow-up consult. Again, there is no cost for the data collection and consult, and there is no obligation. If you would like to take advantage of this offer, please see one of our team members. To everyone, we appreciate the time you took to be here today."*

Many of my clients use this simple format and get an excellent return on the investment of their time. How often the practice holds the office seminar is dependent on the response to marketing measured by attendance and the needs of the practice. A typical event gets ten to twenty attendees, a seventy-five percent acceptance of the call to action, and, of that group, a fifty percent case acceptance of some level of dental care. As an example, if the service is the placement of implants and associated prosthetics, ten attendees would mean four accepted relatively large cases from an investment of a couple of hours – a great return on investment.

Yellow Page Advertising

Yellow page advertising doesn't deserve more than an acknowledgement that it still exists, although in a form hardly recognizable from its heyday of several years ago. Fact is, although phone directories are still printed and circulated, their actual use is so small that they are irrelevant in the world of marketing. It is easier and faster to search online using a phone, tablet, or computer, with access to much more information. For this reason, the Yellow Pages have converted to a mostly online platform that generates poor to modest results, despite the claims from Yellow Pages sales personnel.

Still, there may be some markets, typically rural, where there still exists a positive return on investment from phone directory advertising. The conditions that would warrant this would be availability to purchase full-page or double full-page ("double truck") space in the beginning of the dentist section, a print and online combination package with good reach and frequency, a favorable cost, plus a recent history of effectiveness with Yellow Page advertising in the practice or local market. As with all marketing the key is message, reach, and frequency, plus a cost that works within the practice advertising budget.

Television Advertising

Television advertising, when used properly, can be highly effective. However, the advantages and disadvantages of television marketing for each specific market must be weighed in order to gauge its potential effectiveness.

The pros of television advertising are:

1. Ability to make a powerful visual impression – especially important with cosmetic dentistry and patient testimonials
2. Ability to reach a large population – important because Nielsen reports that U.S. adults watch five hours and four minutes of television per day on average

The cons of television advertising are:

1. Expensive compared to other forms of marketing
2. Challenge to target market a specific demographic
3. Much less effective if there isn't a local television market where the practice is located
4. Less effective if there is a lot of competition with other local dentists using television advertising

Developing a plan that could include television marketing starts with a goal. That goal includes the previously addressed components – reach, frequency, and audience. The prospective television marketer needs to do some research to determine whether these three components, along with the advertiser's budget, make television marketing a viable option to bring a good return on investment.

The most common source of information regarding reach, frequency, and audience for television marketing is Nielsen Media Research, which measures audience size and composition of television programming in the U.S. using a rating system.

Nielsen results are reported in two measurements: ratings points (percentage of viewers in U.S. TV households that were tuned to a program) and share (percentage of households watching TV at that time were watching the specific program in question). Several internet sources list the top Nielsen-ranked television shows and now include more than broadcast television, incorporating streaming platforms like Netflix, Hulu, and YouTube.

Nielsen ratings can also be obtained directly from the television stations in the local market, as well as costs for advertising during specific programming. In addition, the advertiser can use the services of a media buyer. Media buyers work on behalf of the advertiser to search for, evaluate, and negotiate terms for the purchase of media time on television or radio.

The media buyer often claims to be paid out of the discount they are able to negotiate with the television or radio station, although television stations are often able to offer similar pricing if the advertiser deals with them directly.

The potential advertiser should be careful using a media buyer who also has an advertising product to sell. Much like the financial planner who has an investment product for purchase, there is a potential conflict of interest that could result in the advertiser not receiving objective information to make a buying decision.

When making the buying decision, it is tempting to buy time during the highest rated airtime (the highest Nielsen rated show), but this accounts only for reach, not frequency. A better return on investment can be made by blending frequency with reaching the desired demographic.

Once the decision is made to purchase airtime with the television station, an advertising product will be needed. That product needs to satisfy certain parameters in order to accomplish its mission – to create a positive, lasting impression that has the most potential to cause the desired action – to make an appointment.

First and foremost, the message of the commercial must invoke an emotion on the part of the viewer. This can take the form of amusement, sadness followed by happiness, disgust followed by desire, surprise, or trust. If the commercial doesn't have an emotional component, then it is just communicating information. Remember, people don't make big decisions because they know more; they make them because they want more.

The other necessary ingredients are a call to action (for example, "call now," "limited offer," "you can start enjoying your new smile sooner," etc.) and practice contact information.

Who should write the script and produce your television commercial? Let's start with who shouldn't – the advertising dentist. That's not to say the practice owner should not have a vision for the commercial or be involved in every aspect from inception to final product. But the dentist must know their place, and unless they have advanced education as well as extensive experience in television marketing, it is best to leave all the heavy lifting to those who do. The television station may have resources in-house or can refer to an outside agency. Video production companies within the area can be sought out and interviewed. Whoever is chosen to produce the commercial should be able to supply examples of their previous work as a benchmark for their capability.

This television advertising product can take the form of a thirty- or sixty- second spot, a banner ad, or a thirty-minute infomercial.

The *thirty-second commercial* is the most common version. Television, due to its visual and auditory appeal, can leave a positive, lasting impression in this time period. Television programming often has multiple thirty-second commercials combined together during a commercial break. One technique of making sure the advertiser's commercial message is not lost among all the other commercial messages during the commercial break is to "bookend" the commercial. This is where the advertiser claims the first and last spots among the commercials being aired during the commercial break, taking advantage of both the first and last impressions.

The *sixty-second commercial* has more ability to tell a story, but the additional cost may come at the expense of less frequency. When frequency is less, audience (quality and size) and message must make up for it.

The *banner ad* is usually a rectangular graphic display that stretches across the top, bottom, or side of a website, other online advertising, or television commercial. In the context of television advertising, the banner ad is used to highlight a particular event and call to action. An example would be to contact the office today to learn more about financial assistance, or to receive information about a particular service. The banner ad has shown to be effective when advertising the in-office seminar.

The *infomercial* is typically thirty minutes in length and therefore can present a lot of information (hence the name infomercial), but the advertiser must be careful to make the advertisement about the emotion (how the service or product can change the viewer's life for the better), not the information (details and specifics about the service or product). The real advantage to the longer time the infomercial affords is the ability to show multiple testimonials and develop rapport with the dentist.

My own personal experience with using infomercials over several years has shown that patients who come in to the practice as a result of viewing the infomercial feel as though they *know and trust me* before they meet me in person. The credibility that a properly produced infomercial can bestow on a product, service, or individual speaks to the tremendous power of television marketing.

The cost of television advertising is one of the negatives and will be impacted by broadcast versus cable (broadcast is generally more expensive), the time of day (prime time is more expensive), the individual station (the highest ranked station in a market is usually more expensive), the time of year (supply and demand), and the length of the airtime being purchased (the longer the commercial, the more expense). The advertiser must weigh cost, reach, and frequency when determining the options that have the most potential for return on investment.

For example, one would expect the thirty-minute infomercial to be more expensive than the thirty-second commercial, and in many cases that is true. However, a thirty-second commercial in prime time on a broadcast station can cost quite a bit more than a thirty-minute infomercial on a cable channel during non-prime-time.

In fact, I have found that the infomercial airing during a non-prime-time slot early in the morning can reach the desired demographic (for example, implants for the elderly population) much better than a prime-time slot with a broader reach at a considerably greater expense. As with any marketing, the advertiser starts with a goal, including the number of new patients, the budgeted amount, and the desired audience, keeping in mind the necessary frequency needed to generate the intended response. On numerous occasions I have had a new patient from our infomercial say that they watched the infomercial over and over for three years before calling to schedule an appointment.

Radio Advertising

Radio advertising has in the past been a prime marketing strategy for marketing dental practices, and it is still effective in selected markets to this day. The reason for its decline over the last few years is the increase in satellite radio share of the radio market, as well as the overall decrease in radio's influence on the public due to paradigm shifts in the marketplace. Despite the changes in how people access music and talk platforms, radio advertising can still bring a good return on investment given the right market and advertising product.

Getting the listener's attention on radio can be more challenging than television because the listener only has the audio message. This message must be entertaining (humorous or dramatic), informative, or answer a prevalent need. Here, again, telling a story through patient testimonials makes the message resonate more with the listener. The radio advertisement should end with a call to action and contact information for the practice.

As with television advertising, picking the right audience is key. Nielsen Audio (formerly Arbitron) collects listener data on radio broadcasting audiences using ratings. A rating is the percentage of a specific population that listened to a piece of content or ad. Potential radio advertisers can acquire this information directly (Neilsen.com), or indirectly through the radio station or media buyer.

Radio advertising has the most potential to be effective when there isn't a local television market, there isn't much competition with other dentists on radio, and Nielsen Audio ratings are favorable.

Billboard Advertising

Billboard advertising can be a supportive form of marketing, increasing the effectiveness of other, more influential, advertising (word of mouth, internet, or television), under the right conditions. Because billboards are essentially remote signage, if the practice has limited facility signage availability, then a billboard can present an effective alternative.

As with any advertising, the outcome is determined by the right audience, the right message, and the right frequency. With billboards, both the right audience and the right frequency are most impacted by the location of the billboard. The advertiser wants a billboard with the following attributes (in order of decreasing importance):

1. **Memorable message** – If the billboard viewer glances at the billboard advertisement (usually while driving or stopped at an intersection), the advertisement must make a memorable impression within seconds. This requires as few words as possible, not only to make that impression, but also to be large enough to be seen from as far away as possible. The rule is *no more than eight words* for the message itself, plus contact information (website/phone number), and, if space allows, a call to action.

   Obviously, eight words are not a lot, so they must be chosen carefully, but here is a good example of where less is more. A clever or humorous message tends to imbed itself in the viewer's memory. Consider the following examples:

   "I think – therefore iMac"
   "One nation under me – God"
   "I Just Slept with My Dentist – Sedation Dentistry"

   The message can be the "brand" of the practice. Examples such as "Friendly Dental Care" and "Smiles by Design" are phrases or combinations of words that create an identity. Whenever using branded advertising, consider having it trademarked for legal protection against others using it.
2. **Memorable image** – The image can be as meaningful to the message as the words – if not more so. The image of a hammock hung between two palm trees next to a serene beach background complements the words "Relaxation Dentistry – Like A Day at The Beach."
3. **High-traffic count** – Advertising results are a numbers game. The more who see it, the more potential it has to influence the viewer.
4. **Located in a growing, affluent area** – The more the right kind of viewers see the billboard message, the better.
5. **As large as possible** – As with any form of signage, the bigger, the better. This is especially important as the distance from the viewer increases.

6. **As close to the office as possible** – Especially in urban and suburban areas, viewers are less likely to act on the message the farther away the practice is from where they work or live.
7. **At an intersection or other area where traffic is slow-moving** – If the billboard viewer is stationary at an intersection or slower traffic area, then there is more time to view the billboard and let the message sink in.
8. **With as little signage competition as possible** – There should be as little visual noise in the area of the billboard as possible, as other signage or distractions dilute the billboard's potential to make an impression – or be seen at all.
9. **Night-time lighting** – A billboard that doesn't have lighting loses its effectiveness after dark, while night-time lighting accentuates the billboard more than day-time light due to the increased contrast.
10. **Short-term, renewable lease** – The advertiser wants a billboard lease with good terms. Obviously, the advertiser wants to pay as little as possible, but needs to appreciate that the best locations for reach and frequency garner the highest costs. As with any advertising, the cost is only one consideration – return is the other, more significant one.

    If the billboard space has yet to prove its effectiveness, then the advertiser doesn't want to be tied to a long-term lease (more than six months) should the return on investment be ultimately unfavorable. At the same time, if the results are positive, the advertiser wants the option to continue to advertise at that location. If the owner of the billboard space will not extend options to continue advertising on short-term leases less than a year, then it is worth it to sign a one-year lease.

    Billboard space owners in higher populated areas may require advertisers to rotate their space with other advertisers. This means the advertiser may have the desired space for three to six months, then be moved to a less desirable space. This allows the billboard owner to make the most desirable locations available to more advertisers. The advertiser must weigh the advantages and disadvantages of the various locations included in the lease package in order to determine the potential return on investment. In these type of lease packages, the advertiser often has some leverage to negotiate other lease terms such as cost and length of lease.

Electronic (digital) billboards have the added advantage of being more noticeable than traditional billboards, flexibility in changing the message and image, and increased access to prime locations. The disadvantage is increased cost and competition with other advertisers using that same space. As with any billboard advertising, the purchaser of digital billboard advertising must have a unique selling point message, along with sufficient reach and frequency.

Discounted Fee Plans

As mentioned previously, discounted fee plans (for example, Preferred Provider Organizations or PPOs) are a form of advertising. The dental practice owner agrees to perform services at a discounted rate in return for the plan including the practice in its list of participating providers that will be provided to all its subscribers.

The practice owner considering participating should perform a *PPO Analysis* to determine if the discounted fee schedule is profitable and to what degree. The lower the degree of profitability, the more new patients and production from those new patients will be required to make using discounted fee plans as a marketing tool a good return on investment.

Of all the marketing tools discussed to this point, discounted fee plans allow the practice the least amount of control. The marketing message is controlled by the PPO plan, and it seldom separates one practice from another as they are all listed equally on the list of providers. The number of participants in the plan determines reach, and frequency is determined by how often the plan markets the list to its participants. Still, there is the potential for a large number of new patients to come from participating in PPO plans, and as long as the plan discount and the practice overhead allow for profitability, this can be a good marketing tool, despite the relatively high cost involved.

Patient Retention

Paramount to the growth of the prosperous dental practice is not only attracting new patients *but keeping them in the practice for as long as possible.* I know of far too many practices that have a large amount of new patient flow, but have zero net growth, as the new patient flow is negated by patients leaving. These same practices find themselves completely dependent on heavy new patient flow and therefore must invest an inordinate amount of resources on marketing.

According to sources, an *average* dental patient spends between $22,000 (Derek Naylor) and $45,000 (True Dental Success) over a lifetime. If the cost of acquisition is high (more than $300), then the return on investment can be negative or enormous depending on how long the patient remains in the practice. Therefore, retaining patients should be an important part of any practice's plan for growth.

A normal attrition rate of between two and five percent of the patient base annually is to be expected due to patients moving or dying, or changes in their employment or insurance status. Every practice has a portion of their patient base who stays with the practice simply because they don't like changing dentists; the patients will change if they have a bad experience or if another practice offers them something they aren't currently getting. We'll call this group the *fragile portion*. Every practice has another group of intensely loyal patients who are patients for life. Let's call this group the *loyal portion*.

The prosperous dental practice has a very high ratio of loyal to fragile patients, by building loyalty the six following ways:

1. **Treat patients like guests, not customers**. These practices are professional in their dealings with their patients, but they also realize that hard-core loyalty is the result of personal relationships, not working relationships. They make patients feel special. They recognize them by name and show genuine happiness to see them. They know about their patients as well as their dental condition.

   I've always been challenged with remembering names, but could usually remember a face. I could even remember if they had a cusp of Carabelli on their upper first molar. I set out to be better. My practice takes a picture of every patient and places it in in their record, along with some personal notes about family, hobbies, pets, their last vacation, or anything else that comes up in a conversation with them. Each day as I prepare for my appointments, both in my chair as well as the hygiene patients I check, I match the picture with the name and read these personal comments. Recognizing patients by name and mentioning items about their lives makes them feel special.

It's applying the platinum rule – "Treat others like they want to be treated." Patients may not know it, because they don't expect to be treated this way at their dental office, but trust me, they would like to be treated as if they were guests staying in your home. Would you make sure they were comfortable? Would you ask if you could get them anything – a bottle of water, a pillow, or a blanket? Of course, you would – and your guest would appreciate it, return, and tell others.

2. **Provide exceptional treatment**. I've been discussing care, not just treatment, but certainly patients won't continue to patronize the practice unless they are pleased with the outcome of their treatment. Today's patients are more empowered than in the past. They will leave a practice if they feel they've been handled roughly, have unresolved sensitivity following treatment, or must have something redone. Set the bar high when it comes to dental treatment, and consistently exceed those high standards.
3. **Value patients' time**. Nothing says, "My time is more valuable than your time" and therefore "I'm more valuable than you are" more than when the office runs chronically late for its appointments. Most patients have too many choices in dental offices to not feel valued by the office. Seeing that appointment time as a promise made to the patient is a core value of the prosperous dental practice.
4. **Have friendly, competent team members**. The stereotypical demeanor of a dentist is a professional, yet introverted, personality. This can come across as unfriendly, when it is often the result of someone serious about their craft who strives to be at their best to perform difficult procedures. This intensity can be interpreted as a poor bedside manner by the patient who values friendliness. You can overcome this by focusing on improving this aspect of patient interaction and by surrounding yourself with team members who are naturally outgoing and friendly.

   Not a week goes by that a patient doesn't compliment me on my team. We rely on our great team, and their professionalism is a big component of the positive image our patients have of our practice. Our patients are impressed by our team's competence, their attitudes, and their level of concern for the patient experience.
5. **Stay at the forefront (not necessarily the leading edge) of new technology and techniques**. Patients may not mention this as important, but they notice it when it's absent – and especially when it's present. There is simply too much information available to the public about advances in dentistry via marketing and the internet. Patients perceive "updated" and/or "upgraded" as being synonymous with "advanced," and in their minds that means better care. Patients will leave a practice if they feel they can be better cared for somewhere else.

   There's another thing the practice that stays at the forefront of technology and techniques must do. They must let their patients, as well as their prospective patients, know about their expertise. Don't assume your patients know you've been to a continuing education course or have completed a curriculum that changes significantly what you do. Don't expect them to notice a new piece of equipment, often out of their sight, that is a real advancement in the outcome of their treatment. Tell your patients, and don't forget to tell others outside your patient base, via your website and your other marketing tools.

6. **Have a persistent presence in patients' consciousness**. Patients are bombarded daily with messages. If your presence is not reinforced regularly, your dental office becomes lower on their ladder of consciousness, and another dental office's message may supersede yours. Make sure to maintain a persistent presence through your advertising, social media, and direct patient communication.

   Notice than none of the loyalty-building methods mention money. My practice charges fees that are in the top-twenty percentile for our area. The fees you charge have little to do with whether patients repeat and refer. Much more important is how you make them feel.

SIX WAYS TO EXCELLENT PATIENT RETENTION

1. Treat patients like guests, not customers.
2. Provide exceptional treatment.
3. Value patients' time.
4. Have friendly, competent team members.
5. Stay at the forefront of new technology and techniques.
6. Have a persistent presence in patients' consciousness.

PROFITABILITY SYSTEMS

The ultimate objective of any business is to be as profitable as possible, with the definition of profit being the net revenue that exceeds all costs related to operating the business. All the systems described in this book are designed to have an indirect or direct impact on the bottom line. This section addresses those systems that have the most direct effect on profitability.

The Profit Formula

Profit is the direct result of three systems - Production, Collection Rate, and Expenses - working at as high a level as possible. The twelve systems that impact a productive schedule, as well as the financial systems that affect collection rate, have already been covered. In this section, I will address adjustments to production and collections in more detail, as well as the subject of overhead.

Adjustments (Write-Offs)

Negative adjustments to production and collections (aka write-offs) are the silent killers of profitability. "Silent" because they often go unnoticed by the practice owner, and "killers" because they represent production work accomplished that is accompanied by the overhead to perform that work that can never be collected, or in the case of negative adjustments to collections, money returned. Unfortunately, I've encountered many practices that were highly productive and had good collection systems but were unprofitable due to write-offs.

Adjustments need not be silent. They should be tracked by always posting the gross amount of production according to the practice fee schedule, as well as collections, and any adjustment posted in its correct category (for example, PPO, senior discount, marketing, bad debt, etc.). At least once a month an audit trail report that lists all adjustments for that month should be provided to the practice owner and reviewed.

How many write-offs are too many? Generally speaking, eliminating or reducing write-offs as much as possible is the best answer. However, the sum total of write-offs that can be tolerated depends on how much the profitability of the business can tolerate. In other words, the write-off totals that can be tolerated must be considered in light of the practice production and overhead. I work with practices that have a great deal of write-offs yet are extremely profitable due to their high production and low overhead. In some of these practices, their write-offs actually increase their ability to be more productive. Not only can some practices tolerate write-offs better than others, some write-offs are better or worse (better vs. negative write-offs) than others based on their potential to lead to more or less production.

Negative Write-Offs (in order of better to worse):

- **Preferred Provider Organizations (PPO)** – These write-offs represent the difference between the regular practice fees and the fee allowed to be charged by the PPO plan. The advantages and disadvantages to participating in discounted fee plans have already been covered. Ideally, the practice doesn't participate in PPO plans (fee-for-service practice). However, when it makes sense to participate, the practice should maximize the advantages (more patients and production) and minimize the disadvantages (less profit). This includes choosing the right plans to participate in, maximizing production (volume), and, when necessary, limiting the number of PPO patients in each day's schedule. Signs that participating in PPO plans no longer makes sense are a decreasing collection rate each year and decreasing profitability despite increasing production.
- **Employee Dentistry** – A common benefit provided to practice employees is free or discounted fees for dental treatment to the employee and their family. Like most adjustments, many practice owners are not aware of just how much this costs the practice. Like any other employee benefit, limitations should be placed regarding timing of the benefit (both when it starts and when it can be used), who in the employee's family qualifies, the annual maximum, and the amount of discount.

A typical example would be:

  - Three-thousand dollar maximum/employee/year
  - Benefit starting after a successful ninety-day probation period following initial employment
  - All dental work provided at no charge except for any outside costs such as wholesale product and laboratory costs
  - Eligibility for employee's immediate family (spouse/partner and dependent children 25 years or less in age)

- **Charitable** – These write-offs are for charitable causes and selected individuals. It's good to be generous and share the blessings from success achieved. It's even good from a tax-planning basis. One can even argue that it's impossible to be too generous.

One can also argue that every practice expense, including charitable contributions, should be monitored and have a budgeted, planned limit so that they do not negatively impact projected business profitability.

- **Close Personal Friends** – In reviewing clients' monthly reports, I often encounter large amounts of dentistry written off for their friends. When questioned, these practice owners describe large cases with extensive time and cost involved. Sometimes the individual in question is a long-time, close friend, and other times they are closer to an acquaintance than a friend. When I ask these same practice owners if they in turn expect a discount when patronizing any of their friends' businesses, they often say no – and if they receive one, the relative size of the discount they receive pales in comparison to the discount they extend in their dental practice. I'm all for giving a close friend a break, but that discount should be at least within the profit margin of the business. In other words, the practice owner should not lose money when treating friends.

  Consider this: A discount to a friend is like a present. If that friend doesn't think you spent enough on their present, then the friendship needs to be reconsidered.

- **Barter** – Barter is trading dental services for products or services.

  Unfortunately, most of the time when bartering, the dental practice loses. In other words, it isn't a fair trade. The reason for this is that there is less profit margin in providing dental care than most services or products they are trading for.

  My favorite common example is when the practice owner trades dental care for jewelry. The average markup for jewelry is two hundred to three hundred percent, while the average markup for dental practice owners is 27%. If the practice owner is going to trade services for other services or products, then the practice owner should do their homework and make a good (or at least a fair) trade. Better yet, eliminate barter altogether.

- **Senior Discounts** – Somewhere in the past, dental practice owners decided to give a financial break to older patients, most likely because older patients asked for one. Even though some businesses – restaurants during low traffic times, for example extend senior discounts, that does not mean that dental practice owners must do so as well. Every dentist has heard a retired person say, "I'm on a fixed income" when it comes to discussing finances. Fact is, a lot of people are on fixed incomes, not just seniors. Actually, seniors have more financial resources than most young people do.

  In fact, most of the wealth in the U.S. is concentrated in the older population. If practice owners charged their patients based on ability to pay, then their fees would increase with the age of the patient.

  Of course, that's a silly proposition. If so, then why isn't extending discounts to seniors silly as well?

- **Miscellaneous Write-Offs** – I dislike this category because it has no meaning. The practice owner should insist that those posting adjustments eliminate it. Either place the adjustment in an existing category, or when appropriate create a new category and post it there. If you don't know the precise reason for a write-off, you should not accept it.

- **Bad Debts** - These are adjustments for money that is deemed uncollectable from dentistry produced. This is the most negative write-off of all, as it means giving up on compensation for care rendered, which includes both the cost of providing the care and the expected profit. The Financial Systems section of this book reviewed the means of both collecting money within an appropriate time frame and dealing with delinquent accounts.

  Bad debts should be written off only if you believe that continued collection efforts would be more costly than writing off the debt. Whenever debts are written off, the patient's account should be inactivated, the account flagged accordingly, and any patient belonging to the account available for reactivation only on a cash basis along with payment of the written-off debt plus any penalties in advance of the appointment.

Better Write-Offs (in order of better to worse):

- **Pay In Advance** - Let's be clear: this is not a "Pay Today" write-off. Extending a discount because the patient paid at time of treatment makes no sense. That's just a fee reduction. The Pay in Advance courtesy of five percent is for paying at time of scheduling, for scheduled treatment of one hundred dollars or more, and paid by cash or check. Given the nature of the schedule of most dental practices, the discount is applied to appointments often scheduled weeks in advance. The practice may elect to allow the discount for payment up to one day in advance of the appointment.

  There are three advantages to this write-off: 1. The office is assured of being paid. This treatment will not increase the practice's accounts receivable, 2. The office can use the resources from this advance payment (cash flow for operating expenses before treatment is provided, plus any interest accrued), and 3. The likelihood that the patient will miss or reschedule their appointment is much less. Practices who have high Pay In Advance write-offs have higher production and collection rates, and therefore are more profitable.
- **Patient Referral Reward** - The system of using patient referral cards to internally market the practice has already been reviewed in the Growth Systems section. This write-off will include the amounts paid to the referring patient and the referring team member, and the discount for the new patient's visit. While this may amount to more than one hundred dollars per new patient that comes from this system, this cost of patient acquisition is almost always worthwhile in comparison to the value of a new patient to the practice over time.

- **Marketing Offer** - As with patient referral reward write-offs, marketing offer discounts result in more new patients. This adjustment, however, is from external marketing. An example would be a "New Patient Special," a call to action extended by way of print advertising. As long as the write-off amount is reasonable, having large marketing offer write-offs indicates the marketing is working. The reason patient referral reward write-offs are preferable to marketing offer write-offs is that patients that result from internal marketing tend to have more value to the business than those that result from external marketing.

- **Outside Financing** - Write-offs from participating in outside financing programs such as *CareCredit®* can often be as much as a 15% adjustment off of collections. While they are usually less than this, they do affect profitability, and therefore should be reserved for large production cases (for example, more than $3,000). The impact on profitability notwithstanding, these write-offs can lead to bigger cases, and more production. Practices with few outside financing adjustments typically provide less big case-type dental care, and/or do not have an effective means to increase case acceptance. Every large case presented where cost is an objection should include the option of outside financing. The business office (or whomever provides financial arrangements) should know which programs have the best terms for both the patient and the practice and be well-trained in how to present and use those programs to their fullest potential.

- **Refund Overpayment** – These write-offs reflect overpayment, from treatment that was charged and collected for but not provided, treatment that was performed but refunded, administrative errors while posting charges, or any other reason resulting from a difference between charges posted and income collected. While this is a negative collections adjustment, it is positive in the sense that it is "negative accounts receivable" for the period of time the office had use of that income. Practices with high refund overpayment amounts need to research and correct the causes, which may be poorly performing financial systems or dental care that is not meeting the expectations of the patient.

Overhead Control

Managing overhead is one of the three essential components of the Profitability Formula. It is important to understand what overhead is and what it isn't. The standard by which overhead is defined in dentistry is the *percentage of collections paid to operate the business.* Therefore, overhead percentage is the direct result of both practice expenses and collections, and indirectly of practice production. Overhead percentage can be high even though expenses are relatively low if collections are low. By the same token, overhead percentage can be low if expenses are relatively high and collections are high. Some practices have high overhead that is not the result of high expenses, but rather the result of low collections due to low collection rate (high write-offs), or poor collections systems, or inadequate production.

The national average of overhead in dental practices in the U.S. is 73%. The most profitable practices have overhead percentages below 60%. Those practices attain those percentages by being productive, having good collection systems, and having low expenses. We have already covered production and collection systems. This section will focus on how expenses affect overhead.

Managing Expenses

First, what expenses are considered in calculating practice overhead? This sometimes is a point of debate, but it is generally accepted that all expenses that are paid on behalf of the practice are considered in determining overhead. The practice owner's draw before taxes, any other personal expenses paid on behalf of the owner, and equipment depreciation are not considered practice expenses for determining overhead percentage. Therefore, the overhead calculated by these terms may be different from that the practice accountant uses for tax purposes. The two variations have two separate purposes – one is for managing overhead, the other is for managing tax liability.

Since the goal is to spend as little as possible without negatively impacting production, quality of care, and personal preferences of the practice providers, the practice owner and team must have a mindset of keeping expenses as low as possible. This mindset means that the practice questions everything it buys by asking the question, "Is there another product or service and/or another way to buy a product or service that results in savings?"

My experience is that the practice owner establishes this mindset. My experience also indicates that practices with this mindset typically have overhead percentages in the sub-60% range.

The mindset of commitment to doggedly keep spending in check requires planning and action. Planning begins with the practice budget. Each expense line item needs consideration. While a budget is a fluid instrument, the practice should do all that it can to stay within budgeted expense projections.

Fixed Expenses

Fixed expenses are recurring expenses that typically don't change much each month or year and are not affected by how much the practice produces. Examples are loan payments on practice debt, rent, service contracts, janitorial services, and equipment leases. Fixed expenses typically amount to between fifteen and twenty percent of all expenses, and twelve to seventeen percent of overhead. The largest line-item fixed expenses are usually practice rent and debt. The sub-sixty percent overhead practices have fixed expense overhead of around ten percent of collections, give or take one percentage point.

Fixed Expense Categories
Business Insurance
Dues
Equipment Lease
Fixed Miscellaneous
Janitorial
Loan Payments
Phone
Rent
Service Contracts
Taxes
Utilities

Variable Expenses

Variable expenses are tied more to the size of the practice and practice production. Examples are staff salaries, laboratory costs, and clinical supplies. Variable expenses typically amount to between eighty and eighty-five percent of all expenses, and fifty-five to sixty-five percent of overhead.

Variable Expense Categories
Advertising
Bank Charges
Business Supplies
Charitable Contributions
Clinical Supplies
Continuing Education Doctors
Continuing Education Team
Employee Benefits
Equipment Purchase
Equipment Service
Gross Associate(s) Salaries/Wages
Gross Team Salaries/Wages
Laboratory Fees
Legal/Professional
Office Improvement
Postage
Refunds
Travel/Entertainment
Variable Miscellaneous

The largest practice expenses are usually variable in nature – staff salaries and benefits, clinical supplies, and laboratory fees, which often combine for between forty and sixty percent of all practice expenses. Because most practice expenses are variable in nature, managing them has the most potential to reduce overhead percentage. Here's a look at the usual top six practice expenses along with suggestions for managing them:

1. **Staff Salaries & Benefits** – This is every dental practice's biggest expense, and with good reason – investment in the team brings the best return on investment of any expense line item. A dental practice and business cannot expect to reach its potential by being understaffed, having the wrong people in place, or not giving those people what they need to reach their potential.

   One of the most common questions I'm asked when discussing overhead is what percentage of collections the practice should be spending on staff salaries. Many dental practice owners have heard a number (most commonly 25%) that is the percentage they should be aiming for. In their effort to do so, they may understaff, underpay, or under-support, with the end result being underperformance. The right percentage is the percentage that makes the practice the most efficient and effective, and the business the most profitable.

The purpose of staffing is the same as that of the practice (take great care of patients), and the business (be as profitable as possible). The ideal percentage spent on staffing will depend in large part on the type of practice as well as the location. Therefore, the range spent on staff salaries and benefits should be between twenty-five and thirty-five percent. If the practice percentage is at the high end of this range, it should be a practice with very good profitability.

In my many years working with dentists, I have found that only a small percentage of practices overpay good team members. When it happens, it's usually the result of the annual cost-of-living raise mentality with long-term employees. I've also seen it happen as a result of poor leadership – paying someone more than they should because compensation is the only tool they have in their leadership tool belt (more on Leadership in the next chapter).

The practice with high staff salary/benefits overhead percentage is usually not overpaying – if anything, it is underpaying. What's causing the high percentage is under-producing, under-collecting, or under-utilizing the potential of the team – or a combination of the three.

The prosperous dental practice should be staffed with highly capable, highly supported team members who have great attitudes. Their compensation should be at the eighty percentile or higher for the area, and they should be given performance and salary reviews on an annual basis.

Upward salary adjustments should only be made when the practice has proven profitability over the past year, and the employee in question has been a significant part of that profitability. The size of the adjustment should be in keeping with both of those factors.

2. **Associate Salaries** – Associate dentists should be compensated based on their production, their experience and skill set, industry standards, and the overhead of the practice.

   By far the best way to compensate an associate dentist is commission based on collections from dentistry they produce. This motivates them to be more productive, while protecting the business from overpaying the associate when they are not productive. When an associate is new to the practice, and especially when they are beginning a new associate role (rather than taking over from a previous associate), paying a daily stipend for the first six to twelve months is appropriate.

   The commission the associate is paid should be within industry standards. As of the writing of this book, this range is twenty-eight to thirty-five percent of collections from their production. As noted previously, experience and skill set will impact where within the range the associate is compensated. If the overhead of the practice is high, then the profit margin of the practice will be lower, leaving less to pay an associate. The overhead percentage that should be used when determining how much to pay an associate is more than that of the practice without an associate. Paying an associate adds to the overhead of the practice (but not necessarily the overhead percentage), usually anywhere from five to ten percent. Because of this, there is more profitability from the dentistry performed by the practice owner(s) compared to the associate(s).

There are many reasons to employ associate dentists – to increase the profitability of the practice through added capacity and production, as part of a transition strategy, to keep the office open longer hours, to help add and cover hygienists, to perform procedures the owner dentists prefer not to provide, to add additional services, and to help the owner dentists have a more productive schedule by allowing them to focus more on larger-case dentistry. Whatever the reasons, by far the most important one is making the practice more profitable. Unfortunately, I've encountered several practices where the associate dentist is making more than the owner dentist employer. The right associate with the right compensation structure will make the practice more profitable. Associate salaries should be between eight and twelve percent of the practice overhead. There is much more on the associate dentist in the Transitions section of this book.

3. **Laboratory Fees** – Laboratory fees should range from six to twelve percent of practice overhead. Some very profitable practices pay more for lab expenses due to the kind of dental care they provide (for example, fully guided implant placement or same-day prosthesis delivery). Other very profitable practices have low laboratory fees because a sizeable portion of the dentistry normally sent to a lab is milled to a final product or printed by a 3D printer in the office. But when laboratory fees are at the high end of the expected range, or beyond, it is usually due to excessive remakes, fees that are too low, a low collection rate, or using a laboratory with higher than necessary fees.

   Not all dental laboratories are created equal. Labs charge more or less depending on their size, the efficiency of their business, and the quality of the product and service they provide. It is understandable that, when a dentist finds a lab that offers a product and service that consistently results in an excellent and dependable outcome, the dentist becomes a loyal, long-term customer of that lab, regardless of price. But when the price is high relative to the industry standard, it is certainly appropriate to ask for a discount in return for high volume and/or exclusivity. If the laboratory rejects the request, then the dental practice should shop other laboratories who may deliver the same product and service as the existing lab at a lower price. That isn't being disloyal. It's being a smart business owner.

4. **Clinical Supplies** – In general, the most overpaid expense category for dental practices are clinical supplies. A great deal of savings can be accomplished through shopping for the best prices, buying in bulk when appropriate, negotiating deals with suppliers, belonging to buying clubs, having more efficient dental practices, and offering incentives to team members responsible for ordering.

   Oftentimes, the team members responsible for ordering choose the most convenient route – ordering as much as possible from one source. This source is usually chosen because of a relationship the salesperson has developed with the practice or the individual responsible for ordering. But convenience and buying from friends can be a costly choice for the practice. Taking more time and evaluating all of the options usually saves the practice thousands of dollars per year, more than offsetting the extra cost of time and convenience involved. Bulk pricing, while costing more up front, and requiring more storage space for inventory, means lower cost per unit. As with managing dental laboratory costs, the practice should not hesitate to ask for the best price possible and use quoted costs from multiple sources as leverage.

Large practices, and those with multiple locations, use this leverage to order enough volume to negotiate the best deals. Smaller practices can attain similar leverage by becoming part of a buying club. Companies such as *Smile Source* offer clients discounts off supplies and many other practice expenses. The dental practice owner should carefully review such contractual arrangements before joining.

Once the least costly option is determined, that source can become the source where most supplies are purchased, but pricing must be constantly compared to prevent the supplier from capitalizing on a "bait and hook" approach – acquire the practice business with low prices, then raise them and hope the buyer doesn't notice or care.

More efficient and less wasteful measures are also part of managing clinical supply costs. The leadership of the practice must strike a balance between quality of care, preference by dental personnel, and preventing waste.

While it is not uncommon in small practices for the practice owner to order supplies, eventually it makes sense to delegate this role to a team member. Often, one person is designated for the business office and one for the clinical side (perhaps two if the dental and hygiene supplies are ordered separately). These individuals need to have the aforementioned mindset of commitment to doggedly keep spending in check, and they should be rewarded for doing so.

This reward can take the form of wage increases following a performance appraisal and/or a bonus for reaching a certain level of ordering expenses below budgeted amounts. Depending on the practice, clinical supplies should be between five and eight percent of overhead. Some practices that place a lot of dental implants or do a lot of milled crowns in-house will have higher clinical supply costs. Once the practice decides what percentage within the accepted range to budget for clinical supplies, then a tiered level of bonus amount based on percentage savings is established.

As an example, if the practice establishes a budgeted amount for clinical supplies of six percent of collections, and budgets annual collections of one million dollars, then expectations are that practice will spend sixty thousand dollars annually. If instead the practice spends five percent (fifty thousand dollars) while still collecting one million dollars, then that amounts to a savings of ten thousand dollars. The practice could then reward the team member largely responsible for that savings a ten percent, or one-thousand-dollar, bonus. Of course, the bonus levels and amounts are up to the practice owner.

5. **Rent** – If the practice leases their facility space (like more than 80% of healthcare practices in the U.S.), or if they own and pay rent to themselves, rent is a fixed and monthly recurring expense line item.

   I am sometimes asked whether it is better for the practice to own or lease their space. It is tempting to say it is better to own, but this is not always the case. The obvious benefits of ownership are to have equity that can be converted to cash, to have a source of income from leases, and to have more control over everything related to the property, now and into the future. There may be tax advantages as well.

   However, in some cases leasing makes sense. These would be when a prime location with multiple benefits is available for lease but not ownership, when the cost of ownership is prohibitive, when the lease deal is especially attractive from a financial standpoint, or when the practice owner doesn't want all the responsibilities that may come with ownership. The range of acceptable overhead for rent is between three and seven percent.

Negotiating a lease for a prime location toward the low end of this range can save a practice tens of thousands of dollars annually. Depending on the terms presented by the lessor, it may make sense for the practice owner to use the services of a company that works on behalf of business owners to negotiate favorable leases. Terms should not only reflect the monthly lease payment, but also other items including renewal options, increases in monthly rent at each renewal, leasehold improvements, free or reduced rent periods, the right to transfer the lease to another practice owner in the future, and death and disability options.

6. **Loan Payments** – Many practices have some degree of practice debt. Borrowing money to indirectly or directly make the practice more profitable is an acceptable and often necessary action as long as the practice can afford to borrow the money (i.e., the projected collections from the practice budget including the monthly mortgage amount allow for the practice to address both practice and personal financial needs). In addition, the loan conditions must be favorable, including the interest rate of the loan amortization, the term of the loan, and whether there is any penalty for paying off the loan early.

   Having a debt-free practice improves profitability significantly, as most dental practices in the U.S. spend upwards of six percent of their collections on practice debt. Given this, the practice must weigh using financial resources to retire debt as soon as possible versus other practice needs. Whichever makes the practice more profitable in the short and long term is the best decision.

SUMMARY OF KEY POINTS FROM CHAPTER 2 – THE SYSTEMS

1. Any individual desiring to own and grow a prosperous dental practice must maximize production and collection rate, while decreasing overhead.

2. A budget is essential for goal setting, and goals are required for consistent success.

3. The planner must start with the end in mind and work backwards. Personal goals will dictate professional goals.

4. Prosperous dental practice owners dream big. They realize they are unlikely to achieve anything big unless they first envision it.

Production Systems

5. A big part of excelling at diagnosis is being honest with patients and treating them just like you would want to be treated – in other words, having high standards. When dentists embrace this, they diagnose a lot more dental care.

6. The reason commonly-taught selling techniques in dentistry don't work is that people really don't want many of the procedures we perform in dentistry, and people don't buy what they don't want.

7. If you give people what they want, you will never have to sell dentistry again.

8. The key to case acceptance lies with the emotion behind what the patient wants.

9. The patient's personality type reflects how they see the world around them and respond to it. Understanding this is key to how best to communicate with them.

10. There is no better way to make a case for any point than telling a story.

11. A practice with a healthy flow of new patients, and that offers a unique experience that patients aren't likely to find anywhere nearby, has a dominant market presence.

12. You either control the schedule, or the schedule controls you. Patients should be placed into the schedule primarily to accomplish one thing for the business – to accomplish the practice's daily goal.

13. You should not expect your patients to want to keep their appointment any more than you communicate to them the importance of doing so.

14. The biggest impact financial arrangements can have on reducing missed appointments is payment in advance. This one policy can do more than anything else to prevent last-minute schedule adjustments for highly productive appointments.

15. If proper staffing and demand are in place, the best investment a practice can make in tapping its future production potential is adding more treatment rooms.

16. Performing more procedures that are more productive per unit of time is the one thing that has the biggest impact on practice production.

17. Most practices are understaffed, especially in the business office; the most successful practices staff for the schedule they want, not the one they have.

18. Most dentists would rather invest in honing their clinical skills or adding technology or working harder, when investing in the quality of their team would bring a greater return than any of those things.

19. It's nearly impossible to overpay high-quality staff members. If they want more, they will become more. However long it takes, whatever you must do, don't compromise on the quality of your team.

20. The owner dentist doesn't have to be present for the practice to be productive. Adding providers – hygienists and associates – increases the quantity of days worked without the practice owner working more days. This is leverage.

21. If a dentist desires to make more, keep more, and enjoy more, they must understand the concept that dentists in private practice don't make more by providing great dental care, they make more by providing great dental care fast.

Financial Systems

22. While well-defined roles are essential, all business office team members should be cross-trained and able to perform the duties of others in the event of an absence so that no one area falls behind or suffers.

23. Dental practice owners should NOT participate in a PPO plan if they can avoid it. It makes more sense for the provider to be paid their established fee for the care they provide.

24. How is it possible to be highly profitable while participating in discounted fee plans? By outproducing the discount, while keeping overhead low.

25. All payments received after treatment is performed should be limited to insurance payments.

26. The goal of every dental practice should be to not have any overdue (more than 30 days) accounts receivable. All dental practices should pay their accounts payable (expenses) within thirty days, and all income from dental services provided should be collected within the same time frame.

27. The total amount of accounts receivable should be forty percent or less of the average monthly production.

28. Delinquent accounts are almost 100% preventable. Signed financial arrangements plus adhering to the collection systems outlined in this book will keep accounts current and prevent the time-consuming, costly process of cleaning up delinquent accounts.

Growth Systems

29. The formula for effective marketing is: The Right Message, to The Right People, The Right Number of Times.

30. "We're Different" should describe your marketing message. It says that your dental practice is not only unique, but that uniqueness is worth any extra inconvenience and cost.

31. The Million Dollar Question you need to answer is: "Why would someone drive by a hundred other dental offices to come to our practice and pay more?"

32. Effective marketing requires repetition and time. When it comes to marketing, the practice cannot afford to take a day off.

33. Dental practice owners tend to place more emphasis on outside marketing companies and marketing systems, but it's the practice team that makes or breaks any marketing strategy or system.

34. Performing internal marketing at a high level is required before attempting any external marketing, as effective internal marketing is the foundation of effective external marketing.

35. Don't assume that patients make the connection between being impressed with their care and referring a new patient. You must ask for referrals.

36. Team members need to be reminded each day to hand out referral cards, and they need to see the practice owner lead by example.

37. There is no better marketing than the recommendation of an existing patient.

38. Tracking new patient sources is critical to making good decisions regarding getting the best results, as well as the use of ongoing marketing resources.

39. Paramount to the growth of the successful practice is not only attracting new patients but keeping them in the practice for as long as possible.

Profitability Systems

40. Negative adjustments to production and collections (write-offs) are silent killers of profitability.

41. Overhead percentage is a function of both practice expenses and collections. Overhead percentage can be high even though expenses are relatively low if collections are low. By the same token, overhead percentage can be low if expenses are relatively high, and collections are high.

42. The most profitable practices have overhead percentages below 60%. Practices attain those percentages by being productive, having good collection systems, and keeping expenses low.

43. Upward salary adjustments should be made only when the practice has proven profitability over the past year and the employee in question has been a significant part of that profitability. The size of the adjustment is in keeping with both of those factors.

44. In general, the most overpaid expense category for a dental practice is clinical supplies. A great deal of savings can be accomplished through shopping for the best prices, buying in bulk when appropriate, negotiating deals with suppliers, belonging to buying clubs, more efficient dental practices, and incentives for members of the team responsible for ordering.

Chapter 3
The Leadership

Of all the ingredients necessary for a successful dental practice, leadership is unquestionably the biggest. The lack of great leadership is the number one reason dental practices don't come close to realizing their potential, either as a practice or a business. My decades of work with dentists to address the challenges of their practice focuses mostly on leadership. The benefits of great leadership stem from its positive impact on the team, and the team is the most important asset of any practice.

Most practices are leadership deficient for two reasons: 1. Dental practice owners aren't committed to being better leaders, and 2. Dental practice owners don't know how to become better leaders.

LEADERSHIP REQUIREMENTS

1. The Commitment to Better Leadership

Commitment begins with desire. You might think every practice owner wants to be a better leader. After all, the benefits of being a better leader surpass those of being a better dentist – increased harmony among the team, with little turnover; an ownership mentality among team members who take accountability for important roles; a practice owner freed up to focus on fewer tasks; team members all on the same page; a culture of trust in the office; and a more profitable business.

The fact is, despite knowing they need to be better leaders, most dentists loathe working on their leadership skills. I can attest to that: I once taught a leadership class at a dental conference and the attendance at my class was a small fraction of the attendance at a class next door on cosmetic dentistry.

Learning new clinical skills is critical to the development of the dental professional, but in the practice with poor leadership, it's akin to the dental patient with periodontal disease being treated with cosmetic dentistry. The patient is investing in painting the house, while the house's foundation is crumbling.

Perhaps some dentists just don't believe learning to be a better leader is possible for them, believing the phrase "born leader" – you either are a good leader or you aren't. The truth is leaders aren't born; they are built. Is it easier for some? Yes. Those lucky folks have more potential to become great leaders. But I firmly believe, and it has been proven through my experiences, that everyone has some potential to be a good leader, and good leaders can change their destiny and the destinies of those they lead. But, they must want it badly enough to put forth continual effort to truly change.

2. The Path to Better Leadership

One of the premises that this book began with was that "Success is the Result of Great Team Members Implementing Great Systems in The Presence of Great Leadership." Leadership, like most things, can be reduced to a system – a series of logical steps that when connected result in the desired outcome. In this case, the desired outcome is becoming the best possible leader.

Step #1 – The leader must have a purpose. The purpose is why they exist. I've already alluded to the book, "*The On-Purpose Person: Making Your Life Make Sense*," by Kevin McCarthy. I also highly recommend the follow-up book by the same author, "*The On-Purpose Business Person: Doing More of What You Do But More Profitably*." After reading these short but powerful books, lights went on inside me. All of a sudden, I had the answer to why I exist – my purpose. Without purpose, the full potential of leadership cannot be realized.

Purpose drives passion, and without passion leadership will be limited. Passion is contagious. It inspires others, because people want to be a part of something that matters, instead of just going through the motions to earn a paycheck.

Early in my career the practice of bleaching teeth began; as the movement gained momentum, it became a bigger part of the cosmetic dentistry services that we provided. From a practice standpoint it made perfect sense – everyone wanted whiter teeth, and we could easily and safely make that happen. It also made sense from a business side – the overhead and time involved in providing that service, although not a big-ticket item, had a relatively high profit margin and often led to other cosmetic procedures.

There was only one problem – we weren't doing nearly enough of it. Try as I might to influence our team to present it, and to encourage those who were interested to have it done, we just weren't doing much of it. Then, we became involved with a charity for children with cancer. I showed the team a video produced by the charity of young kids without hair fighting a deadly disease. For a period of time, all the proceeds from our bleaching would now go to supporting that fight. Our bleaching presentation and case acceptance increased by four hundred percent. We had a purpose, one that both our team and our patients were passionate about.

You know you've found your purpose when you've found the passion. My purpose? "To Lower Other People's Handicaps." I know that sounds like a metaphor for golf or a description of physical disabilities, but it's really about helping dentists and their teams be more successful. I just liken the level of a golfer's game to the level of a dentist's game.

Step #2 – The leader must have a vision. It's one thing to have a purpose and be passionate about it, but it isn't meaningful until you know where you want that purpose to take you. That destination is your vision. Once you know your purpose, you then must decide what you are going to do with it. The simplest way to find your vision is to *Dream Without Limits*.

What would you do if there were no obstacles standing in the way? What if money, or time, or physical ability, or anything else you can think of that might keep you from becoming or doing what you truly want, was not standing in your way? Most people don't come close to realizing their vision because they can't see what they want because of what they allow to block their view.

Most amazing accomplishments happen not because of incredible talent, but because of incredible effort fueled by incredible desire (See Key Concept of Law of Attraction).

Once you have a vision, you need to share it with others you are leading. You won't get there by yourself. Share your vision passionately, commit to it wholeheartedly, and show others what your vision will mean to them. If you have the right people, in the right culture, they will adopt your vision and play an important role in making it a reality.

Revisit the vision often. It helps to have a visual depiction either in words or in an image that you see frequently to remind you of your vision.

THE KEY CONCEPT

The Key Concept of Outcome Visualization – To your brain, visualizing success is as real as actually achieving success. Once your brain believes in the outcome, the outcome becomes more possible and, when practiced regularly, inevitable. Denis Waitley said, "When you visualize, then you materialize."

Step #3 – The leader must have a mission statement. Because a vision is often a long distance away and may take a considerable amount of time to accomplish, it is helpful to break the ultimate goal into smaller goals that can be accomplished in shorter periods of time.

For example, a country at war may have a vision to win the war, but that vision will require multiple steps, or successful missions, to accomplish. The leader and the team need to define their mission in *The Mission Statement*, a formal summary of the aims and values of a company, organization, or individual.

My team and I took the following approach in constructing our practice mission statement. First, we involved the whole team. They had insights I didn't have, and they were more likely to *own* the mission statement if they played a role in writing it.

We then asked everyone to think about and contribute words or phrases that describe what we aim to accomplish, each day, that will lead us to the vision. These are values and philosophies that define who we are and who we want to become. Once everyone's contributions were collected, a group of four individuals assembled the words and phrases into a single paragraph.

The mission statement must be long enough to be comprehensive, yet short enough to be easily read, displayed prominently in the office, memorized, and frequently recited (typically three to five sentences).

Our practice mission statement goes as follows:

"The Team at Dental Wellness of Lexington Pledges to Deliver You Quality, Courteous Care in a Clean and Comfortable Atmosphere. Our Team Will Offer Efficient and Experienced Service,

Always Listening to You and Being Respectful of the Time That You Spend with Us. We Promise That We Will Always Present You With Exceptional Dental Care. We Are Your Home for Professional Dental Excellence."

Step #4 – The leader must have goals. Goals are well-defined, objective, measurable, and connected to a period of time (hours, days, weeks, months, etc.). They are steppingstones along the path to the common vision of the enterprise.

Goals are the difference between winning and losing, between success and failure, and in the presence of good leadership, goals are worth doing whatever it takes to accomplish them.

The overwhelming majority of practice owners and their teams go to work every day without goals. And many of those who do have goals aren't committed enough to making them a reality. They figure they tried their best, and it just didn't happen.

What I know is that if the right people have the desire, determination, and commitment to an unrelenting pursuit of a goal, those people will attain their goals.

Step #5 – The leader must have the right people on the team. It does no good to have a purpose, vision, mission statement, and goals if you don't have the right people on the proverbial bus. Refer to the first chapter section on "The Individual," and the three As – Aptitude, Ability, and Attitude – as well as the section on Team Quality in the "The Production Wheel" in Chapter Two.

Leadership is something that is pervasive among the team. Everyone plays a leadership role and exhibits leadership traits. However, the practice owner is the ultimate leader of the dental practice. The owner is primarily accountable for determining the vision, communicating it passionately, setting goals, assembling the highest quality team possible, and creating a culture within which that team will flourish.

CREATING THE PROSPEROUS TEAM CULTURE

The word "culture" is often overused or misused. It seems to be a mysterious concept that most individuals on a team want (a good culture, that is), even if they can't articulate what it means.

Team Culture is about the entire team sharing in common values, beliefs, attitudes, and behaviors, and working together toward a common vision.

We've discussed values and beliefs, and we've covered the qualities the individual needs to have, but a group of great individuals does not necessarily translate into a great team. That takes a whole new set of essential ingredients, and this list starts with *Trust*.

Patrick Lencioni, in his quintessential book about team culture, "*The Five Dysfunctions of a Team: A Leadership Fable*," describes the fundamental causes behind team failure. He calls absence of trust the biggest and most significant dysfunction. Without trust, teamwork is impossible, as team members must trust that their fellow team members' intentions are good. Absence of trust prevents honest, open communication and extra effort; it encourages gossip and fosters low morale.

Ravi Kumar, in his article titled, "Absence of trust – The foundational dysfunction in any team," describes the characteristics of members of trusting teams:

- Admit weakness
- Ask for help
- Accept questions and input about their areas of responsibility
- Give one another the benefit of the doubt before arriving at a negative conclusion
- Take risks in offering feedback and assistance
- Appreciate and tap into one another's skills and experiences
- Focus time and energy on important issues, not politics
- Offer and accept apologies without hesitation
- Look forward to meetings and other opportunities to work as a group

How do team leaders develop trust among the team? First, they need to start with themselves. The phrase "Trust Is Earned, Not Given" is very true. Good leaders never give anyone on their team a reason for distrust. They walk their talk, are true to their word, and admit when they fall short in any way. They demonstrate genuine empathy toward their team members.

In "*The Five Dysfunction of a Team*," Lencioni talks about a simple but effective exercise: During a team meeting, members of the team take turns answering questions about their childhood, siblings, favorite hobbies, work experience, and other personal experiences. This simple exercise encourages greater empathy and understanding of one another, which discourages poor and inaccurate impressions among team members.

Once the team trusts one another, it's about influencing others so that they work together toward the common goal – the practice vision. This is often referred to as getting the team on the same page or getting them to buy in. We've already discussed involving team members in the mission statement, passionately sharing the vision and what that vision means to them. Let's expand on what's in it for the team member by examining what the team members of the prosperous dental practice want.

WHAT THE TEAM MEMBERS OF THE PROSPEROUS DENTAL PRACTICE WANT:

#1. Direction

Team members want to know what's expected of them, i.e., the responsibilities of the position. The prosperous dental practice team members want to know even more: what do they have to do to perform exceptionally (to win)? These expectations can be communicated in a variety of ways, but the standard is the written *Job Description*. This document can also be used in the search and selection process, and as a measurement tool for performance evaluations.

Whenever new job descriptions are created, existing team members should be involved in the process. While the team leader and practice owner have the ultimate say, it is helpful to have team members involved in the process for their valuable insight and to create additional buy-in. Each team member should be required to read and signify their understanding and agreement with their signature. The documents should be revisited and updated periodically. Job descriptions for most practice positions can be found in the Glossary.

#2. Support

Now that team members know *what* to do, they need support through training in *how* to do it. Even if team members have years of experience, they need to know how to apply that aptitude within the systems of the office. Whenever there is a gap between expectations and performance, team members need the support of their fellow team members, their team leader (if applicable), and the practice owner. This support may be as simple as in-office training, or it may require continuing education outside the office.

#3. Feedback

One of the biggest and most frequent deficiencies in dental practice leadership is feedback. Team members want to know how they're performing (good or bad) from their leaders in the practice. They want to know where they stand relative to what is expected of them. This is formally accomplished through performance evaluations but should occur more often in a less formal format in one-on-one conversations during the course of a day in the office.

The Performance Assessment

Both the team member and the practice owner (or team leader if applicable) must approach the assessment with a good attitude. Most dentists don't appreciate the value of this meeting and it shows. Team members dread or even fear it. The practice owner or team leader needs to set the example, openly expressing the importance and looking forward to the time to meet with the team member. After all, this is a time where team members can receive validation, direction, and information; can exchange ideas; and can learn how they measure up to practice standards and expectations. Well-done, a performance assessment leaves the team member motivated, appreciated, respected, informed, and committed to the team's objective – winning.

Both participants should come to the meeting prepared. Two weeks prior to the performance assessment, both team leader and team member are given the assessment form, so they have ample time to research and consider the evaluation. An example of performance review for the team leader is included here:

PERFORMANCE ASSESSMENT TITLE: TEAM LEADER					Page 1
	Below Expectations	Needs Improvement	Meets Expectations	Exceeds Expectations	Team Member Initials
Takes accountability for his/her team					
Interviews, hires, and recommends termination					
Disciplines team members when needed (verbal & written)					
Answers and reports to office manager &/or practice owner					
Holds monthly team meetings					
Participates in monthly team leader/ Doctor meetings					
Responsible for knowing each team member's job descriptions and makes sure it is getting done properly					
SWOTs team members 1-2 times a year and discusses improvements needed to be made					
Listens to requests of team members and helps find solutions for issues being addressed					
Takes requests for further CE courses, dates, cost, and course description					
Researches request information and presents to doctor with cost and date information					
Supports his/her team					
Supports doctor(s), office manager, and other team leaders					
Is available to team members for requests and challenges					
Is a problem solver					
Handles conflict among team members and other teams					
Motivates team members to be the best version of themselves					
Performs 89-day and annual performance reviews for team members					
Takes accountability for challenges facing team and assures doctor/office manager they won't happen again					
Helps set goals for team and office					
Accountable for training new team members and associate dentists					

PERFORMANCE ASSESSMENT
TITLE: TEAM LEADER

Page 2

Areas Needing Improvement and Plan for Correction

The following areas noted in today's performance appraisal need improvement.
Develop an action plan to bring about the desired result,
and a target date to complete and review.

1. ____

____

Target Date ____________________ Review Date ____________________

2. ____

____

Target Date ____________________ Review Date ____________________

3. ____

____

Target Date ____________________ Review Date ____________________

4. ____

____

Target Date ____________________ Review Date ____________________

____________________ ____________________
Reviewer's Signature Date

____________________ ____________________
Team Member's Signature Date

Here is a suggested agenda for the performance assessment meeting:

1. Begin with praise and acknowledgement of the employee's contributions. This sets a positive tone for the meeting, puts the team member at ease, and disarms any negativity.
2. Review and compare the Performance Assessment form that both team leader and team member have filled out. This should be a conversation, not a presentation, and certainly not a lecture. The team member should be encouraged to do most of the talking.
3. Compare the results from the last assessment (if applicable). Don't forget to praise and applaud if the team member is performing to and especially when exceeding expectations.
4. When the team member is not performing to expectations, and/or has regressed from a previous assessment, the meeting should still be positive and the feedback constructive. At the same time, the team leader's perspective should be uncompromising when it comes to the standards of the practice. The deficiency must be clearly described and agreed upon by both parties. The team leader should ask what support the team member needs, and a plan to eliminate the gap between expectations and performance, complete with a deadline, should be agreed upon.
5. The next meeting should be scheduled – in one year if the team member is performing to or above expectations, three to six months if not, and one to three months if the team member's performance gap is severe enough to warrant dismissal if not corrected.

Key points to remember about the performance assessment meeting:

1. Always be positive – Unless the primary purpose of the assessment is disciplinary in nature, all communication should be colored with encouragement. If team members perceive these meetings as a time where they get criticized, the assessment will be dreaded and its usefulness will be negated.
2. Be specific – Good results are the culmination of precisely identifying any area of the team member's performance that needs improvement. Then and only then can constructive progress be made.
3. Don't get personal – When the assessment concentrates on the individual, the individual gets defensive. When it addresses behavior, the exchange becomes two people on the same side working toward a solution.
4. Put everything in writing – Carefully document the details of the meeting, including all areas of the team member's performance deemed less than satisfactory. All agreed-on decisions need to be described in writing with both the leader and team member's initials and signature. The infrequent nature of these meetings, along with their possible implication in an employment dispute, mandate thorough documentation.
5. Privacy is paramount – Performance assessments can be held within or outside the office as long as they are in a private setting. If held outside the office (such as a restaurant during lunch), plenty of time should be allowed for travel to and from the location so that the meeting is not rushed.

#4. Appreciation

In the many exit interviews I've participated in over my career, the number one reason an individual was looking to be employed elsewhere was because they were feeling underappreciated. While the primary goal of an employee may be to make a living doing their job, they will not continue for long in an environment where they don't feel valued beyond merely being paid for what they do.

The simple yet powerful act of saying "thank you" may seem like a little thing, but it acknowledges the act that preceded it and recognizes the individual with respect. And when that respect is extended, it is often returned.

Praise goes one step further, expressing approval or admiration for someone. Thanking someone communicates respect, but praise makes someone feel better about themselves, and more self-esteem unleashes more of that someone's potential. The acronym for P-R-A-I-S-E that I believe best describes what the word means is: Personal Recognition And Instilling Self Esteem. Through *genuine* acknowledgement of someone or their actions, team leaders have an opportunity to nourish team members' belief in themselves. I've received numerous thank-you notes over the years, and I've kept every one of them. The simplest one is perhaps my favorite of all – it reads, "*Thank you for believing in me.*"

Still, expressing praise is not something that comes naturally to me, and I believe that is true of many dental practice owners. However, like anything else you really want to change, you can do it. It's simply a matter of establishing new habits.

While I can't recall the source, early in my career someone told me about "*The Ten Dimes.*" Placing ten dimes in one's pocket at the start of each day, and removing a dime each time you express praise for someone doing something really well, is a useful way to remind yourself of the need to take time to express appreciation and recognize good performance. When I did this, I found myself not only praising team members when they performed at a high level, I found myself *looking* for opportunities to praise. The team noticed a difference, and I noticed a difference in their level of performance, because positive acknowledgement of behaviors encourages more positive behaviors.

#5. A Path to Advancement

When I talk to practice owners who have high turnover, and review what their team members want, owners are not surprised by team members wanting more compensation or appreciation. But they are often taken aback by team members desiring a path to advancement. In their minds, hygienists will remain hygienists for the remainder of their career, as will assistants. Someone in the business office may become an office manager, but otherwise the concept of advancement is relegated to learning more. (By the way, this is often how dentists think of their own career.)

Dental office personnel who experience burnout and consider career changes often have at the root of their dissatisfaction the belief that they are in a dead-end job. Prosperous dental practice team members are ambitious and need a path to grow in their career. The military gives us an excellent example of this career ladder, with increasing rank as a means to instill a desire to aspire to the next step or promotion.

This path can take the form of increasing knowledge and skill sets through continuing education, giving accountability over key functions (for example, ordering supplies, OSHA compliance, social media marketing), and giving increased leadership roles in the practice (departmental leaders). Each team member should have a plan for advancement, constructed collaboratively between the team leader and team member, taking all of these options into consideration.

This path of advancement can make the difference between an employee mentality ("I have a job to pay my bills"), and an *ownership* mindset (a feeling of personal responsibility for everything in the organization).

Kenneth Acha in his article, "Owner vs. Employee Mentality" writes, "Because they have an owner's mindset or paradigm, they automatically start seeing things and paying attention to detail in ways that someone with an employee mindset doesn't do even if he wanted to. Just like a mother develops maternal instincts that someone without a child may not have, a person with an owner mentality develops owner instincts about the business that people with an employee mentality don't have." They will step in and do whatever is needed. Their work isn't limited to their job description. They make sacrifices to ensure that the business succeeds.

Leadership Structure Models

In the prosperous dental practice, leadership is pervasive throughout the entire team. Everyone exhibits leadership qualities such as integrity, active listening, delegation, problem solving, decisiveness, self-motivation, humility, passion, resilience, accountability, empathy, and empowerment. As the size of the practice grows, some team members will answer the call to lead *and manage* practice departments within the office.

The distinction between manager and leader is not just semantic in nature. The two terms are different in their meaning and purpose. Simply put, managers are responsible for making sure *things are done the right way*, while leaders are responsible for making sure *the right things are being done*. Leadership is more about making sure the vision is being worked on, while management is more about working the vision. Both roles are vital to the success of the practice and the business, and all members of the practice, including the practice owner, will be called upon to be both managers and leaders. The size of the practice dictates whether the practice owner plays both roles, or whether departmental managers are needed.

In order to give some guidance as to when to adjust the organizational structure of a dental practice to reflect the changing needs of the growing practice, it is helpful to divide practices into levels depending on the size and makeup of the team.

Level One practices consist of fewer than three members in each of the three departments (assistant, hygienist and business office). Business offices should expand to three members before the assistant or hygienist department does. The expansion of the business office is necessary for the growth of the assistant and hygienist departments. In the Level One practice, the practice owner/dentist acts as the practice leader and manager. As the practice grows, the increasing managing responsibility placed on the practice owner starts to lead to a diminishing return on efficiency and productivity, as well as emotional stress. I have heard practice owners say hundreds of times over my career, "Dentistry is easy. What I hate is managing the staff." This is the result of both leadership failure on the part of the practice owner and an inadequate leadership structure for the number of team members in the practice.

Level	Size & Makeup of Team	Accountable for Management	Accountable for Leadership
One	Less than three team members in each of the office departments (assistant, hygienist, and business office)	Practice Owner	Practice Owner
Two	Three or more members in all three departments	Practice Owner manages Team Leaders & Team Leaders manage members of their department	Practice Owner supported by Team Leaders
Three	Multiple dentists or four or more members in all three departments	Practice Owner manages Office Manager who manages Team Leaders who manage members of their department	Practice Owner supported by Office Manager and Team Leaders
Four	Larger Group Practices with multiple practice locations	COO manages Office Managers who manage Team Leaders who manage members of their department	Practice Owner & CEO supported by COO, Office Managers and Team Leaders

Team Leaders – The Next Level of Leadership

Level Two practices have three or more members in all three departments (assistant, hygienist, and business office). The Level Two practice benefits from designating a leader of each department to take over most of the management duties of the practice owner. The **Team Leader** accepts accountability for the success of their department. The Team Leader should support individual team members to reach the potential of their aptitude and ability, and influence the team to contribute significantly to the overall vision of the practice. The Team Leader must also manage the implementation of systems within their department.

The Team Leader takes ownership of their department; the practice owner should give the Team Leader what they need to succeed in their role. This includes allowing the Team Leader to formulate a strategic plan for their team, to train to performance standards, to conduct performance assessments, and to recruit, interview, and recommend selection, correction, and termination of team members. Team Leaders, in essence, operate a business within a business.

Many practice owners are uncomfortable delegating this much responsibility to a team member. They argue that a team member is not qualified enough, nor can they care enough, to have this much responsibility and perform these roles as well as the owner would. While this view reflects the mentality of many dentists, my personal experience has proven this view to be incorrect.

If I had to choose one word that best describes the professional personality of a dentist, it would be "perfectionist." In the DISC Profile personality system, every good dentist I know has a high degree of "C" (Conscientiousness). This, in part, made them want to be a dentist. It was not only reinforced in dental school but was required for survival of the curriculum. Perfectionism requires its possessor to control as many of the variables of a task or endeavor as possible in order to assure the best and most predictable outcome. While this may make for good dentistry, it can make for poor leadership, stifling delegation and crippling the growth of the practice and the business.

It's true that a team member may not perform some things the same way as the practice owner would. But – does it really matter? I recall a client whose perfectionist tendencies prevented him from delegating the responsibility of escorting a patient from the reception room to the clinic area because he couldn't find a team member who did it exactly the way he wanted it done. This practice owner had aspirations of growing larger, but never grew beyond a small practice and experienced the continual stress of constant staff turnover. I was never able to get through to him that a dental practice cannot grow beyond the practice owner's willingness to go from a "means justifies the end" to an "end justifies the means" mentality.

I'm not saying that performance standards should be compromised, nor that a high level of control should not be maintained by the practice owner through the leadership and management team. Never delegate a responsibility to someone who cannot do it well. But notice that I didn't write, "do it perfectly." No one should be held to that standard, not even a dentist. Doing so leads to frustration, stress, and unhappiness. Dentists and their teams should recognize perfection as something they should continually work toward, but not feel like failures when they achieve really good results yet fall short of perfection. Vince Lombardi said, "Perfection is not attainable, but if we chase perfection, we can catch excellence." Don't let perfectionism get in the way of excellence.

Once the practice owner gets over the hurdle of a team leader having too much responsibility, the next challenge is determining *who* should be a team leader.

The Seven Requirements of the Team Leader Position:

1. **They must have the highest standards and be the best example of a team member possible**. They must have an exemplary attitude and should have the highest aptitude and ability among their team. Simply put, they should be the example that the rest of their team aspires to.
2. **They must have the respect of those they are asked to lead**. This ties in to the first requirement, except it adds the quality of integrity. For the team leader to have respect, they must walk their talk, asking no one on their team to do something they haven't done well repeatedly, and aren't willing to do when necessary.

   One may ask where experience fits in to the list of requirements of a team leader. It's not listed here as a requirement because performance is so much more important than experience. In fact, the two aren't necessarily related. Certainly, the team leader must have some degree of experience to be the top performer on a team, but this is not a position of seniority. Respect doesn't necessarily accompany experience.

   A team leader should not be hired but developed within the team in order to garner the respect of the team they are leading. If there isn't a suitable team leader on the existing team, then a new hire must be made with the idea of developing that new team member into a team leader. Such a process should take, at the minimum, three months.

3. **They must have an ownership mentality**. They must be sold completely on the practice vision and their department's important role in accomplishing that vision. They must understand the goals of the practice and the business and strive to reach the goals of their department. As with the owner, failure is not an option with the team leader.
4. **They must select themselves to be a team leader**. In other words, they must really want to be a team leader. No matter what other boxes they may check off on this list, they shouldn't be forced or coerced into taking on this role.

   The process of appointing a team leader starts with the practice owner assessing who among that team is most qualified based on the previous three requirements – standards, respect, and mentality. If there is an obvious individual, the practice owner should approach that team member and explain the concept and the role; how the team leader will be supported, rewarded, and empowered; and why the owner feels the person is qualified to succeed in that position. The person also needs to know that while this is a promotion, it shouldn't be accepted unless they understand that no one succeeds as a team leader unless they really want the role. If interested, the person should see a job description for the Team Leader. The person may accept or reject the offer immediately, or may want time to consider. A job description for Team Leader can be found in the Glossary.

   Should the selected team member choose not to accept, or there isn't a clear choice among the existing team, then the practice leader should approach the team as a group. Here's a sample dialogue:

   "In order for our practice to grow, our team needs to grow. Once a team gets to a certain size, we need to reorganize so that we can communicate better and operate effectively and efficiently. We want to grow so that we can take even better care of our patients and extend that care to many more. But in the process, we don't want to lose the quality of that care nor harm the culture that is often easier in a smaller workplace. Therefore, we have decided to organize the practice into smaller groups or departments. Each department will meet on a regular basis and work on matters specific to that group. There will be a hygienist department, an assistant department, and a business office department. For each department to function at its highest level, and to coordinate with other departments as well as myself, we will be appointing a team leader for each group. While everyone in the group is responsible for the success of that department, the team leader will be accountable. We want someone who is not only qualified, but desiring to do this, which is the reason I'm putting it out there for all of you to consider. We can choose only one person, so if you're interested and/or want to know more, please let me know individually, and I will be happy to discuss this with you."

   Parts of the preceding explanation to the team can be used to introduce the concept to the entire team if departmental team reorganization is being undertaken for the first time.

5. **They must be supported in their role**. A new team leader is often overwhelmed with being accountable for the actions of others. They may never have been placed in a leadership role before. The practice owner must support them through training from within and outside the practice. There are many resources in the form of online materials and courses, textbooks, offsite continuing education, and onsite training. Leadership is a continual journey rather than a destination.

One of the biggest reasons a team leader fails, and in the process that department suffers significantly, is because the practice owner doesn't have the team leader's back. If the team leader position is just a title with more work, then it will lead to the team leader taking on more responsibilities, but not being able to succeed. This is a sure way to lose a good team member.

An example of this is a team member going around their team leader directly to the practice owner with a problem or a request, and the practice owner making a decision regarding the matter. This is an end-around, and it completely undermines the team leader's authority. When faced with a situation like this, the practice owner should remind the team member that the proper channel for ideas or opinions is through their team leader. If the team member says they have already addressed this with the team leader, then the practice owner should respond by saying that he/she will discuss it with their team leader.

Practice owners should completely support the team leaders; if they don't, they should have a very good reason. That reason should be addressed with the team leader. If the team leader is no longer the right person for the role, then the practice owner must take appropriate action.

6. **They must be compensated and rewarded appropriately for their role**. It should go without saying that the team leader should be the highest paid member of their team. Not only do their qualifications warrant that, but the additional responsibilities they will be undertaking justify it.
7. **They must be empowered by the practice owner**. While the title of Team Leader can be bestowed upon someone, the title doesn't make them a leader. It is essential that the leadership role be awarded by the practice owner to the team leader in front of the group at large.

   The practice owner might say, "*I am pleased to announce that Susan will lead the hygienist team. As Team Leader, Susan has agreed to be accountable for the team, as well as take on additional responsibilities. Susan has my full support in her new role and will require the full cooperation of everyone on her team for the hygienist department to be even more successful than it currently is. Susan will be working not only with the hygiene team, but also the other team leaders and myself so that the result will be an even better practice and business. Thank you, Susan.*"

The practice owner may encounter the following questions:

Question - "*Is the team leader my superior?*"

Answer - "*No one in this practice is superior to anyone else. For purposes of improving organization and communication, as we grow larger, we need to use departments with team members designated to lead those departments.*"

Question - "*Is the team leader my boss?*"

Answer – "*The team leader is the leader of your department, and in that role will take into consideration everyone's input, but the team leader does have a say as to who performs tasks and how tasks are done within the team.*"

It is important to distinguish between a boss and a leader. While the leader performs the role of a boss when defined as someone who manages a group, there is often a negative connotation associated with the word "boss." Bosses are often seen as demanding and authoritarian, establishing methods and goals without involving others. This is the exact opposite of what the team leader should be. Instead of demanding, team leaders should coach. They should foster goodwill, building unity by involving everyone, giving credit where it is due, and maintaining the standards of the team.

Question - *"Do I answer to you (practice owner) or to the team leader?"*

Answer – *"You answer to your team leader. If you feel your inquiries are not being dealt with appropriately, then you may address them with me, but the proper channel is to go through your team leader first."*

Team leaders as a group should meet with the practice owner at least once a month. At this meeting each team leader presents a departmental report. In this way, the various team leaders and practice owner form the core leadership of the practice. In my experience, these meetings accomplish the most important business of the practice. More details are contained in the section on Team Meetings.

The Office Manager – The Leader of the Team Leaders

Without a doubt the most inappropriately used title and role in a dental practice is that of Office Manager. Some Level One practices appoint an office manager to run the office. The word "run" in this context usually means the administrative duties and staff management/leadership that the practice owner doesn't want to do. For this the office manager has some authority to manage the office and make practice decisions but most often is just someone with the most experience and ability in the business office who has a title and an inflated salary. Those administrative duties could be delegated to any member of the business office or a bookkeeper.

Team department leaders should be appointed before an office manager is considered when the Level One practice becomes a Level Two practice.

In the ***Level Three*** practice, where the practice has multiple dentists, or four or more team members in each department, then a separate role that truly fits the definition of managing the office can be considered.

This position oversees human resources and payroll, acts as team leader for the team leaders, and serves as a direct liaison between the team leaders and the practice owner. The office manager also oversees all practice and business metrics, including recording and interpretation. The office manager plays a key role in making sure all departments are working together to meet all business objectives. The Office Manager job description can be found in the Glossary.

The Chief Operating Officer (COO)

In the ***Level Four*** practice the Chief Operating Officer has similar responsibilities as an office manager, but on a larger scale, accountable for day-to-day operations of larger group practices with multiple locations. Depending on the size of the team, each location may have a dedicated office manager. The COO leads the office managers or team leaders of the practice(s) and answers directly to the practice owners.

The COO for a dental practice may or may not have a background in dentistry. They should at least have experience as a COO in the service industry, including recruiting and training new employees and marketing for growth of a business. Because they are accountable for a large business, COOs should have an advanced degree in business, such as an MBA, which typically requires a relatively large salary. The COO job description can be found in the Glossary.

Other Executive Positions - Human Resources Director, Chief Financial Officer, Chief Executive Officer

As Level Four practices expand, so do management and leadership requirements. As such, the need for other specialized positions addressing human resources, financial operations, and executive-level leadership may be necessary.

The Human Resources (HR) Director handles all matters related to recruiting, screening, and training staff, and administering employee-benefit programs. They are also the chief compliance officer when it comes to governmental regulations. This individual has an appropriate educational background, as well as experience. While experience in dentistry is helpful, it is not necessarily a requirement. The HR Director answers directly to the practice owner(s), or the Chief Executive Officer if applicable.

The Chief Financial Officer (CFO) is the senior executive responsible for managing the financial actions of the business. The CFO's duties include tracking cash flow, financial planning, analyzing the business's financial strengths and weaknesses, and proposing corrective actions. The CFO is the direct liaison between the business and outside accounting agencies. The CFO should have a degree in accounting and should be a certified public accountant (CPA). The CFO answers directly to the practice owner(s), or the Chief Executive Officer if applicable.

The Chief Executive Officer (CEO) role may be filled by a practice owner who acts as a managing partner, or an individual with a business background familiar with the dental industry. The CEO is accountable for the success of the business, is involved with searching and acquiring additional practices, and oversees business legal needs as well as strategic planning and execution. The CEO answers directly to the practice owner(s).

#6. Compensation

Of all the factors that make up what team members want in order to be happy and fulfilled in their role on the team, compensation is often the first thing that comes to mind. But it is not necessarily the most important. For that reason, it is mentioned last among the other factors: direction, support, feedback, appreciation, and a path to advancement.

High-quality team members are unquestionably the most valuable assets of the prosperous dental practice. A cohesive team, all on the same page, passionately working toward a powerful vision, is an unstoppable force.

Compensation must be commensurate with value to the practice and the business. As such, high-quality team members will be at the *eighty to one-hundred-plus percentile* for similar roles in their region of the country. The compensation range for a particular position in the practice region can be determined from online information and local sources.

Within that range, compensation will be dictated by experience, responsibility, aptitude (skill and knowledge level), and marketplace forces. The latter come into play in an employee market, when a position is being recruited and qualified applicants are scarce. This is simply a supply and demand issue, requiring the business to adjust compensation not only for the new hire, but for other members of that department as well. The same can also apply conversely, in an employer market, where there is a ready supply of qualified applicants for that position. The practice owner should have a range in mind before advertising the position.

Personal experience and working with hundreds of dentists have taught me that it is best not to offer someone I am considering hiring less than they ask for. While this may appear to leave room to overpay someone unnecessarily and raise the largest expense item a dental practice has, any benefits of negotiating lower compensation with a qualified applicant are short-lived.

First, it starts the working relationship off on the wrong foot. High-quality team members earnestly believe in themselves and the value they bring to a practice. If the practice owner starts out by sending the message they don't believe in that value to the same extent, the team member understandably questions if the owner ever will.

Secondly, I've found high-quality people tend to rise to the level at which they are rewarded. I know that whenever I raise my fees, I feel responsible for adding even more value to the services I provide. Remember my advice from earlier chapters: "If you want more, you must become more." With good people, getting more causes them to become more. I've said many times to surprised audiences that it is nearly impossible to overpay a good team member, because good team members will rise to the level of their compensation.

Finally, team members who feel they are undercompensated will likely be open to, or downright seek, other employment opportunities. In short, they are not fully committed to the practice and its goals, because they feel the practice is not committed to their goals. If the practice owner doesn't believe the applicant is worth what they are asking, or they cannot afford to pay someone what they request, the practice owner should move on to other applicants.

Practice owners and many consultants talk about controlling employee salaries by keeping the total amount to twenty-five percent or less of collections. While it is always best to keep overhead as low as possible, this rule of thumb often gets in the way of what is really important – developing the best practice and business possible. If paying employees thirty percent of revenue means the service they provide their patients is better, and the profit from doing that is increased, then thirty percent is a better number than twenty-five percent.

I've had numerous practice owners literally agonize over offering a team member one dollar an hour more in compensation, as if that one dollar would mean the difference between profit and financial ruin. Let's do the math: If the employee or applicant in question works thirty-six hours a week, then that one-dollar increase will mean approximately $156 more per month (not including payroll taxes and benefits), or $1,872/year. You have to ask, "Are the benefits of having a high-quality team member worth an additional $2,000, or $3,000, or even $10,000 a year to the practice, or is it better to risk losing that individual and finding someone who will work for $2,000, $3,000, or even $10,000 less?" The answer should be obvious.

It is important to know what a qualified applicant is asking for in regard to compensation. However, it isn't appropriate for the departmental leader or office manager performing the interview to ask this question, as compensation for all team members is information only the practice owner should have (or CEO when applicable). The applicant may willingly offer salary requirements or ask about compensation. The team leader or office manager should respond by saying that the practice owner will handle the discussion of compensation and benefits.

Hourly Wages, Salary, or Commission?

Over time, I've seen just about every possible compensation structure possible. Nearly all have merit, and good reasons exist both for and against their use. Before I examine the pros and cons of the three main methods, let's check that we are not missing the forest for the trees. The compensation structure works for the success of the practice and the business. In other words, the end, in this case, justifies the means.

Hourly Wages – This is the most common method of compensating dental practice employees. The pros are that team members are paid for the time they work – not more, not less. As long as the hourly wage is correctly set, neither the practice owner nor the employee feels taken advantage of. The cons are that the risk falls primarily on the employees, as they may not be guaranteed a certain number of hours per pay period in order to meet their needs, and they may not be granted permission to work beyond an allotted maximum number of hours per pay period.

Salary – The pros of salary compensation are that employees are guaranteed a certain amount of compensation per pay period; if they don't work a full typical pay period, they are not penalized. The pro to the employer is that if the employee needs to work more than the typical pay period in terms of hours, the employer does not have to pay additional wages. The cons are the exact opposite: If the employee works more or fewer hours than a typical pay period, either the employee or the practice owner feels taken advantage of.

Commission – If the commission is set properly, the employer has no risk in the arrangement. From the employee's perspective, they have the freedom to earn more if they do more. One disadvantage to the employee is that they are not guaranteed a set amount of compensation. Another disadvantage of this method is that employees, given what amounts to an unlimited ceiling on pay, may sacrifice quality of work to make more money. This is sometimes seen with commissioned hygienists who shorten their time with patients in order to produce more and make more.

Combination of Base play Plus Commission – This achieves the advantages of both methods, while minimizing the disadvantages of both. However, the disadvantages of both still exist, and this combination method involves more complicated payroll and bookkeeping.

My recommendation is that, given the pros and cons of each of these methods, the disadvantages of hourly wages are less than those of the other methods. The risk is minimal to both sides when the hourly wage is set correctly. When combined with an effective bonus system, this form of payment can achieve some of the benefits of commission compensation.

Bonus Systems or Profit Sharing?

Just about every bonus system used in dental offices ultimately fails to do what it was designed to do – motivate and reward team members for exceptional performance. Instead, the business owner eventually resents the bonus system, because it becomes an *operating expense*, an increase in wages, and not a reward from profits.

Team members come to expect the bonus, so it becomes a regular part of their compensation, and they even adjust their lifestyle as a result. When the bonus isn't reached, either because the potential for additional production has been maxed out, or bonus levels have increased, it results in demotivation – "Where's my money?" Over time, the business owner may begin to feel trapped, and may eliminate the bonus altogether (which will make employees feel like they have taken a pay cut) or make it easier for employees to reach bonus levels (which will negatively affect practice profitability).

My recommendation is to stop relying on a bonus system for a *sizeable portion* of any team member's compensation. While the concept of commission sounds like it protects the business owner AND motivates the team member, it often accomplishes neither. There will be months when the schedule just doesn't allow for consistent production and/or collections. Many team members live paycheck to paycheck. The risk of not getting a paycheck sufficient to satisfy their obligations is not one that most team members can afford.

To the business owner, a commission-based pay structure doesn't always mean profit. The reason? Overhead. There will be months when the practice doesn't make money, even when collections are high. Yet most bonus systems will still generate bonuses and make profitability even more negative. As a result, and rightfully so, the owner may raise the bonus level. The team member now feels that the carrot is further away, just so the owner can pay less bonus money and take home a bigger piece of the pie that the team member feels they were a big part of making.

Instead, owners should pay team members a higher-than-average hourly rate. Make it impossible for a valued team member to go anywhere else in the local market for more money. Then, if the owner feels compelled to do so, implement a bonus system that will result in bonuses the practice can afford, because they come from profit, taking into consideration the three components that control profit – production, collection rate, and expenses. The bonus amounts will likely be more modest than a previous failed bonus system, but the outcome will properly compensate an employee who receives a bonus when two things happen: 1. The practice profited, and 2. The team member contributed meaningfully to that profitability.

Years ago, I developed a program for my *Sunrise Dental Solutions* clients to address all of these concerns. The instrument, the Sunrise Team Achievement Rewards (STAR) Program, was designed to be a fluid instrument that can be personalized and modified periodically to the individual needs of the practice. Once it is set up properly, it requires a designated individual to enter daily practice provider production and collection numbers, keeping a running tally of each team member's total monthly bonus amount to date as long as certain practice benchmarks are met.

First, a word of caution: Most practices which replace their previous bonus system find this bonus system pays out smaller bonus amounts. This is because most dental practice bonus systems overpay employees by basing the bonus on the wrong parameters (production and/or collections), paying bonuses for performance that is expected (in the job description) instead of for performance that goes above and beyond what is expected, and paying everyone the same amount.

The Sunrise Team Achievement Rewards Program (STAR)

Rules of the Game

1. The bonus system must allow for the practice owner to benefit financially, not just the employees.
2. The bonus system must be based on profitability, not production or collections. Regardless of effort or performance, no bonus will be paid unless the practice reaches a profitability threshold.
3. Everyone's individual contribution to reaching that profitability threshold must be measured and rewarded (or not). Paying everyone the same bonus amount is socialism, and socialism doesn't work any better in a dental practice than it works in government. It penalizes those who perform well and rewards those who don't.

Setting Up the Program

1. Set up an appointment with a *Sunrise Dental Solutions* analyst to establish the program. This appointment should be with the practice owner, even if a team member will be assigned record-keeping duties related to the program.
2. Before the call, familiarize yourself with the concept by reviewing the "SDS Team Rewards Program – Rationale & General Mechanics" available through Sunrise Dental Solutions.

The appointment will accomplish these objectives:

1. The spreadsheet that records and calculates the program's rewards will be reviewed.
2. Any questions the practice owner has regarding the program will be addressed.
3. The amount of money available to pay bonuses from practice profit will be determined using the *Profit Available For Bonuses Per Practice Production* worksheet. An example of this worksheet is included in the Glossary.
4. Teams and team members, daily goals, daily rewards, monthly collection percentage threshold, monthly super level, and super rewards will be established.
5. Daily and end-of-month management of the program will be reviewed. An example of the *Sunrise Team Achievement Rewards Program* spreadsheet is included in the Glossary.

Here's a review of team members' wants:

WHAT TEAM MEMBERS OF THE PROSPEROUS DENTAL PRACTICE WANT:

1. Direction
2. Support
3. Feedback
4. Appreciation
5. A Path to Advancement
6. Compensation

They also need something else – Team Communication. We've covered one-on-one communication through support and feedback (Performance Assessments), but the team as a group needs an effective system for group communication and interactions.

TEAM COMMUNICATION

There is no more crucial ingredient of extraordinary leadership than communication. How you **communicate** to your fellow team members will determine the success or failure of your business enterprise. And there is no better opportunity for effective communication than meeting together with members of your team.

Team Meetings

Most dentists do not have effective team meetings. In fact, many dentists have told me they literally dread these encounters and are even intimidated by them. Even more alarming are the comments I've heard from team members who consider these events to be useless, boring, and morale-destroying.

The missing ingredient in team meetings is leadership. Your team meeting should empower each of your team members with an action plan. It should provide an open forum to applaud successes and address shortcomings. It should motivate and inspire participants. It should inform the team about its progress toward fulfilling the organization's vision, mission, and goals. Your leadership can ensure the success of the Ultimate Team Meeting.

The Ten Parts to the Ultimate Team Meeting are:

1. Attitude

Attitude is everything. One hundred percent of the time, a good attitude toward yourself, your team, the meeting, and its objectives will produce a positive outcome. A great attitude does not just happen. It is not the result of good things that have been happening lately. It is the result of a conscious decision on your part to choose to be positive and enthusiastic about your circumstances. You can't always change your circumstances, but you have complete control over your perspective.

As the leader, your attitude will be reflected by your team. Regardless of what might be going on in your professional or personal life, you must come to your meeting with enthusiasm. It has been said that what made Thomas Edison such a great inventor was that his unlimited enthusiasm conveyed the feeling that he would press on until he succeeded.

This must be genuine. Look at yourself in the mirror before you go into the meeting. Does your face and body language emanate enthusiasm? Remember, we don't smile because we're happy, we're happy because we smile. You can decide to create team meetings that have a positive outcome. Make it office policy that everything that is done or said will be done or said in a positive way.

The team meeting is not a place for someone to vent frustrations. Solutions to problems should be presented as *requests*. Approaching challenges in this way compels each individual to evaluate the request before it is made. Each participant must ask the question "Is this request meaningful to the success of the business?"

We have a rule in our office: ***No whining***. Whenever someone tries to be negative, everyone in the office has the right to call him or her on it, even if that person is you, the leader.

A leader can't lead without followers. And no one will follow you unless they trust you. A humble attitude goes a long way in winning the trust of your team. Don't ever pass up the opportunity to admit when you're wrong. Six of life's most important words are: "I admit I made a mistake."

2. Integrity

You, the leader, must model the way for others to follow. You must send the signal loud and clear that positive, productive team meetings are a prerequisite to the practice's success. Your team members will observe and then follow your lead regarding the manner in which you conduct yourself prior to, during, and following every encounter.

For example, if your office policy states that attendance at all team meetings is mandatory, and you as the team leader never miss a meeting, then your team members will likewise make every effort to be present. Likewise, if you are always on time for the meeting, and you start the meeting on time, then your team members will respond in kind. Again, don't expect others to put any more effort into your meetings than you personally demonstrate.

3. Preparation

The Romans had a saying, "If you want peace, prepare for war." Never come to a meeting without a very good idea of what the meeting is about and how it should proceed. The goal here is to control the meeting without anyone knowing it. You will accomplish this with careful forethought and planning.

If employees are compensated by a defined unit of time worked, say per hour, then they should be compensated for time spent in team meetings. Team meetings are work. You require the full attention and participation of your employees, and they should be paid for it. As an employer, you want to get the best return for your investment in time and money. Make the most of every minute you spend in a team meeting.

For a team meeting to be efficient, each member must come to the meeting prepared. An agenda must be distributed at least a day ahead of time. In the absence of an office manager, the practice owner should prepare the agenda. Each team member should prepare reports or bring information related to any agenda items related to their responsibilities.

At Morning Meetings, for example, require that each provider and assistant review all patient charts for that day ahead of time. This way, you can accomplish a lot in a short time.

4. Participation

There's a reason they're called ***team*** meetings. Just as each member of your team fulfills an important role within the office, each member must play a role in the meeting for the meeting to reach its potential.

The tendency in most meetings is for the practice owner to dominate the discussion with a few others participating. This leaves many team members, who may have valuable insights to share, on the outside looking in. In time, they will just stop trying, instead spending their time glancing at their phones and daydreaming. These members never reach their potential, and never feel empowered.

Each team member should be informed ahead of time of his or her expected role in the meeting. For example, in your Annual Goal-Setting Meeting, an individual from each department of your office should have prepared a report outlining the last year's accomplishments and the coming year's objectives and strategies.

Each team member's job description should include meeting participation. Likewise, each performance evaluation should evaluate the quantity and quality of a team member's participation in team meetings.

You can draw some conclusions if, after you have established the importance of participation in team meetings, a team member does not participate. Your team member either has no interest in the subject matter or has nothing valuable to add to the matter at hand. The former speaks to attitude, the latter to ability.

You as the leader can encourage participation during the meeting by asking for opinions and input. Show genuine interest in your team members' responses. Once team members feel their participation is not just expected, but valued, they will participate willingly and effectively.

5. Recognition

The Ultimate Team Meeting applauds successes and addresses shortcomings in a motivating and inspiring way. This meeting empowers everyone and redirects the entire team to its ultimate purpose.

The five most important words in the English Language are, "*You did a great job.*" Many dentists don't have any idea how those five spoken words can form the foundation of a loyal, potential-reaching team.

People want to be noticed. They want credit for personal achievements and appreciation for their contributions. Constructive appraisal has a place, but not in a team meeting, and not in front of one's peers. Recognition, on the other hand, is much more effective if given in a group setting.

Recognition strengthens an individual's self-esteem and positively reinforces behavior. Public acknowledgement also educates others. It establishes what is important to you and the standard of service you expect. Recognition and appreciation create an environment of friendly, constructive competition among your team members.

Once a year, my office has an "I Appreciate You" Meeting. Each team member takes a turn in the "warm seat," The other team members direct statements of appreciation to every individual in the "warm seat." A selected team member records the appreciation statements on a sheet of paper and gives it to the esteemed team member. The effect of this session on team morale and cohesiveness is immeasurable.

In every group encounter, search for a way to communicate how much you appreciate your team. When appropriate, single out individuals, but try not to focus on the same ones at every meeting, for this can build resentment.

Recognition is a method to build people, and people are your business' most valuable asset. Every leader wants to bring out the best in the team. And every leader knows that encouragement is the way to do it.

6. Information

The Ultimate Team Meeting informs the team of its progress toward fulfilling the organization's vision, mission, and goals. Many dentists mistakenly feel that they must withhold business performance figures from their team in order to maintain their position of power and insure confidentiality.

I call this the "Mushroom Farmer Theory of Management." This management style says you treat your team like you're growing mushrooms. You keep them in the dark and feed them manure. These managers seem to always have personnel problems, and marvel at the lack of buy-in on the part of their employees.

Your team has a right to expect that you will keep them in the loop, communicating not only the changes that need to take place but also the reasons behind those changes. People become uncertain when they feel that they are being left in the dark. They become distrustful of you, their leader.

Nothing involves people and sustains credibility more effectively than providing and discussing all organization performance figures with your team members. This does not mean that your team should have access to the business checking account. What it speaks to is the importance of sharing the business statistics that are needed in order to accomplish the practice's objectives.

7. Focus

Another very common characteristic of the misguided team meeting is the tendency to get off track. A good leader will sense this and remind the team about the meeting's purpose, in a courteous, respectful manner. Priorities must be established through the agenda, and religiously adhered to.

Contributions should be concise and to the point. Great leaders are often highly eloquent, but eloquence is not a requirement of effective communication. In most situations, all that is needed is a leader who communicates clearly, succinctly, and efficiently.

8. Respect

You cannot lead without followers, and no one will follow you unless they respect you. No one will respect you unless you first respect him or her. You demonstrate respect for your team by showing courtesy, genuine interest, and sincere appreciation.

Treat your team members as equals. Don't make the mistake of equating personal value with income, socio-economic status, or an educational degree. Three important words are "If you please," and two additional important words are "Thank you." Courtesy will reward you with respect.

Actively listen to your team. Ask for their opinion. Anthony Eden considered Winston Churchill's outstanding leadership characteristic to be his willingness to listen; he never cut off a suggestion with a curt dismissal but encouraged elaboration. Listening demonstrates concern and respect, and it shows that you value your team and their abilities. Without respect, you will never be able to lead.

2. Financial Coordinator – gives yesterday's collection totals, informs the team about patients with outstanding balances that he/she needs to address before the patient is seated
3. Hygienist – reviews his/her schedule
4. Dentist – in the absence of the office manager, facilitates the meeting, and interjects only where appropriate
5. Dental Assistant – reviews the dentist's schedule

If everyone cannot be present, a representative from each area of the practice must attend. That person should be prepared to present information to the meeting on behalf of their department, and to forward information from the meeting to their department members. The following form can be used for this vital information:

Practice Name ______________________ **Date** ______________

Yesterday	Production	+/- Goal	Comments/Opportunities
Hyg. 1			
Hyg. 2			
Hyg. 3			
Dr. 1			
Total			
Today			
Hyg. 1			
Hyg. 2			
Hyg. 3			
Dr. 1			
Total			
Tomorrow			
Hyg. 1			
Hyg. 2			
Hyg. 3			
Dr. 1			
Total			
Positive Thought for Today			

The meeting should last no more than fifteen minutes. This underscores the importance of being prepared and succinct.

Departmental Meeting

The Departmental Meeting's objective is to deal with specific issues and requests pertaining to that department. The department's strengths and weaknesses are reviewed, and role-playing (when necessary) is accomplished to better prepare everyone for specific situations.

The Team Leader will need to prepare agendas and reports for each meeting, and present those reports at Team Leader Meetings, Total Team Meetings, and the annual Goal-Setting Meeting.

The Departmental Meeting can be held at any time during the day at a private location within the office or off-site. They can be held one or two times each month depending on needs and should last 45 minutes to an hour.

Team Leader Meeting

The objectives of Team Leader Meetings are to inform the leaders of the practice about what is going on in each department and to address practice concerns. The real leadership and management decisions are often made during these encounters.

The Office Manager (or dentist in the absence of an Office Manager) facilitates the meeting. Often the Office Manager is the team leader of the Business Office Department.

Each team leader gives a report of their departmental meeting. Requests are acted upon, and progress toward office goals is charted.

These meetings can be held at the beginning of the day or mid-day, either on-site or off-site. There is real value in holding at least half of these meetings off-site for privacy, to reduce distractions, and to enhance creativity.

They are held twice a month, once during a week where there are no departmental meetings, and once prior to the Total Team Meeting. They typically last 45 minutes to an hour.

Total Team Meeting

The Total Team Meeting is where the entire team comes together with the objective to inform, problem-solve, influence, and unite the team toward the goals of the practice.

Attendance and participation are mandatory. The goal is for everyone to leave the meeting feeling positive about the office and their role in its success. This meeting is first and foremost a team-building event. Additionally, it is a mastermind session to address practice concerns. The Office Manager or Practice Owner facilitates the meeting.

The Total Team Meeting can be held at the beginning of the day, in an extended lunch hour, or on a weekday when the office is not seeing patients. The advantage to holding it when the office is closed to patient care is that there aren't interruptions like incoming calls and patients dropping by. When held when the office is closed, it can be held off-site.

This meeting should be held once or twice a month, depending on need and the size of the practice. For larger teams, once monthly is preferred. Generally speaking, the more people involved in a meeting, the more difficult it is to manage. Larger practices tend to get much more accomplished in departmental and team leader meetings.

There are five rules for the total team meeting:

1. There will be no whining. Everything will be phrased in a positive manner. Each team member is given permission to "call" the offending party on this and redirect them to the positive.

2. No one will be allowed to bring up any request without also offering two solutions, one of which is to cost little or no money.
3. The meeting will start on time and end on time.
4. Preparation and participation are mandatory.
5. An agenda will be prepared in advance and given top priority.

The agenda is prepared by the office manager or other designated member and posted at least one day prior to the meeting. The order of the agenda shall be:

1. The agenda begins with the mission statement: why our organization exists. Everything we do must be directed toward and be graded by how well we accomplish this mission.
2. After the recitation of the mission statement by a team member (who is often rewarded by some form of compensation), the floor is opened to discussion of instances where we are achieving this purpose. This may be a patient compliment, an instance where we as an office overcame an obstacle, etc.
3. Next, departmental reports are presented by each team leader.
4. This is followed by miscellaneous agenda items that are addressed through the collective mastermind of the total team.
5. Finally, each individual team member is allowed time for remarks and requests. The total team meeting typically lasts 90 minutes to two hours.

Delinquent Accounts Meeting

The objective of the Delinquent Accounts Meeting has already been addressed in the Financial Systems portion of this book. This once-a-month, 30-minute to one-hour meeting has been very instrumental in saving dental practices thousands of dollars in uncollected money and collection-related costs. It can be held any time during the normal workday, at any private location, since sensitive information is discussed.

The Financial Coordinator leads the meeting. He or she prints up a delinquent accounts report in descending order from highest balance to lowest balance. The Financial Coordinator then reviews the status of each account and asks for input when needed, as well as addresses any questions from the other participants, which include the scheduling coordinator(s), office manager, other business office personnel who collect money, and the dentist(s). Strategies are devised for collecting the outstanding balances.

Goal-Setting Meeting (aka "Annual Year-End Review & Goal-Setting Meeting")

The objective of the Goal-Setting Meeting is to review the past year, to set new goals, to devise strategies to accomplish these goals, and to plan the coming year's calendar. The meeting is designed to motivate, inspire, and unite the entire team toward the ultimate goal, the vision of the leader. Each team member should leave the meeting feeling great about being a part of a successful organization, their role in that success, and what the future holds for the practice. Speaking from personal experience, I know that the potential of this meeting is that it is the most enjoyable, and arguably the most productive, day the practice has each year.

It is usually held annually within a couple of weeks after the end of the fiscal or calendar year, whichever is applicable. It can be held on-site or off.

A slide presentation is helpful to guide the team expeditiously through the office performance figures, goal setting, team reports, and calendar. This presentation should cover:

1. The past year's office statistics
2. Last year's goals
3. Team reports
4. This year's goals
5. Strategies
6. Calendar

Each team leader is accountable for preparing their departmental report and presentation for their respective departments, involving all members of their team. The practice owner supplies all the office statistics and, in the absence of an office manager or team leaders, is accountable for organizing and facilitating the meeting.

One more thing: This meeting should be fun for all involved. Team members should look forward to it each year. Sadly, the exact opposite occurs in many practices because team members see it as a boring, poor use of time that usually results in criticism, asking everyone for more without any realization of why or what "more" means.

How do you make it fun? Years ago, I decided to ask each department to present their report and perform a skit, a short comedy sketch related somehow to last year's accomplishments and/or this year's goals. At first there was some hesitation, but after that first meeting, the laughter and fun made the exercise something they looked forward to preparing and presenting at each annual meeting. Participants dressed in costume and even poked a little fun at management. We soon began to vote on which department skit was the best and awarded prizes to the members of that department. While this may sound corny to some, it has made a huge difference in our team's outlook on what can be an intense four-to-six-hour meeting.

CONFLICT RESOLUTION

Conflict within any group of people is inevitable. No matter how good the chemistry, how positive the culture, how talented the team, or how in tune they are with the vision of the practice owner, a group of human beings will encounter conflict. How they address conflict may make the difference between overcoming it or being overcome by it. Years ago, I came up with the following rules for addressing conflict. I posted it in my office and referred to it whenever conflict reared its ugly head. There are nine *Conflict Resolution Rules*:

THE RULES OF CONFLICT RESOLUTION

1. **Think Win/Win** – Search for resolution where no one loses.
2. **Listen** – Show respect and set the stage for a constructive discussion.
3. **Seek First to Understand** – Don't expect others to understand you until you make them feel completely understood.
4. **Attack The Behavior, Not the Person** – It's the two of you against the problem, not the two of you against one another.
5. **Manage Emotion** – Emotions obscure objectivity and invoke an equal and opposite emotional response.
6. **Think Big Picture** – Personal ego takes a back seat to the objectives of the organization, which benefits everyone.
7. **When Possible, Negotiate** – If your values and the values of the organization aren't at risk, then seek a compromise. Be willing to give a little.
8. **When Necessary, Accept Mediation** – If the process stalls, seek mutually agreed upon outside perspective.
9. **Commit to Resolution** – Make a personal commitment to complete resolution.

DISMISSING A PATIENT

Knowing the proper way to dismiss a patient from the practice is a leadership attribute. Along with dismissing an employee, this can be the most unpleasant occurrence that a practice owner must experience. However, both events, when undertaken with the right mindset and implemented appropriately, can also be liberating, even practice-building, experiences. There are four components to the process:

1. Perspective & Prevention

Perspective

The dentist/patient relationship is a complicated one that involves the patient's needs, desires, past experiences, emotional and physical state, resources, and expectations. On the dentist side, there are their skills, knowledge, experience, resources, team support, emotional and physical state, and expectations. Any one or more of these factors on either side of the relationship can negatively impact the relationship and, ultimately, its success.

Some relationships do not work out. Try as they may, dentists cannot be all things to all people. Some working relationships will not be successful, and they will have to be ended, for the best interest of all involved. Much like terminating an employee relationship, the end of the doctor-patient relationship allows both parties the opportunity to seek success where they are currently failing. Of course, the fewer times this relationship termination happens, the better, which is where the skill of patient selection comes in.

Prevention

With the complex nature of the dentist-patient dynamic in mind, both the dentist and the patient need to carefully consider selecting the right person to work with for the delivery of care. Almost always, the patient puts a lot more effort into the selection process than the dental professional. The dental professional must keep in mind that it is their right, and sometimes in their best interest, to not treat a patient. *The cost of treating a patient can be much greater than the cost of not treating them.*

Practice owners sometimes say, *"If I had only listened to my gut," or "If I had only paid attention to those red flags, I would never have taken this patient on."* The dentist should lean on their experiences as well as these gut instincts to determine the likelihood of a successful outcome of care. Remember, the definition of successful outcome is whether the professional standard of care is obtained, and the *receiver of the care is satisfied*. It is essential to determine the patient's expectations of the outcome of treatment *prior* to any treatment.

A telltale sign that the patient is going to be hard if not impossible to please is when they have had an unsuccessful outcome somewhere else and they blame the previous dentist. That is not to say that the blame wasn't warranted, but you should take some time to evaluate the treatment and the patient's reasons why they feel the treatment was unsuccessful.

If the patient's needs are more advanced than the provider's training and skill level, or if the patient's health prevents them from being safely treated at the existing facility and/or by the dentist and team, or for any other reason you do not feel you can trust the patient and their intentions, you should not accept the patient.

Effective language for declining a patient might be:

"I am not the right dentist to provide your care.

Some dentists and patients work better together than others and your care is too important to not have the best possible working relationship with the dentist and staff that is providing your care."

or

"Your treatment needs are beyond the training and experience that I and my staff have.

Because of that, I will not be providing your care."

2. Making the Decision

When it is apparent that the patient should not be accepted for treatment or it is obvious to the practitioner that the dentist/patient relationship has deteriorated to the point of being non-salvageable, it is time to cut the cord. The decision is better made earlier than later. Backing out later is still possible, but the price is higher, because of the time invested and the potential argument the patient may raise regarding being abandoned during treatment. Whenever possible, complete all treatment that is incomplete. This doesn't mean the entire treatment plan, just the parts of the plan that have been started but not completed.

3. Preparation

The practice owner should contact his/her liability insurance carrier for guidance in properly executing the dismissal. This can be invaluable, especially if for any reason the liability insurance carrier will need to act on the part of their client.

The practice owner should mentally prepare themselves for what they intend to say and be steadfast in their resolve to follow through despite objections. All patient records should be properly documented. A decision should be made about when (sooner the better) and where to inform the patient. If money is to be refunded, it should be delivered upon notification of dismissal.

4. Execution

The message should be delivered in a respectful and unapologetic manner. A modified version of the language described in the first step of the dismissal process can be used:

"I've come to the conclusion that I am not the right dentist to continue providing your care. Both the experience during your treatment as well as the outcome afterward are dependent on a good doctor/patient relationship, which we clearly do not have. Because of that, I have decided to discontinue any further treatment. Once you choose a new dentist, let us know where to forward your records."

It is best to decline to go into specifics if pressed – this likely makes things worse, just as when an employee is dismissed. The practice owner should simply say that the patient would be better off with another dental office. Neither should the practice owner react negatively to any negative response from the patient but be respectful even if it is not deserved. There is no way to avoid some negative fallout, but every effort should be made to minimize it.

Referring the dismissed patient to another practice is usually not a good idea, as any relationships with that office could be damaged if they are referred a patient that has had at least one unsuccessful doctor/patient relationship in another office.

The account should be flagged in the practice software, so that everyone accessing the patient's account in the future is aware of its status in the practice. When documenting the conversation in the patient's record, words should be chosen carefully. The patient may request the clinical notes and may be entitled to them. Make sure the words are professional in their tone and content.

TIME MANAGEMENT

Efficient use of time is a quality of good leadership. Many practice owners waste time, which negatively impacts both the practice and the business. Good leaders value time as the one asset that is finite. Each year has three hundred and sixty-five days and fifty-two weeks, each week has seven days, each day has twenty-four hours, each hour has sixty minutes, and each minute has sixty seconds. It's the same for every living person, so how do some accomplish so much more than others, in shorter time, garnering a greater return on their resources?

I'm often asked how I manage to run a full-service coaching and consulting company, lead a large dental practice, teach courses throughout the year all over the country, and perform other projects, manage to do them all well, and still take what amounts to a two-week vacation every month. And, I might add, with no more intelligence and talent than the dentists I coach who struggle with managing time. It comes down to *Leverage*.

"Leverage" has many meanings, spanning the world of physics to finances. It can also mean, as it does here, the exploitation of available resources to accomplish tasks more efficiently. The effective time manager can use the leverage principle through organization, preparation, and surrounding yourself with a great team.

Organization

The leader with effective organizational skills brings clarity to the job at hand, allowing ready access to necessary information and addressing crucial tasks that are time sensitive. I can look at someone's desk and get a good idea of their organizational skills. While some can juggle multiple tasks all at the same time and function effectively in a chaotic environment, most of us benefit from a methodical and orderly workplace and taking the time each day to maintain that sense of order.

Early in my career as I took on more obligations, I found myself bogged down and frustrated, feeling burdened with more and more responsibilities. My desk became more cluttered, my days became longer, and meeting deadlines became more uncommon. Thankfully, I happened upon a principle that became critical to improving my time management skills – The Four Ds. *The Four Ds* are Delegate It, Dump It, Delay It, and Do It.

Delegate It - I've referred more than once in this book to dentists' general aversion to allowing other people to do things they can do legally and do to reasonable standards. Whether the practice owner enjoys the task, doesn't believe anyone else can do it as well, doesn't want a team member to have access to practice information, or just wants to have control over everything possible, the limitations imposed by not delegating are inversely proportional to the practice owner's ability to grow, have more freedom over their time, and accomplish more.

I ask dentist clients to ask themselves before doing anything in a typical day, "Is there someone else who can legally do this, and can be trained to do it as well as I can?" If the answer is yes, and that person is on their team, then delegate it. If they aren't on their team, then find that person. The feeling of freedom from letting go of something is truly liberating. *Just Delegate It.*

Dump It - Most people do things every day that don't need to be done. They do them out of habit, or in the belief that they do matter in some way, but when it comes down to it, these things have nothing to do with obligations made or the vision one should be working toward. Ask yourself, "What would happen if I didn't do this?" If there would be no untoward consequences, *Just Dump It.*

Delay It - People who are always struggling to meet deadlines, or asking for extensions, or performing below standard, lack focus and clarity in prioritizing their time. If you were to make a list of all the things that you should do (and I highly recommend it), it would be clear that you aren't going to be able to complete all those things today. You can, however, make significant progress on what's most important and what's most time sensitive. Everything else will have to wait if you are to make the best use of your time. For many things that are competing for your attention, *Just Delay It.*

Do It - After the other three Ds, what remains are those obligations that only you can do and that have a deadline attached to them, plus those things that have a high priority due to their connection to your vision. Both are important, but the obligations with deadlines can sometimes monopolize all your time. If these obligations are not related to the realization of your vision, look for ways to minimize or eliminate them.

Time management is all about keeping the main thing the main thing. At some point, usually unknown to us, our time runs out. What will be left behind are the things we got done (part of our legacy), and those we didn't. Use your time wisely. The imprint on the world you leave depends on it. When it comes to what matters most, *Just Do It.*

Preparation

Now that you have your desk (literally and figuratively) organized into four piles, you need a plan for tackling the Just Do It pile. Average people go to work each day without a plan. They just start working and plan as they go along. This wastes valuable minutes, which over time become hours, weeks, months, and years. Taking just fifteen to thirty minutes to plan the current day, or the next day, can not only save time, but also give you focus and the peace of mind that accompanies preparation.

Some will do better planning the next day the night before. Oftentimes, the subconscious mind works through challenges, and the solutions become apparent the next morning. There really is something to the saying, "I'll sleep on it."

Others, like myself, do better planning in the morning for that day. I've always arrived at the office at least one hour before my morning meeting which is scheduled for 6:45 a.m. My mind is fresh, and I'm by myself without any distractions as I plan out the day, both in the practice and for my other professional interests. This allows me to operate at a high level of efficiency and keeps me grounded on focusing on my obligations and my priorities. Daily preparation is an essential component of effective time management.

Surround Yourself with a Great Team

No one in this world accomplishes anything of significance by themselves. Two other natural conclusions to that statement are: The more people you have working on your behalf, the more you will accomplish; and the higher quality those people are, the more you will accomplish.

Throughout this book I have referenced the importance of a great team to build a more prosperous dental practice and business. The same principle applies to time management. I've heard the excuses before: More people, more stress. More people, more expense. More people, more time to manage them, which defeats the purpose. There are two ways to approach getting things done – excuses and results. Results come from being committed to success combined with the premise of this book: The key to success is "*A Great Team* Implementing *Great Systems* in the presence of *Great Leadership*."

Before I leave the topic of leadership, I want to remind you that leadership is a continual journey, not a destination. The journey is not a straight line but is accompanied by setbacks. Everyone experiences leadership fails from time to time. Fortunately, the biggest variable in the leadership journey is also the variable you have most control over – yourself.

SELF-TALK

I'm mindful of the following saying and how true I have found it to be in my life:

"Watch your thoughts, for they become words. Watch your words, for they become actions. Watch your actions, for they become habits. Watch your habits, for they become character. Watch your character, for it becomes your destiny."

Ultimately, your thoughts determine your destiny, and that's good news because you get to choose what you think about. Therefore, since you control your thoughts, you control your destiny. I understand it's not as simple as thinking your future into existence, but your thinking and your future are inexorably linked.

It all starts with your thoughts – what you choose to think. What you think about, you bring about. Successful people think about success. Non-successful people think about other stuff.

Walter Hailey was the first to teach me about "self-talk" – having a conversation with yourself about the right thoughts to set you up for success. It is part of my daily routine during the time each morning I spend preparing myself for the day. Each individual must choose how that conversation goes, but it is likely to include positive phrases that have the most meaning for them to focus on. Here are a few of my favorites:

"People don't care how much you know until they know how much you care." – Theodore Roosevelt

"Ask and it will be given to you; seek and you will find; knock and the door will be opened to you." – Matthew 7:7

"You dominate a conversation by talking. You control a conversation by asking questions." – Unknown

"Our goal is not to make a sale. Our goal is to create a customer." – Unknown

"Whatever you can vividly envision, ardently desire, earnestly believe in, and expectantly act toward, with God's help, must inevitably come to pass. That which you are seeking is seeking you." – Paul Meyer

"When it comes to success, nothing can take the place of persistence. Talent will not; nothing is more common than unsuccessful people with talent. Genius will not; unrewarded genius is almost a proverb. Education will not; the world is full of educated derelicts. Persistence and determination alone are omnipotent." – Calvin Coolidge

"The pessimist sees the difficulty in every opportunity, while the optimist sees the opportunity in every difficulty." – Winston Churchill

"You can have everything in life you want if you will just help enough other people get what they want." – Zig Ziglar

"Things may go to those who wait, but only what's left over from those who hustle." – Abraham Lincoln

"Whatever the mind can conceive and believe, it can achieve." – Napoleon Hill

"When you are faced with decisions, make that decision as wisely as possible, then forget it. The

moment of absolute certainty never arrives. And above all, remember that God helps those who help themselves. Act as if everything depended on you and pray as if everything depended on God." - SH Payer

"If you really want to do something, you'll find a way. If you don't, you'll find an excuse." - Jim Rohn

"I always do what I ought to do, whether I want to do it or not - no debate" - Unknown

"When someone offends you, or wrongs you in some way, weak people seek revenge, strong people forgive, intelligent people ignore." - Albert Einstein

THE KEY CONCEPT

The Key Concept of Positive Affirmation - "Affirmations are proven methods of self-improvement because of their ability to rewire our brains. Much like exercise, they raise the level of feel-good hormones and push our brains to form new clusters of "positive thought" neurons. In the sequence of thought-speech-action, affirmations play an integral role by breaking patterns of negative thoughts, negative speech, and, in turn, negative actions." - Dr. Carmen Harra

SUMMARY OF KEY POINTS FROM CHAPTER 3 - THE LEADERSHIP

1. The benefits of being a better leader include increased harmony among the team with little turnover; ownership mentality with team members taking accountability for important roles, freeing the practice owner to focus on fewer tasks; team members all on the same page; a culture of trust in the office; and a more profitable business.
2. Without purpose, the full potential of leadership cannot be realized.
3. Once you know your purpose, you then must decide what you are going to do with it. This is your vision, and the simplest way to find your vision is to Dream Without Limits.
4. Share your vision passionately, commit to it wholeheartedly, and show others what your vision will mean to them. If you have the right people, in the right culture, they will adopt your vision and play an important role in making it a reality.
5. To the team of the prosperous dental practice, goals are the difference between winning and losing, between success and failure, and are worth doing whatever it takes to accomplish.
6. Team culture is about the entire team sharing common values, beliefs, attitudes, and behaviors, and working harmoniously together toward a common vision.
7. Team members want to know what's expected of them, i.e., the responsibilities of the position. The prosperous dental practice team members want to know even more: What do they have to do to perform exceptionally (to win)?
8. Team members want to know how they're performing from their leaders in the practice. They want to know where they stand relative to what is expected of them. This is formally accomplished through Performance Evaluations but should occur often in a less formal format in one-on-one conversations during the course of a day in the office.
9. The simple yet powerful act of saying "Thank you" may seem like a little thing, but it acknowledges the act that preceded it and recognizes the individual with respect. And when that respect is extended, it is often returned.
10. The prosperous dental practice team member is ambitious and needs a path to grow in their career.
11. Managers are responsible for making sure things are done the right way, while leaders are responsible for making sure the right things are done. Both roles are vital to the success of the practice and the business, and all members of the practice, including the practice owner, will be called upon to be both managers and leaders.
12. Team Leaders accept accountability for the success of their department. This requires them to be leaders in two ways: to support their individual members to reach the potential of their aptitude and ability, and to influence their team to contribute significantly to the overall vision of the practice. It also requires them to manage the implementation of systems within their department.

13. People want to be noticed. They want credit for personal achievements and appreciation for their contributions. Constructive appraisal has a place, but not in a team meeting, and not in front of one's peers. Recognition, on the other hand, is many times more effective if given in a group setting.

14. The efficient use of time is a quality of good leadership. Effective time managers use the leverage principle through organization, preparation, and surrounding themselves with a great team.

Chapter 4
The Transition Options

In the initial interview with a new dentist client, I usually surprise them with the following question, "What is your transition plan?" Unless the client is within a few years of transitioning their practice, they don't typically have a plan.

I maintain that every dentist should begin their career with a plan for how they want their career to evolve, up to and including how they want it to end. It's never too early to envision your future, no matter how far away that future may appear. You can always make adjustments along the way, but having a plan allows you to make decisions so that your preferred outcome is more likely to happen. Yogi Berra said it best, *"If you don't know where you are going, you'll end up someplace else."*

Wise mentors have taught me that the ultimate purpose of owning a business is to sell that business. That serves as a reminder of the following:

Profit from a business comes not only in the form of cash flow, but also through equity. Prosperous dental practice owners are always looking for ways to increase the value of their equity in the business, even if that means decreasing their percentage of ownership.

In the past, transitioning a dental practice meant owning until retirement age (this age used to be late 50s or early 60s, but by 2019 the retirement age for dentists had risen to age 70), then selling the practice to a younger dentist. More times than not, as the practice aged it declined, and in some cases the dentist merely walked away, recommending a colleague to his (pronoun intended) patients to take over their care. Of course, this was during the heyday of dental insurance, when there was little competition, no discount dental plans, shorter life spans, and no dental school debt.

As the dental economy and marketplace changed, so did transition strategies.

Now it is incumbent for dental practice owners to make the most of the equity they have accumulated in order to sustain their chosen standard of living – whose costs have risen along with a longer life span. To complicate these objectives further, dentists have a higher debt load both from education debt and from the rising cost of starting and operating a dental practice. Dentists are retiring later, and using innovative strategies to increase both the cash flow and the equity of their practices.

RETIREMENT PLANNING

While not innovative in nature, the timeless strategy of planning and funding retirement as early as possible has never been more important. I started my practice in 1983 upon graduation in my hometown of Lexington, Kentucky. Lexington, having a dental school at the University of Kentucky, was overcrowded with dentists, many of whom grew up in other areas of Kentucky but decided to stay in a nice, relatively affluent community. Not coming from affluence, I borrowed most of the cost of dental school, and graduated with an educational debt of $30,000. I know that seems ridiculously small compared to today's average dental student debt of nearly $300,000, but to me it was huge. Due to some advance word-of-mouth marketing, my first week in practice, working out of one rented operatory, without any staff, I produced $6,000 of dentistry. The first check I wrote from that money was a retirement savings check of $600. I've been saving at least ten percent of my earnings ever since.

I made a commitment to save, realizing that just as important as the amount someone puts away – if not more important – is when they start and how diligent they are in their commitment to saving. In fact, investing money carefully and allowing it to grow at compound interest will allow someone to accumulate a significant amount of financial wealth. You can use the *Rule of 72* to determine how long it would take for your money to double at any rate of interest. Simply divide the interest rate into the number 72.

THE KEY CONCEPT

The Key Concept of Compounding Interest - Compound interest is considered one of the great miracles of all of human history and economics. Albert Einstein described it as the most powerful force in our society. When you allow money to accumulate at compound interest over a long enough period of time, it increases more than most people realize.

The next strategy is to utilize both financial and practice consultants to create a financial plan and to support you in implementing that plan.

Everyone who appreciates the importance of a financial vision – financial freedom – needs their "number." The number is the amount of money they will need upon retirement to support their chosen lifestyle until their anticipated time of death.

Traditionally, the phrase "financial independence" has described the end game of accumulation of retirement income – that point in time at which having more money was no longer a concern. Lifestyle, while part of the financial independence equation, was secondary, but a paradigm shift has taken place in financial planning to place more priority on using savings for quality-of-life choices. Today's financial plan should address that shift from accumulating retirement income to achieving financial independence and maintaining the desired lifestyle – without having to worry about finances.

Financial consultants can assist with determining the financial and lifestyle freedom number. A very simple, yet relatively accurate, method that I use for a quick calculation of this number is the *Retirement Savings Worksheet*. It incorporates all the most important variables in the calculation – present age, retirement age, anticipated number of years of retirement income, average annual income, and inflation rate. It uses the general rule of thumb that seventy percent of the retired individual's present annual income will be needed in retirement.

It does not calculate compounding interest from existing or future retirement savings, as this can be highly variable. Therefore, the retirement amount calculated by the Retirement Savings Worksheet will err toward calculating an amount larger than needed. Despite this, I've found that using the worksheet results in a number that is very close to a more detailed analysis performed by a financial professional.

Retirement Savings Worksheet	**Name**	**Dr. Smith**
Present Age	62	
Years of Saving	8	
Retirement Age	70	
# of Yrs. Ret. Income	25	30 years of retirement income is used as a default, but may be adjusted up or down given genetics and/or health considerations.
Avg. Annual Income	$ 750,000.00	Anticipated increases or decreases in future annual income should be taken into consideration.
% of Annual Income Needed at Retirement	70%	70% is the default percentage but is based on your existing house being paid off by retirement, or selling existing house and downsizing. If you have two or more children and/or would like to assist them and their children, or figure to up-size in housing, use 100% here.
Inflation Rate	1.77%	The average inflation rate from 2010-2019 was 1.77%.
Annual Income Needed in Retirement	$ 525,000.00	This is the average annual income multiplied by the default percentage of income needed at retirement.
Retirement Account Needs Before Inflation	$ 13,125,000.00	This is the retirement income needed accounting for the number of anticipated years of retirement, before inflation.
Retirement Account Needs After Inflation	$ 13,357,312.50	This is the amount of income needed in retirement that accounts for inflation rate.
Existing Retirement Savings	$ 9,000,000.00	
Amount Needed to Save/Year Until Retirement Age	544,664.06	

Another strategy to make the most of your retirement income potential, while obvious but seldom employed, is to grow the practice all the way to the sale of the practice. In other words, instead of a practice value being less than its peak value some time (often years) prior to its sale, the practice value is at its height of value at the time of the sale. I've consulted with many dentists who have purchased practices at 10-20% of their appraised values from just a few years before. These practices had decreased dramatically in value because the practice owner had essentially retired before the sale of the practice, decreasing their interest and time spent working both on and in the business.

Continually growing the practice until its sale requires the practice owner to operate the practice at high levels, which includes updating technology, upgrading and refining systems, attending the finest continuing education available, marketing the practice, and investing in the attraction and retention of the best team possible. Many practice owners believe they won't make a return on these investments so close to the sale of their practice, but my experience is that the declining practice sells for pennies on the dollar, while the ascending practice sells for multiples of dollars on the dollar.

An additional trend transitioning practices are utilizing to grow their practices and increase equity is adding providers as both employees and owners. By adding additional dentists, the practice adds capacity for additional production, allows the practice owner to practice less and focus more on certain procedures, and creates a built-in transition from associate dentist to owner dentist.

In fact, the phrase "*Retire in Practice*" describes how many dentists are continuing as owners, while working less chairside, and in some cases working only in a managerial role. This way they can continue to participate in the cash flow and equity of the practice even after they end their clinical dentistry career.

For a growing percentage of practice owners, due to their financial needs, it doesn't make sense to sell all of their practice until much later than the traditional retirement age.

Regardless of when practice owners sell a portion or all of their practice, they need an accurate valuation so that both seller and buyer have an idea of the market value of the practice. Because so much is at stake to both parties – no one wants to sell for less, or buy for more, than the true value – the decision regarding what type of valuation, who performs it, and ultimately how much the practice is sold for is critical.

PRACTICE VALUATIONS

Practice valuations come in all shapes and forms, from the most informal to the most elaborate. Generally speaking, the more formal and elaborate, the more credibility the valuation has with sellers, buyers, advisors, and financial institutions.

Informal valuations are arrived at through industry standards based primarily on practice parameters such as production and collections, along with trends, geographic location, potential for additional capacity, and other practice metrics.

For many years, the industry standard was that a single-owner-owned dental practice was worth 70% of its average annual revenue over the last three years. Amazingly, no matter how intricate a formal appraisal was performed, the number from that appraisal nearly always ended up within 10% of that standard. Therefore, this standard is useful as a starting point guestimate for purposes of preliminary planning.

It is important to note that this industry standard may change as marketplace conditions change. For instance, in 2018 the demand driven by a Dental Service Organization (DSO) buying frenzy of practices increased the value of dental practices to eighty to one hundred percent of average annual collections. For group practices, the value exceeded one hundred percent of average annual revenue, and for multiple location practices, the value soared to multiples (3-5 X) of EBITDA (Earnings Before Interest, Taxes, Depreciation, and Amortization). EBITDA for a dental practice is, for all practical purposes, equivalent to operating cash flow after the owner's salary is deducted. Once the COVID-19 pandemic arrived in early 2020, marketplace conditions driven by the reversal of demand and increased supply drove practice values back to 2018 numbers.

As stated previously, the industry standard will be impacted (increased or decreased by as much as ten percent) by individual practice characteristics. The following is a list of such characteristics in order of having the most to the least effect:

Practice Characteristics that Affect Valuation

Characteristic #1 - Practice Is Declining or Increasing

A practice whose production and collections are trending up will hold more value, whereas the opposite is true if these metrics are trending down.

Characteristic #2 - Selling Doctor Transfers Trust to Buying Doctor

If the selling doctor continues seeing patients in an associate relationship for at least six months after the sale, then this is more likely to secure the biggest asset transferred in any practice acquisition – the goodwill of the patient base.

When a practice is sold, existing patients are not automatically transferred to the new owner. They have a choice of remaining or finding a new dental office (perhaps that of their spouse, or friend, or one that is more convenient to where they work or live). During this transition period, the selling doctor communicates with the practice base about how they hand-selected the buyer, how impressed they are with the dental care the new owner provides, and how much trust they have in the new owner to continue their care.

I have seen multiple situations where the selling doctor remaining in the practice can be a hindrance to the success of the buying doctor. This can occur if there are differences in practice philosophy that may include diagnosis, treatment planning, team management, collection systems, or more. Should these differences prove irreconcilable, then the selling doctor transferring trust to the patient base need not remain with the practice any longer than six months.

In addition to face-to-face communication between the selling doctor and the patient base promoting the buying doctor, written communication (posted and/or electronic mail) should communicate the same message in a more detailed manner. This communication should go out as soon after the sale of the practice as possible. Here is an example of such a communication to the patient base:

<SELLING DOCTOR'S HEADER>

<Date>
<Selling Doctor's Name>
<Selling Doctor's Address>

Dear <Personalized Name of Selling Doctor's Patient>,

Greetings! I hope this letter finds you and your loved ones doing well during this holiday season <or whatever time of year>. The holidays always prompt me to stop and consider my blessings, many of which revolve around the privilege of providing dental care to the people of <city, town> and surrounding areas for the past <number> years. While watching over your dental health all these years, I've seen many of my patients grow up, graduate from high school and college, get married, and bring their next generation to me for dental care. For allowing me to be a part of that, I am grateful. I want you to know I've always endeavored to provide you with the best care possible.

– cont'd

<SELLING DOCTOR'S HEADER> – cont'd

Now it's time for me to move on and pass the torch to the next generation so that you can continue to receive the very best dentistry has to offer. I am pleased to announce my retirement from dentistry, and even more so to recommend that you continue your dental care with one of those former patients who grew up in my practice and went on to establish himself as one of the most successful young dentists in this area of the country.

Dr. <buyer's name> is a <year> graduate of the <name of school> College of Dentistry. He and his <relationship, name> along with their <number if appropriate> of children reside in <city, town, or area>. <Buyer's name> has been recognized by many national and international organizations for his many accomplishments, including <list accomplishments here>. He is an active member of many professional organizations and has taken more than <number> hours of continuing education since graduation, providing the very latest in advancements in the dental profession. He and his highly skilled team of professionals provide the most technologically advanced care in a clean, safe, comfortable environment.

My biggest concern upon retirement was finding just the right dentist to continue your care. Dr. <buyer's name> has addressed that concern. Please join me and my family in continuing your dental care with Dr. <Buyer's name>. Your records have already been transferred to his office and you can expect to hear from <his or her> professional staff in the next few weeks with a special introductory offer the first time you visit them. If you need attention before that, you can reach <Buyer's name> office at <phone number>.

Once again, I want to thank you for your loyalty and patronage all these years. I wish you health and happiness this holiday season and into the new year.

Yours truly,

<Seller's name>

Characteristic #3 - Team Stays After the Sale of the Practice

Also important to the transfer of trust from past ownership to the new owner is the familiarity and likeability of the existing staff. These team members have built relationships with the patient base and can maintain that continuity, so that existing patients feel more comfortable with the transition to new practice ownership.

Characteristic #4 - A Healthy Hygiene Department (active patient base)

A healthy hygiene department is a leading indicator of the health of the practice. Healthy in this sense refers to a hygiene department that has at least 1.5 full-time hygienists per full-time doctor, increases production commensurate with the overall office increase in production, produces at least twenty-five percent of office production, and has an appropriate mix of preventive and periodontal treatment procedures.

The most important asset that a seller has to sell, and a buyer wants to buy, is the goodwill of the patients, so knowing the number of active patients is crucial. The hygiene department figures prominently into this calculation. The industry standard for determining the number of active patients is the number of patients that have had a hygiene appointment within the last twelve months.

Characteristic #5 - Geographic Location

Location can figure favorably into the value of a practice when appraised. Practices located in growing, affluent areas tend to attract more affluent patients who have the potential to spend more money at those practices, and are more highly valued.

Characteristic #6 - Condition of Facility

Modern, clean, visually appealing, and technologically advanced facilities will garner a higher appraised value. Conversely, facilities that require major remodeling and upgrades will have a lower value.

Characteristic #7 - Profitability

Obviously, profitability is a key characteristic. The better the bottom line of the practice, the higher the value (and less risk to the buyer and the lending institution).

Characteristic #8 - Potential for Additional Capacity

Practices that can add facility space and providers have more potential for growth, making them more likely to appreciate in future value, which increases their present value in the mind of the buyer and the appraiser.

Choosing the Appraisal Type and Appraiser

Formal valuations give both buyer and seller more confidence that the true value of the practice has been determined as a result of their in-depth analysis of practice characteristics and marketplace conditions. If nothing else, the substantial volume of material collected, analyzed, and calculated by a certified appraiser operating according to industry standards gives credibility to the outcome of the appraisal. For this reason, formal valuations are almost always required by lending institutions.

The appraiser chosen for the formal valuation should be a valuation professional, and preferably one who has valued a significant number of dental practices. These individuals have had substantial training and experience in business valuation and should have one or more of the following credentials:

- ASA (Accredited Senior Appraiser), sponsored by the American Society of Appraisers
- CVA (Certified Valuation Analyst), sponsored by the National Association of Valuation Analysts
- ABV (Accredited in Business Valuation), sponsored by the American Institute of Certified Public Accountants
- CBA (Certified Business Appraiser), sponsored by the Institute of Business Appraisers

I cannot stress enough the importance of choosing an appraiser or valuation firm that is working within the standards of one or more of the above organizations. Unfortunately, practice brokers will sometimes misrepresent themselves as accredited appraisers, and not disclose when they have a conflict of interest in the financial transaction.

I have also seen instances where the seller's accountant, without significant dental practice valuation experience or valuation credentials, performs an appraisal. As well-meaning as these professionals may be, their product may not be up to the standard the parties to the transaction deserve. Oftentimes, these appraisals come back much lower than the value should be.

The seller supplies the appraiser practice data from a list of requested documents which includes tax returns, profit and loss statements (P&Ls), historical production and collections reports, and payer-by-source reports, among others. The appraiser analyzes and organizes all the data and places it into a financial model that converts it into information.

Next, the appraiser works with the dentist to establish the net income from the business and applies valuation methodologies, weighing each one based on certain qualitative aspects of the business. After establishing the value, the appraiser compiles a document detailing the methodologies and academic theories used to obtain the estimated value of the practice.

In my experience, the cost of formal practice evaluations ranges from $6,000 to $30,000. At the low end of the cost range are valuations that are done remotely, meaning there is no on-site visit by the appraiser.

Traditionally, the seller pays for the appraisal. Unless there are major changes in the practice statistics, appraisals should be relevant for up to two years after they are performed. In some cases, the buyer and seller agree beforehand to split the cost of the appraisal, feeling that this should be a shared expense by both parties. This can also make the appraisal appear more independent. Occasionally, both parties may agree to a second appraisal, typically because one or both sides were expecting a significantly different appraised value. In this case, the two parties may agree that the practice value is the average of the two appraisals, with the additional appraisal paid for by both the buyer and the seller.

THE TRANSITION TEAM

A well-planned and executed transition plan is not something the practice owner should attempt on their own. Utilizing the experience and expertise of a team of professionals is more likely to result in a successful outcome. Each member of the team plays an important role in acting on the behalf of the practice owner.

The team should consist of the following:

- A practice consultant, who is knowledgeable about the practice owner's practice and able to support the owner in developing goals, refining practice systems, and providing leadership and advise through the transition process
- An attorney, who can prepare and advise the practice owner about the legal documentation required, protecting the owner's interests
- An accountant, who can advise the practice owner as to the tax consequences of transition transactions

One may ask where the *Practice Broker* fits into the transition team. A practice broker may work independently or as an agent of a transition company. These individuals usually advertise their services as all-inclusive, implying that they handle every aspect of the dental practice transition for the buyer and/or seller from start to finish, including practice valuation, search and selection, negotiations and contracts, and implementation.

My experience, and that of many others who have shared their experience, is that practice brokers may play too many roles in which they are not as fully qualified as specialists in those roles. For example, they are many times ill-experienced, often having never worked in a dental practice, or if they have, unsuccessfully, so they are not qualified to act as the practice consultant. Their lack of credentials in accounting or law makes them also unqualified to act as the accountant or the attorney. Even if they have accounting or legal professionals in their brokerage firm, there is the question of conflict of interest, when they play the role of valuator, advisor, and broker within the same transaction. Finally, unlike the transition team outlined above, the practice broker is usually paid a percentage of the transaction, much like a real estate broker. This percentage of the transaction can be multiples of what a transition team consisting of a practice consultant, attorney, and accountant would charge the practice owner while supplying a superior service.

All the members of the transition team should have significant experience in the transition of dental practices. Everyone should be on the same page regarding the best interests of the practice owner and how to plan and execute the mutually-agreed-upon and approved plan. Occasionally, there may be one member of the team that isn't qualified, or committed, or capable of working within the framework of the practice owner's approved plan, requiring replacement of that team member with someone who meets these requirements.

TRANSITION MODELS

Transitioning is about how the practice and business evolves over time to meet the objectives of the practice owner. Traditionally, that meant preparing the practice for and executing its sale. The contemporary meaning of transition incorporates not just the sale, but the changes over time that support the ultimate purpose of the business owner – to achieve lifestyle as well as financial freedom. There are different models for the transition process, all of which may accomplish this objective.

The Walk-Away Sale

In the walk-away sale, the practice owner advertises the practice, connects with the buyer, negotiates terms, completes the transaction, and retires completely from the business. This is the traditional method by which most practice owners transition from active clinical practice to retirement. In many instances, the practice owner works reduced hours leading up to the sale. This can be a desirable model for the sole owner who has properly prepared financially in advance, so that the sale of the practice assets is the final piece of the financial puzzle, allowing the practice owner to walk away after the sale confident that they can live their desired lifestyle for the rest of their life. It is also the simplest model for transitioning a practice, which usually means less effort and less likelihood that something will not go as planned.

I have already discussed financial planning, including the importance of beginning as soon as possible once becoming a practice owner. The plan requires diligence, commitment, and constant assessment and adjustments. Advisors who can assist the practice owner with profitability systems and financial planning should be engaged.

Unfortunately, this level of planning and commitment, especially in the first half of the owner's career, is uncommon. For this reason, only 6% of dentists can retire and enjoy their pre-retirement lifestyle after retirement. This, plus market conditions, has pushed back the retirement age of retiring dentists by several years and forced many to look at other transition models.

Searching for the Buyer

Advertising for a buyer is much like advertising the sale of any major asset, or, for that matter, advertising for new patients or new team members to the practice. The same principle applies to finding the right buyer - the right message, to the right people, the right number of times. As with these other examples, identifying who the right person (or right people) is should come first, as this will have a large impact on the message and the search process.

The right person could be any dentist who agrees to the purchase terms and can qualify financially, making the population of potential buyers large. However, the practice may be a specialist practice, or perform advanced procedures, or require a certain amount of experience in dentistry in order to handle the workload or team size in a walk-away sale transaction. In addition, the seller may have preferences regarding the buyer related to maintaining the quality of care to the patient base at the same level or higher.

The right way to advertise for the buyer often depends on the seller's sense of urgency. I'll break down the search into three different levels. If the urgency is less, the seller may want to spend less on the search process in the beginning, spending more only if they don't get a response within a certain period of time. The seller who wants or needs to make the transaction faster will be willing to spend more as a tradeoff for reaching more people in less time to generate more buyer leads.

Advertising for Associate and Partner Dentists by Different Levels of Cost, Reach, and Time to Results

Level One	Level Two	Level Three
Least Cost Least Reach Greater Time	More Cost More Reach Less Time	Most Cost Most Reach Least Time
Dental Educational Institutions Local Dental Suppliers Local Dental Laboratories Local Colleagues	Dental Trade Journals Online Search Sites	Headhunter Services

Level 1 is all about getting the word out to the local market. There is no cost involved, but this type of advertising may take a long time to bring results. It involves notifying nearby dental educational institutions, local dental suppliers, laboratories, and, if the seller is comfortable with the idea, local colleagues.

If the seller is inclined to offer the purchase opportunity to a less experienced dentist, then contacting dental schools, general practice residency programs and, if applicable, specialist residencies within the state and adjacent states, may generate good quality applicants. Most, if not all, of these institutions have a contact person or department that deals with such offers and may even assist with placement of its graduates. If the seller knows such an individual, or at least can reach out with a personal phone call to the individual, they can describe the opportunity and the type of individual they are seeking. The next best thing is to send a letter describing the opportunity, addressed to a specific person, marked Personal & Confidential. The letter should be followed up by a phone call.

Example of Dental Institution Letter:

Dear <Name of Individual>,

I am writing to inform you of an associate opportunity with our general dentistry practice that may be of interest to one or more of your general practice residents.

There is an immediate opening available of <number> days a week for an associate in our busy, progressive general dental practice. Our office is located in <city and description of location>. The practice has enjoyed significant growth in terms of production in each of its <number of years> years of existence. Our business enjoys a high collections percentage and low accounts receivable, and is not affiliated with any form of managed care. There is a very healthy influx of new patients every month, most of which are referred from the existing patient base. However, the practice does market extensively its unique services. There is currently a staff of <#> well-trained, experienced employees in a modern, <number> operatory, <#>-square-foot facility. Our practice performs every discipline of dentistry with an emphasis on <description of services>.

The associate dental practitioner compensation/benefits package would include a generous paid commission on collections from production, continuing education, insurance, all supplies and equipment, as well as the support of a talented team. The opportunity to become a partner is available to the right individual(s).

We are looking for an individual who is hard-working, ambitious, clinically competent, and people oriented. Should this description fit an individual or individuals whom you are familiar with, please forward to them this opportunity. We would very much like to meet and discuss this wonderful career opportunity.

Please feel free to contact me with any questions or recommendations. Thank you for your time and consideration,

<Practice Owner Name>

<Practice Owner Signature>

Local dental suppliers and laboratories may know dentists in the area who want to purchase a practice or someone who is considering relocating to the area. Even if they don't, these individuals are now aware and become referral sources should they hear of someone who may be interested in purchasing a practice.

Level 2 advertising for a buyer utilizes advertising that involves some cost but reaches beyond the local market. It employs local, state, and national dental trade journals and online employee search sites such as DentalCareerNetwork.com, MyDentalJobs.com, DentalPost.net, and DentalGrind.com, among others. This level allows practice owners to post advertisements locally, regionally, and nationwide for buyers searching for opportunities that match desired characteristics such as location and practice type.

Level 3 advertising uses headhunter services. These organizations have a team dedicated to advertising for and matching potential sellers and buyers. They tend to have a nationwide reach and use questionnaires and interviews to determine key characteristics for the best match between seller and buyer. They have a vested interest in the success of the transaction because they are partially or wholly compensated when the deal is consummated. They may charge a flat fee when the contract is signed to retain their services, or they may charge a percentage of the purchase price when the deal is made, or a combination of fee and percentage. Fees and percentages vary widely. Examples of headhunter organizations include ADA Practice Transitions, ETS Dental, and Dentistheadhunter.com, among others.

The right advertising message communicates what makes the practice attractive – what sets it apart from other opportunities. In other words, the right advertising message communicates the practice's unique selling point. This is where a lot of sellers miss opportunities. The typical ad in a dental trade journal goes something like this:

Dental Practice for Sale Trenton. Grosses $1,000,000 in four ops. Great location, equipment in good condition.

It's as if the practice owner is trying to use as few words as possible to save costs. And there will be five or six others almost identical to that ad. Now consider the same practice being advertised for sale:

Dental Practice for Sale Trenton. Tremendous opportunity for the right buyer! Highly profitable practice located in a growing area with high visibility. Wonderful facility with modern equipment and technology, along with an amazing team that works well together and wants to stay after the sale supporting the new practice owner, while continuing to provide superior care to a high-quality patient base.

Which practice are you more interested in considering for purchase? I ask my clients advertising for a buyer (or an associate) to go further in creating a compelling message in the form of a marketing piece that is sure to get more attention. I request they come up with five to ten bullet points that describe what makes their practice such a great opportunity for purchase (or to associate with). It is important that the practice owner participates in this process, as the owner will end up having to use these points to close the deal. Those unique selling points are put into paragraph form, with some images and graphic artwork to create a compelling marketing piece.

Example of an Associate/Partner Brochure (courtesy of Dr. Jim Sparaga)

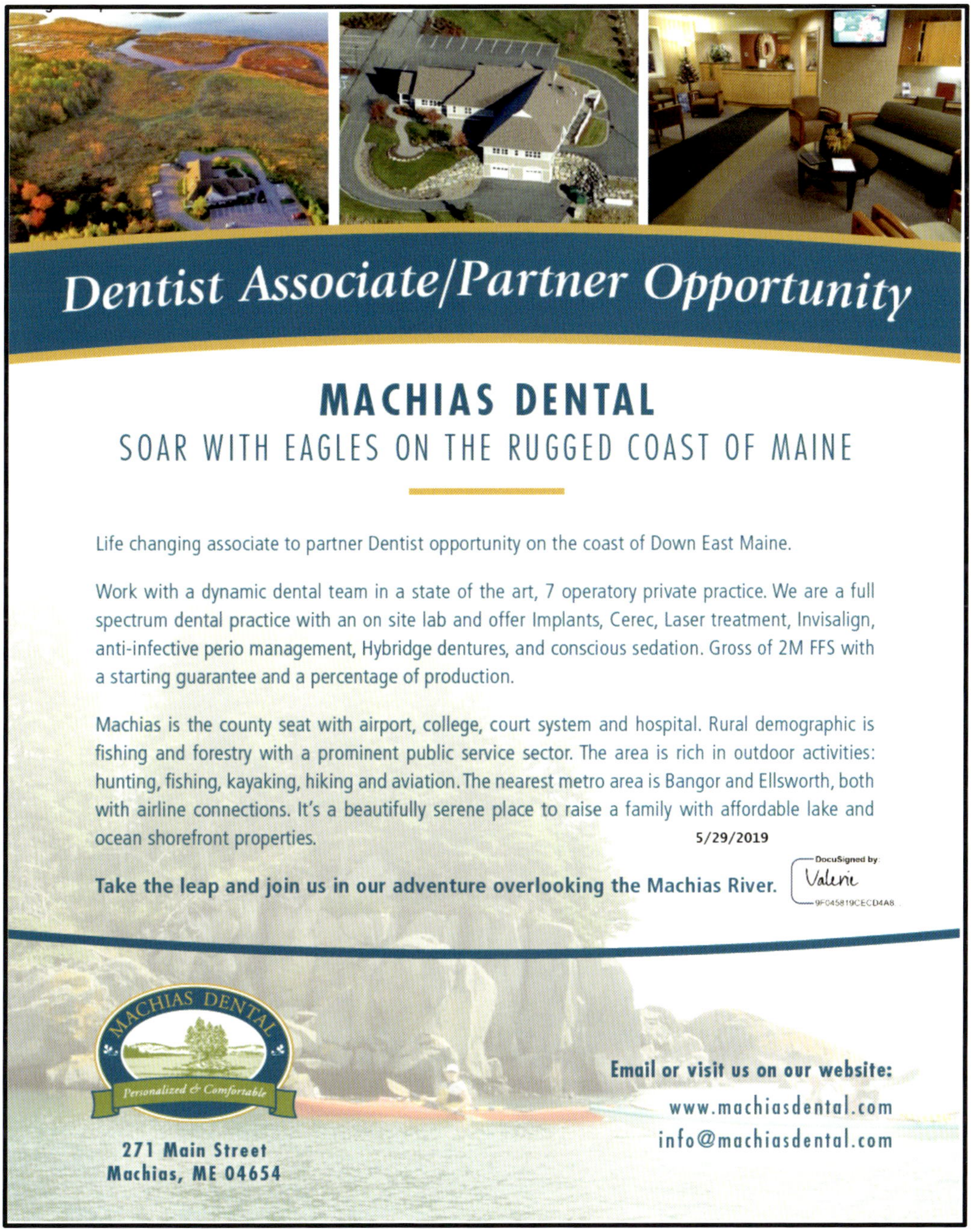
Dentist Associate/Partner Opportunity
MACHIAS DENTAL
SOAR WITH EAGLES ON THE RUGGED COAST OF MAINE
Life changing associate to partner Dentist opportunity on the coast of Down East Maine.
Work with a dynamic dental team in a state of the art, 7 operatory private practice. We are a full spectrum dental practice with an on site lab and offer Implants, Cerec, Laser treatment, Invisalign, anti-infective perio management, Hybridge dentures, and conscious sedation. Gross of 2M FFS with a starting guarantee and a percentage of production.
Machias is the county seat with airport, college, court system and hospital. Rural demographic is fishing and forestry with a prominent public service sector. The area is rich in outdoor activities: hunting, fishing, kayaking, hiking and aviation. The nearest metro area is Bangor and Ellsworth, both with airline connections. It's a beautifully serene place to raise a family with affordable lake and ocean shorefront properties.
5/29/2019
DocuSigned by:
Valerie
Take the leap and join us in our adventure overlooking the Machias River.
MACHIAS DENTAL
Personalized & Comfortable
271 Main Street
Machias, ME 04654
Email or visit us on our website:
www.machiasdental.com
info@machiasdental.com

Once potential buyers contact the practice owner, the main determinant as to who to sell to in a walk-away sale comes down to who makes the best offer, with the goal to sell for the asking price, usually the practice valuation. When a prospective buyer wants to negotiate a lower price, the seller must determine if they can accept the reduced price or not. The funds from the sale may be critically important to the seller's retirement plan.

There are other parts to the sale that can be negotiated that may allow the seller to sell for the desired price. For instance, the seller may offer to work for three to twelve months to help transition the practice to the new owner, seeing patients and transferring trust from the patient base to the new owner. In addition, the seller may offer to finance the sale, and offer attractive terms to the buyer.

Execution of the sale involves the entire transition team: the practice consultant to advise on terms, the accountant to run financial scenarios and address tax implications, and the attorney to draw up the buy-sell agreement. All members of the transition team, together with the seller, need to work together to create the sales agreement that best reflects the seller's interests.

Sale to an Existing Associate Dentist

As opposed to the walk-away sale, selling to an existing associate involves more advanced planning, preparation, and time to search for, select, and mentor a dentist in the practice who, if appropriate, is offered an opportunity to purchase part or all of the practice. In contrast to the outright sale to a buyer, the practice owner grooms the associate for their eventual purchase and successful transition to owner and supports them in building a loyal following among the patient base. The advantage of this transition method compared to a walk-away sale is that the practice owner acquires all the benefits of having another dentist in the practice, such as:

1. Additional production, collections, and profitability
   a. increased capacity for the doctor schedule
   b. the ability to add and support additional hygienists
   c. keeping the office open when the practice owner is away
   d. extended office hours
   e. more productive schedule for the practice owner (the owner performs more productive procedures while the associate performs procedures the practice owner prefers not to perform)
2. Option for the practice owner to work fewer days
3. Higher practice value than a sole practitioner office
4. Second set of eyes and hands to consult with on selected cases
5. Potential built-in transition strategy

The number-one reason to have an associate is to increase cash flow to the practice. The prosperous practice owner should continually review practice statistics to ensure the owner-associate relationship is a profitable one for both parties.

Prior to the sale to an associate, the practice should have a successful practice owner-associate working relationship of one to five years. The definition of a successful working relationship is when the associate meets the expectations of the practice owner, and the practice owner meets those of the associate. From the perspective of the practice owner, these expectations usually involve quality of dentistry and productivity, as well as interactions with team, patients, and the practice owner, among others. From the perspective of the associate, these expectations usually center on compensation, autonomy, work environment, and the relationship with the practice owner.

In my decades of experience, I have found the success of the practice owner-associate working relationship to be abysmally low – around 20 percent or one in five. The reasons for this are twofold:

One, even the best arrangements for the associate pale in comparison to that of an owner. The associate, even if well compensated, is taxed as an employee, unlike the owner who can deduct practice expenses. In addition, the associate often has less autonomy regarding how they practice, what procedures they do, and their office hours compared to that of a practice owner. Also, the associate doesn't have the built-in job security that an owner has. Finally, and arguably the most meaningful, is that the associate is not building any equity as they work. In fact, they are building equity for the practice owner. For these reasons, many associates leave the practice they are working in to pursue a practice ownership opportunity for themselves.

The second reason most practice owner-associate relationships fail is that the practice owner chooses the wrong person for the associate position, or the associate chooses the wrong practice owner to work with.

The Six Steps to Hiring the Right Associate Dentist

I developed this process many years ago. It is an orderly, logical sequence of steps designed to assist the practice owner through the exercise of associate selection from initial screening to drawing up the contractual agreement.

The Six Steps to Hiring the Right Associate Dentist	
The Search	**1. Discovery** a. Envisioning Who the Associate Is b. The Seven Boxes c. Associate Financial Analysis **2. Advertising**
The Selection Process	**3. Review of Resume & Initial Phone Interview** **4. On-Site Visit** a. In-Office Observation by Associate Candidate b. Candidate/Owner Meeting c. Owner/Team Assessment Meeting d. Social Visit - Family Assessment **5. Personality Testing**
The Agreement	**6. Negotiations & Contractual Agreement**

The Search

Step 1: Discovery

The search for the right associate starts with the practice owner determining who the right associate is. By determining as specifically as possible the characteristics this individual should possess, the owner can better advertise, as well as recognize the right associate when that person appears.

For instance, is this person someone young and just out of school or someone with a certain number of years of experience? Is there a minimum requirement of a residency or other post-doctoral education degree? Will they be a full or part-time associate? Will they have a local background? Will they have certain skill sets? These are all questions the practice owner must determine according to individual preference. However, from the perspective of the owner, there are certain characteristics (or "boxes") the associate needs to possess in order to assure the most successful outcome. Therefore, *they are not optional*. I call these *"The Seven Boxes."*

THE SEVEN BOXES

Seven Essential Requirements for Associate Selection

1. They have outstanding production potential. They care less about what they want to do, and more about being really productive.
2. They are ambitious. They want to do big things and be a part of something big.
3. They are hungry. They are willing to work hard.
4. They understand that future growth and success in the business is a ladder. (They start at the bottom step, pay their dues, then they get to take the next step.)
5. They are a great dentist, or at least a good dentist on their way to becoming great.
6. They have good communication skills. They are likeable and well spoken, and they listen as well as they speak.
7. They see the world the way the practice owner sees it (share core values).

THE KEY CONCEPT

The Key Concept of Like Likes Like – In high school chemistry class we all learned this concept: Chemicals with a similar structure when mixed together form a solution. The same applies when choosing people to work with. Choose those individuals who mix well with you – those who, in the most important ways, see the world as you do.

The associate candidate must check off all seven boxes. Remember, this person will be treating the patients from the practice, and the practice name will be associated with them. They may even enter into a business marriage with the practice owner. As such, the practice owner must choose wisely, without compromise.

In addition to determining who they want and what qualities a candidate possesses, the practice owner also needs to discover the financial impact of bringing in an associate, and what they can afford to pay them. This requires a financial analysis that calculates the net take-home income before taxes for both the practice owner and the associate based on days worked, percentage of collections paid to the associate, practice overhead, and collection rate. Examples of the *Senior Doctor* (practice owner) *Net* and *Associate Net Take-Home Income Before Taxes* spreadsheets can be found in the Glossary.

You can pay associates two basic ways – fixed rate (salary or per diem) or commission. For less financial risk for the practice owner, as well as more motivation on the part of the associate to produce more, commission wins out. Still, most associate arrangements allow for a per diem payment for the initial period (six to twelve months) of the associate's tenure in the practice, especially when the associate is filling a new associate position. This allows the associate to be paid enough to cover living and lifestyle expenses while building their schedule. To further incentivize the associate, you can pay the per diem rate or the agreed upon commission percentage of collections, whichever is greater.

Commission should be based on a percentage of collections from dentistry produced by the associate. When commission is based on *production*, adjustments off that production can negatively impact the practice owner who will have to pay the associate on production that cannot be collected.

For years, the practices I have coached have relied on *Senior Doctor Net* and *Associate Doctor Net Take-Home Income Before Taxes* spreadsheets as the primary determinant of the percentage of collections off production to pay associates. To use these spreadsheets, the practice owner decides on a reasonable amount of production per day that the associate should be producing at the point their compensation becomes commission based (usually six to twelve months after starting). The ideal point for the compensation percentage paid to the associate is when the senior doctor takes home one dollar for every dollar the associate takes home.

The *Net Take Home Income* spreadsheet analysis provides a useful, quantifiable method to determine what the practice can afford to pay an associate. However, other factors need to be taken into consideration when determining associate compensation. These include market standards, practice overhead, supply and demand, and sense of urgency on the part of the practice owner.

Market standards for associate compensation vary from time to time, and by area, although not by more than a few percentage points. The national average range is between twenty-eight and thirty-five percent of collections from associate production. At the higher part of the range, the associate usually has more experience and ability, plus a track record of being productive. They may also be asked to pay for more of their practice or professional expenses.

A lack of supply and a higher demand for available associates may require a higher percentage of compensation. There are parts of the country where the pool of potential quality associate candidates is small. Whenever competition for (demand) and the sense of urgency is high, compensation rates will also increase.

To soften or reduce the financial risk to the practice owner, a couple of alternative methods can be attached to the higher compensation rate. One way is to have the associate pay the same percentage of the lab fees related to their production as they are paid on their collections from their production. In other words, if they are paid thirty-five percent of collections from their production, they pay thirty-five percent of their lab bill.

Another way is to pay a lower percentage of collections from their production until they reach a certain production level, then pay at a higher percentage. For example, the associate could be paid at thirty-two percent of collections until their monthly production reaches $75,000/month, at which point they could receive thirty-five percent. The combinations are nearly endless, and consultation with a consultant, coach, mentor, or other advisor can be helpful in arriving at the right combination.

There are other advantages of having an associate dentist that can factor into the compensation paid to the associate. Even if the practice owner just breaks even on what they pay the associate, the benefits to the practice owner of adding capacity, keeping the office open when the practice owner is away, enabling a better practice schedule for the owner, increased equity value, and a potential transition strategy all make adding an associate advantageous for the practice owner.

Step 2: Advertising

Now that the practice owner knows who they want and the terms they can offer, they are ready to get the word out. Advertising for the associate uses the same elements as advertising for the potential buyer. This includes all three levels of advertising previously mentioned, as well as creating the advertising message and marketing brochure.

Here's an example of advertisement copy for an associate:

> **Seeking Full-Time Associate Dentist** for large, patient-centered, progressive practice with opportunity for future partnership. Excellent position for young dentist desiring to be mentored by experienced owner of a growing, successful practice, with a generous compensation package with incentives for above-average production. Looking for someone with good communication skills who is a great dentist, or a good dentist on their way to becoming a great dentist. Visit our website at <your practice website>, watch our vision video, and read our patient testimonials. If you're passionate about what we're passionate about, then send a resume to <your practice email address>.

The Selection Process

Step 3: Review of Resume & Initial Phone Interview

If an individual's resume fits the characteristics the practice owner seeks, then an initial phone screening is arranged. During this conversation, the practice owner should be familiar with the applicant's resume and have interview questions prepared in advance that help in determining if further consideration is warranted for this individual.

During the interview, the practice owner should talk less and listen more. Telling the applicant what they are looking for or describing the opportunity before the applicant speaks may taint the applicant's responses.

Interview Questions

The information the practice owner needs from an associate candidate can be categorized into four areas: Personality, Vision, Culture, and Skills. The best candidate will be a close match in all four of these areas.

INITIAL PHONE INTERVIEW FOR ASSOCIATE CANDIDATE

Personality - The first screening questions should address how this person thinks. If the practice owner is going to work in the trenches side by side with someone, sharing patients and staff, without having to explain and justify their decisions, they need someone who sees the world similarly to them. They don't have to be close friends with this individual, but they do need to enjoy each other's company. High school chemistry taught us that "like likes like." If they are oil, don't try to mix with your water. The practice owner needs an associate that will make their life better, not one that will be a thorn in their side. Questions like these will help you assess an applicant's personality:

1. What does an ideal day in a dental practice look like to you?
2. Have you taken any personality tests in the past? If so, what did you learn about yourself?
3. If you had to rate the following four items in terms of what matters the most to you, how would you rate these four things on the order of 1 through 4?
    1. Reaching professional goals
    2. Having fun
    3. Building relationships with people
    4. Being the most skilled and knowledgeable dentist you can be

The third question places the individual in one of the four personality types of the DISC Personality Profile.

Vision - Aside from questions that uncover the candidate's basic personality traits, the practice owner is looking for someone who will help them fulfill their vision. Is this person to be only an associate or an associate with future partnership potential?

4. Where do you see yourself in 1 year, 5 years, or 10 years?
5. What would you do to build this practice?
6. What is your definition of success in dentistry?

Culture - The next set of questions should address how this person is likely to fit into the unique culture and environment of the practice's location.

7. What do you like to do when you're not working?
8. What type of local environment do you and your spouse (if applicable) like best, and why?

Skills - Finally, the practice owner needs to determine if the applicant has the skills and aptitude to meet the needs of the practice.

9. What are your favorite dental procedures to perform?
10. What type of continuing education have you had? Or, if a recent graduate, what were your favorite procedures in school?
11. Are you open to learning and performing procedures that you have not had much experience or interest in before now?
12. What procedures, if any, are a definite "no" when it comes to dentistry?
13. On a scale of 1 to 10, how would you rate your current proficiency in restorative, prosthetic, endodontic, cosmetic, and surgical areas of dentistry?

This interview will help determine if the practice owner likes the individual. There's no use moving forward unless the practice owner and associate candidate can click. This is a hard concept to describe, but in the process of asking them questions about their background, the practice owner will formulate an impression of this person regarding their personality, their likes and dislikes, their confidence, their energy level, and their enthusiasm. If at any time during this meeting the practice owner feels that this is not the right person, then end the meeting by thanking the applicant for their time, explaining that you are looking for someone with different qualifications, and wishing them good luck.

If the practice owner likes the person they're talking with after this initial phone interview, the owner should tell the person about themselves and their practice, answering the same questions they just asked of the associate candidate. Questions about compensation should not be addressed at this point. The applicant should get an overall view of the screening process as outlined here, and should be assured that all questions will be answered in time and in the right order. The practice owner should end the meeting by asking the associate candidate if this sounds like the kind of situation they're looking for, and if they are interested in further pursuing this opportunity. If both parties agree, an on-site visit to the practice should be arranged.

Step 4: On-Site Visit

A date for an on-site visit by the associate candidate should be chosen at the earliest time available that is suitable for both associate candidate and practice owner. It serves no purpose to wait longer than necessary, since waiting makes the meeting less likely to result in a successful outcome and wastes time.

The associate should plan a visit of one to three days – one if they are local or within a reasonable driving distance away. This visit includes visiting and observing the practice for at least a half day, a professional meeting with the practice owner, and a social meeting (dinner for example including spouses/significant others if applicable). A second day would be needed if the associate candidate is not from the area of the practice and needs to fly in. In this case, a third day would be reserved for exploring the area and its attractions.

Who should cover expenses of the on-site visit, including travel, lodging, and meals? That depends on the circumstances surrounding the associate search. If you are evaluating multiple candidates who have reached Step 4, and/or they are local or within driving distance, then the candidate should pay all expenses except for meals with the practice owner. If the candidate needs to fly in from a distant location to the meeting, then the practice owner should pay for travel and/or lodging.

The office visit should include the office morning meeting. The team should be briefed ahead of time with basic information about the individual, and instructed on their role in the visit. Their role is to be available to answer questions from the candidate and learn something about the candidate so that they can contribute their thoughts on them after the visit. The associate candidate should spend time shadowing the practice owner and other providers, visiting with team members, and observing the facility and general flow of patient care. No financial or other practice data should be shared at this time.

After the site visit, the associate candidate and practice owner should meet for a couple of hours. During this meeting the associate should share their impressions of their observations of the practice and be allowed to ask any questions about the practice, as well as the employment opportunity itself. The practice owner should be prepared to address questions about the number of days/week the associate will be required to work, the hours/days, types of treatment the associate will perform, and other responsibilities. The practice owner should have a job description for the associate candidate. The Associate Job Description can be found in the Glossary.

The topic of compensation or practice statistics may come up in this conversation. It is best that specifics regarding compensation be addressed in Step 6 (Negotiations & Contractual Agreement). The practice owner should not be seen as avoiding this question, so should respond by saying that specifics regarding compensation are in large part based on the outcome of the candidate review procedure, which is still incomplete, but that the compensation will include an initial per diem rate, followed by a commission-based payment structure. The amount of commission will be based on a practice financial analysis, candidate experience and qualifications, and industry standards.

At some point soon after the associate candidate visit, the practice owner should meet with the practice's team members (or core group of team leaders, if applicable) to solicit their input regarding the candidate. Team members can provide a unique perspective which the practice owner often does not have. If nothing else, inviting them to give input gives them the sense that their opinions are valued, and that they have some say as to the new dentist they will end up working with. General, open-ended questions are best: "Was there anything you heard, saw, or noticed about the candidate that left an impression on you, favorable or otherwise?" Or, "During your interaction with the candidate, what is your opinion as to whether he/she would be a good fit for our practice?"

During the on-site visit of the associate candidate, a dinner should be planned at a restaurant or other dining establishment outside the practice owner's home that includes the practice owner and their significant other, as well as the associate and their significant other, if applicable. No one else should be invited to this dinner, which should be social in nature. In other words, this is not an interview, but a get-together of couples (if applicable) who want to get to know each other better. Explore and share information about family, outside interests, and favorite vacation destinations, for example. The practice owner can discuss the local area of the practice if the associate candidate is not familiar. While addressing practice questions is not off limits, the idea is to assess who this candidate is as a person, not just as a dentist.

One of the lessons I learned early in my consulting career was that my client was not only the practice owner who hired me, but also the practice owner's *family*. In other words, I was hired to fulfill the needs of a practice, but also to fulfill a *personal vision* that involved the partnership between a practice owner and their significant other. In the majority of cases, the significant other was essential to the decision to hire me and was a big part of the coaching relationship. I came to see this as not only necessary, but preferable. Most practice owners need the perspective, wisdom, and support that their life partner offers. After all, who knows the practice owner better than their significant other? Since it is essential that the practice owner and associate (possibly a partner-to-be) have key characteristics in common (core values, the way they see the world, etc.), the significant other's input is as valuable to the selection process as any other factor.

After the social dinner, the practice owner should ask for the unbiased opinion of their significant other: "Based on what I've shared with you, as well as what you observed during our dinner with the candidate, do you believe we are a good match, and why or why not?"

If the associate candidate has successfully passed steps 3 and 4, then they are ready for the next step, a personality profile test that will offer a deeper understanding of who they are and how that matches who the practice owner is.

Step 5: Personality Testing

Earlier in the chapters on The Team (Team Selection) and The Systems (Production Systems, Team Quality), I discussed personality tests that determine how an individual (team member or potential team member) sees the world, and cognitive ability tests to determine mental ability. The *Caliper Personality Profile* is a test that accomplishes both, and I have found that it is the best assessment of an individual who is going to be highly compensated and accountable for major responsibilities within the practice. It provides insight into individuals' motivators, behaviors, and personalities by way of 22 personal attributes. The test consists of more than 100 questions in five sections and includes an abstract reasoning component. It takes between 75 and 90 minutes to complete and is not timed.

The Caliper Personality Profile is not inexpensive to take, and since the practice owner will be paying for it (plus their own if they've never taken one before), then it must be determined that the associate candidate is serious about the available opportunity. It should be explained to the associate that the test is used to gain more information about them and how well suited they are to succeed as an associate in the practice. The practice owner should not use the phrase, "how well you match with me," as this may influence the associate to answer questions through what they believe to be the eyes of the practice owner. The practice owner can share with the associate that the test measures leadership, persuasiveness, problem solving, decision-making, interpersonal and service orientation, and personal organization and time management abilities.

The results are formulated by the Caliper organization into a report that includes a quantitative analysis with metrics for each trait measured and a written analysis and overall recommendation of the candidate's suitability for the position. In addition, Caliper provides a follow-up phone conversation with an analyst to explain the results as well as their recommendation.

I've found that while the report's recommendation and follow-up phone call with the analyst are helpful, a side-by-side comparison of the practice owner's and the associate candidate's numbers for each attribute via a spreadsheet is extremely revealing and useful. The *Caliper Profile Comparison Spreadsheet* has columns for percentage differences in the attributes and comments from the evaluator. I've learned that, as both a coach to the client (knowing them better than the analyst does) and as a dentist myself (knowing what's required of the role in question), my assessment of the results of the test for the practice owner-client is beneficial.

Comparison of Caliper Personality Profiles for Practice Owner and Potential Associate Dentists

Characteristic	Practice Owner	Associate Candidate #1	% Point Difference	Associate Candidate #2	% Point Differnece
Leadership:					
Assertiveness	76	2	74%	83	-7%
Aggressiveness	54	16	38%	88	-34%
Ego-Drive	84	25	59%	66	18%
Empathy	68	68	0%	20	48%
Ego-Strength/Resilience	26	1	25%	94	-68%
Risk Taking	99	7	92%	73	26%
Urgency	85	47	38%	85	0%
Cautiousness	5	38	-33%	1	4%
Openness	16	68	-52%	19	-3%
Interpersonal:					
Empathy	68	68	0%	20	48%
Sociability	26	1	25%	60	-34%
Gregariousness	52	6	46%	52	0%
Accommodation	24	90	-66%	43	-19%
Skepticism	48	48	0%	65	-17%
Ego-Strength	26	1	25%	94	-68%
Problem Solving/Decision Making:					
Abstract Reasoning	52	52	0%	63	0%
Idea Orientation	77	12	65%	77	0%
Thoroughness	12	12	0%	9	3%
Flexibility	42	25	17%	33	9%
Cautiousness	5	38	-33%	1	4%
Risk Taking	99	7	92%	73	26%
Urgency	85	47	38%	85	0%
Level-Headedness	41	16	25%	94	-53%
Personal Organization/Time Management:					
Self-Structure	20	31	-11%	65	-45%
External Structure	5	26	-21%	36	-31%
Urgency	85	47	38%	85	0%
Thoroughness	12	12	0%	9	3%
Risk Taking	99	7	92%	73	26%
Cautiousness	5	38	-33%	1	4%
Energy	60	1	59%	60	0%
Comments:		This is a poor match for a partner, and a border-line match for an associate. Candidate lacks the assertiveness to be an effective leader, and the confidence, sociability and energy to be a highly productive dentist. His low ego strength means that he would not respond positively to constructive appraisal. The results of the Caliper were further demonstrated in the phone interview. Candidate wants the benefits of ownership, with the limited demands of being an employee dentist.		This an excellent match on characteristics for both an associate and partner. I see some conflict from being so alike but the conflict will be tolerated well by Candidate as long as there is a common vision and both doctors are clear on the future path of Candidate. Candidate is not someone who will tolerate being an employee dentist for a long time.	

The comparison groups and color-codes the differences between the practice owner and associate candidate into three sections: Similarities (differences of 33% or less, and shaded green), Differences (differences of between 34 and 66%, and shaded yellow), and Major Differences (differences greater than 66%, and shaded red).

One might assume that the green shaded areas, the more alike the two individuals are, would generally be the most desirable. However, if one were to assume this is always good, that assumption would be incorrect. It depends on the attribute in question. If the difference reflects the associate being strong in an attribute the practice owner is weak in (yellow or red), then this major difference may be good. Likewise, if both practice owner and associate are similar in their weakness in an attribute (green), then this may not be good. If the associate is weak in a category compared to a practice owner by a major difference (red), this could be a source of major conflict. Over the years I've been able to reliably predict the outcome of the associate/practice owner working relationship using the *Caliper Profile Comparison Spreadsheet*.

Once the tests are taken, the report is in hand, and the *Caliper Profile Comparison Spreadsheet* has been prepared and reviewed by the coach with the practice owner, it can be determined if the associate candidate is a prospect or a suspect. The practice owner should contact the associate candidate to review the results of the profile and, if applicable, initiate Step 6. The test is the property of the practice owner who paid for it, and it should not be sent to the associate candidate.

The Agreement

Step 6: Negotiations & Contractual Agreement

If the associate candidate has passed steps 3, 4, and 5 in the selection process, then the practice owner should initiate the discussion of working relationship terms. Sharing practice statistics at this time is appropriate after the associate candidate has signed a Non-Disclosure Agreement (NDA).

NON-DISCLOSURE AGREEMENT

THIS AGREEMENT is made and entered into as of <Insert date> ("Effective Date"), by and between <Insert Practice Name> ("the Disclosing Party") and <Insert Associate Name> ("the Recipient") (collectively, "the Parties").

Purpose for Disclosure ("Business Purpose") <Insert Purpose – for example "Evaluation of Dentist Associate Working Relationship">:

The Parties hereby agree as follows:

1. For purposes of this Agreement, "Confidential Information" shall mean any and all non-public information, including, without limitation, technical, developmental, marketing, sales, operating, performance, cost, know-how, business plans, business methods, and process information, disclosed to the Recipient. For convenience, the Disclosing Party may, but is not required to, mark written Confidential Information with the legend "Confidential" or an equivalent designation.
2. All Confidential Information disclosed to the Recipient will be used solely for the Business Purpose and for no other purpose whatsoever. The Recipient agrees to keep the Disclosing Party's Confidential Information confidential and to protect the confidentiality of such Confidential Information with the same degree of care with which it protects the confidentiality of its own confidential information, but in no event with less than a reasonable degree of care. Recipient may disclose Confidential Information only to its employees, agents, consultants and contractors on a need-to-know basis, and only if such employees, agents, consultants and contractors have executed appropriate written agreements with Recipient sufficient to enable Recipient to enforce all the provisions of this Agreement.

- cont'd

NON-DISCLOSURE AGREEMENT – cont'd

Recipient shall not make any copies of Disclosing Party's Confidential Information except as needed for the Business Purpose. At the request of Disclosing Party, Recipient shall return to Disclosing Party all Confidential Information of Disclosing Party (including any copies thereof) or certify the destruction thereof.

3. All right, title and interest in and to the Confidential Information shall remain with Disclosing Party or its licensors. Nothing in this Agreement is intended to grant any rights to Recipient under any patents, copyrights, trademarks, or trade secrets of Disclosing Party. ALL CONFIDENTIAL INFORMATION IS PROVIDED "AS IS." THE DISCLOSING PARTY MAKES NO WARRANTIES, EXPRESS, IMPLIED OR OTHERWISE, REGARDING NON-INFRINGEMENT OF THIRD PARTY RIGHTS OR ITS ACCURACY, COMPLETENESS OR PERFORMANCE.
4. The obligations and limitations set forth herein regarding Confidential Information shall not apply to information which is: (a) at any time in the public domain, other than by a breach on the part of the Recipient; or (b) at any time rightfully received from a third party which had the right to and transmits it to the Recipient without any obligation of confidentiality.
5. In the event that the Recipient shall breach this Agreement, or in the event that a breach appears to be imminent, the Disclosing Party shall be entitled to all legal and equitable remedies afforded it by law, and in addition may recover all reasonable costs and attorneys' fees incurred in seeking such remedies. If the Confidential Information is sought by any third party, including by way of subpoena or other court process, the Recipient shall inform the Disclosing Party of the request in sufficient time to permit the Disclosing Party to object to and, if necessary, seek court intervention to prevent the disclosure.
6. The validity, construction and enforceability of this Agreement shall be governed in all respects by the laws of the state of <Insert State>. This Agreement may not be amended except in writing signed by a duly authorized representative of the respective Parties. This Agreement shall control in the event of a conflict with any other agreement between the Parties with respect to the subject matter hereof.

IN WITNESS WHEREOF, the Parties have executed this Agreement as of the date first above written.

______________________________, on behalf of Disclosing Party

______________________________, on behalf of Recipient

Before the terms of the contractual arrangement for the associate are discussed, the practice owner should consult his/her transition team of advisors. This team will review the most important elements of the associate contract. I have participated in literally hundreds of associate contractual exercises, and all "good" contracts, on behalf of both parties, include the following terms (or close variants of):

1. **Employment And Term** – This includes the beginning date of employment, which will also be the date of renewability for successive annual terms, unless either party gives written notice (usually thirty to sixty days) of intention not to renew.
2. **Exclusivity of Professional Duties to the Practice** – It is best that the associate *works only for the practice owner's practice.* This means the associate is committed to the practice, is less likely to leave for an opportunity in another practice where they are also employed, and is less likely to share proprietary information with potential competitors. However, if the associate is employed only part-time by the practice, then the practice owner needs to accept that the associate may need to work an accumulated full-time week to meet their personal needs.
3. **Business Hours** – These are the normal work hours of the associate. Additional or altered work hours may be required for completion of patient care, and in the interest of the practice and business. Such exceptions are expected to be uncommon.
4. **Compensation** – This is based on the percentage of adjusted collections (net collections after refunds or other write-offs) from dentistry produced by associate. This amount has been predetermined based on the Associate Compensation Analysis and in consultation with the practice owner's transition advisory team. As has already been discussed, it is common and acceptable for associate contracts to have a guaranteed per diem rate for the first six to twelve months.
   It also needs to be determined what the professional duties of the associate entails. For example, will the associate be compensated for performing hygiene exams? What about x-rays or other treatment performed by auxiliaries (whose wages are paid for by the practice)? In most cases, the associate is compensated for these services if they perform the hygiene check and if the patient whose treatment is performed by the auxiliary is scheduled in the associate's column.
5. **Items To Be Provided By Owner** – These usually include malpractice liability insurance coverage to the same amount as the practice owner, clinic attire, *unpaid* vacation (usually the equivalent of two to three weeks days annually), *unpaid* sick days and holidays (because the associate is a commissioned employee), instrumentation and equipment, staff support, supplies, continuing education budget and terms, and health insurance to the same extent offered to other team members.
6. **Allocation And Scheduling of Patients** – Patients are allocated at the discretion and direction of the practice owner. This will be based on patient care needs, the ability of the associate to address those needs, and the needs of the practice and business.
7. **Termination Without Notice** – This refers to unlikely occurrences such as license revocation, unprofessional conduct, failure to follow directions, failure to follow provisions of the contract, conduct harmful to the practice, failure to work harmoniously with staff or patients, willful breach of contract terms, or conviction of felony or serious misdemeanor.

8. **Emergency Services** – Coverage for after-hour emergency care is scheduled in advance and is at the discretion of the practice owner, who will take into consideration the associate's availability.
9. **Records** – All patient records are the property of the practice. The associate is expected to thoroughly and conscientiously keep records of patients they treat up to date.
10. **Retreatment** – Any patients who the associate treats, and who at the discretion of the practice owner must be retreated, may be retreated by the associate or another practitioner (including the practice owner). If the associate retreats the case, it will be performed at no additional compensation to the associate. If someone else performs the retreatment, it will be at the expense of the associate.
11. **Covenant Not to Compete** – It is essential that the practice owner protects himself or herself from creating a future competitor through the significant investment in resources (time, money, knowledge, proprietary practice information, and mentoring) that occurs when an associate is hired. This covenant has two elements – time and distance. Time refers to the number of years after the associate leaves, and distance to the number of miles away the associate is restricted in practicing during that time period. Of the two, time is more important than distance from the office. A typical contract states two to three years of time, and a distance of ten to twenty miles. The covenant also covers solicitation of employees and patients.

There are usually some negotiations regarding the terms outlined above; the practice owner should enter the discussion of terms prepared for this. The impact on both the practice and the business should determine which items are negotiable and to what extent. The quality of the applicant and the urgency of need should also be considered. It should be kept in mind that the end goal in the negotiations with the associate is not to win, as winning means that someone lost; ultimately the best negotiations are when both sides win or lose – they are different sides of the same coin.

When the practice owner and associate candidate are in agreement about the contract terms, the attorney on the practice owner's transition team draws up the first draft of the legal contract (the practice owner pays for the legal contract to be drawn up). The practice owner presents the contract to the associate candidate with the following instructions:

"This contract represents the terms that we agree upon, plus typical contractual language. This legal agreement also represents a document that has stood the test of time as a standard contract in nearly every state for many years. You should have an attorney representing your interests review the contract. You should also know that your attorney will look for ways to not only protect your interests, but also gain an advantage for you. They feel that is their job. However, that is likely to cause you and me to renegotiate terms which we've already settled on, which will at best cost both of us time and money, and at worst jeopardize our working relationship before it begins. Therefore, my recommendation is that you inform your attorney that the terms have already been agreed upon, and that your attorney should review the contract and make only the recommendations they feel are absolutely necessary."

An example of a typical associate contract can be found in the Glossary.

Integration of the Associate into the Practice

A successful associate working relationship is not only about choosing the right person, but also about both the practice owner and the associate following a systematic approach to creating an environment that the associate can thrive in. Successful implementation involves seven things:

1. **Preparing both Associate and Team** – First, the associate and practice owner need to define what a successful associateship means. Like any team member, the associate needs to satisfy the job description for their role. The associate dentist has significant responsibilities as a provider of care, leading the team in the operatory during procedures, and representing the practice. The patient may not know the associate is not the practice owner, and if they do it doesn't matter relative to how pleased they are with their treatment. In other words, the associate might as well be the practice owner in the mind of the patient. The associate needs to understand their journey is like moving up the steps of a ladder. They start at the first step of the ladder and, with time and performance that meets or exceeds the standards set for them (see associate job description in the Glossary), they earn the right to take the next step. The practice owner defines the steps. The top step may be a partnership arrangement.

   The associate needs to appreciate that success is closely tied to their ability to work harmoniously with the team. One of the biggest mistakes a new associate makes is entering a new practice with the mindset that their dental degree means they are more important to the practice than a team member without a dental degree. I tell every new associate that the most important thing they can accomplish in their first few months in the practice is to win over the team – to earn their trust and respect.

   The associate also needs to understand that they will be working within the systems that are already in place in the practice. They will be using the same equipment, supplies, and techniques as the senior doctor unless otherwise determined. The team doesn't need to practice one way with the practice owner, and another way with the associate.

   The associate dentist should spend two to three days in the office prior to their official start (at their own expense) shadowing the practice owner, observing how he/she communicates to patients and team members, observing treatment, and asking questions of team members so that they understand as much as possible about the delivery of care. The associate also should spend time observing how the business office operates, learning about scheduling, financial, and other systems the business office performs.

   The team needs to be prepared for the associate's new role in the office. The practice owner should explain the role, revisit the benefits, and solicit the help of everyone on the team to support the associate in being a successful team member of the practice.

   The team needs to understand the limitations and boundaries of the associate's position. Despite this, it is important for the team members to not portray the associate to the patients of the practice as less than the practice owner. For this reason, it is not advisable to refer to the associate dentist in front of a patient as "the associate." The insinuation is that the associate is second rate. Instead, the team should refer to the associate dentist as *"Dr. _______," who was hand selected by Dr. __________ (the practice owner) and is an exceptional dentist that we are very pleased to be a part of our practice."* This is necessary to build confidence in the associate dentist on the part of the patient base.

The team and the associate need to understand that, when it comes to scheduling, the practice owner runs the show. This means that the associate's scheduled production is not meant to be at the expense of the practice owner's scheduled production.

The practice owner should remember that the number one reason to employ an associate is for profit, and more profit results from dentistry the practice owner performs compared to what the associate performs. This is because there is higher overhead on the associate's dentistry because in addition to all the other overhead that is paid on the delivery of that care is the associate's salary. The only exception to giving preference to the owner's schedule is during the first few months when the associate may need help in building their schedule.

2. **Addressing Staffing** – Part of the arrangement with the associate dentist involves providing support staff. The practice owner should make sure the associate has a qualified dental assistant to support them. An additional assistant should be hired for the associate dentist if utilizing the existing dental assistants will adversely affect the practice owner's schedule and production goals.

   The practice owner can assign assistants to work with the associate in a couple different ways. One way is to utilize all the existing assistants, and rotate which assistant works with the associate. The second way, and the one I recommend, is that the associate has a dedicated assistant. The advantage is that the dedicated assistant and associate form a team that works efficiently together.

   One of the reasons to hire an associate is to expand the hygiene department, so if the practice has been holding off hiring an additional hygienist because the practice owner didn't have the bandwidth to do more hygiene checks, then the addition of the associate can allow for an additional hygienist.

   Finally, depending on the staffing of the business office, an additional team member may be needed there as well.
3. **Addressing Facility, Equipment, and Supply Needs** – If the associate dentist is to be productive enough to warrant their presence, they need at least one operatory (in the beginning) to work out of that doesn't negatively impact the other providers' schedules. In addition, any additional equipment or supplies for a full associate schedule should be added.
4. **Creating a Schedule for the Associate**
   a. Scheduling systems – The types of procedures that the associate can and cannot perform need to be identified so that patients can be scheduled appropriately. Also, the time the associate will need for procedures will need to be discovered. If the time the associate wants for a procedure is excessive compared to that of the practice owner, then the reason for this needs to be known and addressed so that the associate's clinical efficiency is not a deterrent to a productive and profitable schedule.
   b. Marketing – If the associate position is a new position on the team, then an additional schedule of production needs to be created. In other words, there is an additional mouth to feed. The practice needs to determine the number of additional new patients needed (new patient analysis spreadsheet) and create a marketing plan to attract these patients (using previously discussed marketing plan criteria).

5. **Establishing Policies Related to the Associate** – Specifically related to examining existing and new patients, it will need to be determined if the associate will be responsible for performing any scheduled treatment diagnosed at those appointments. Typically, if the associate checks a patient normally seen by another dentist in the practice, then that treatment is performed by that other dentist. If the associate checks a patient new to the practice, then the associate performs any diagnosed and treatment planned care on that patient, unless that treatment is something they normally don't perform.
6. **Setting Up a Continuing Education Plan for the Associate** – Before the associate begins working in the practice, the practice owner should identify and create a plan to address all areas in which the associate is deficient. The practice owner should prioritize those areas they want the associate to be proficient in. For new dentists not far removed from dental school, basic skills such as diagnosis and treatment planning should be addressed early in the continuing education plan.
7. **Providing Mentoring, Feedback, and Support** – The practice owner must accept the responsibility for mentoring the new associate. Depending on the age and experience of the associate, this could be a minor or major responsibility. If closer to the latter, it will require considerable time and effort. Like any endeavor, it must begin with a plan that includes clear-cut objectives coupled with time-associated goals, regularly scheduled meetings, feedback, and support.

Transition of the Associate to Partner

The transition of associate to partner can be likened to dating before getting married. Not all dating relationships become marriage relationships, nor should they. An associate is like a boyfriend/girlfriend. You like them enough to spend time with them, but that time can be limited or long-term, based on how the relationship dynamics work out. If they don't work, then it may be a little messy, but there usually aren't ties that keep both sides from moving on. But if the two do get married and things don't work out, then a break-up is a bigger deal, which means a divorce, including attorneys and asset separation. The same issues impact the associate versus partner relationship. Therefore, a partner must be carefully selected and, in almost every instance, a partnership should be preceded by an associateship.

The length of this trial period will vary depending on a multitude of factors – age of the practice owner and associate, experience and skill level of the associate, time until anticipated retirement of the practice owner, and others. It is typically not less than six months and not greater than five years.

Before the transition from associate to partner, both parties must be convinced it is in their best interest, meaning there is a shared vision for the partnership and an agreed-upon path to partnership. The purchase price is arrived at through the practice valuation process previously described.

Partial Buy-In by the Associate - The percentage of transfer of ownership can vary from twenty-five to one hundred percent. Less than twenty-five percent ownership will usually mean less income than the buying-in partner would make as an associate. The percentage of ownership purchased is often tied to the percentage of dentistry (of the combined amount of the practice owner and associate) produced by the associate. For example, if the practice owner is producing on average $150,000/month, and the associate is producing $50,000/month, then the associate can purchase twenty-five percent of the practice ($50,000 is twenty-five percent of the total $200,000/month produced). A large portion of the reason for the purchase percentage being tied to the production percentage of the associate is due to financing requirements. If the purchase involves less than one hundred percent, then the remainder may be purchased in increments at agreed-upon intervals of time. The sale price of future increments is usually based on the original valuation.

Total Purchase by the Associate - A variation of the Sale to Existing Associate is when the associate acquires one hundred percent of the practice, and the former owner works as an associate for the new owner. The success of these working relationships is largely dependent on the attitude and commitment of both parties, the alignment of the vision of both owner and associate, and the terms of the contractual agreement.

The advantages of this arrangement to the seller are that they can continue to do something they enjoy while making income, usually on working terms (time and treatment) that suit their desires. They also have some freedom as to how long they continue as an associate.

The advantage to the buyer is that they have a proven practitioner who has an existing relationship with the team and patient base. This can make for a more streamlined transition of ownership for the buyer, rather than having to take on all the dentist provider responsibilities with the schedule or adding a new associate dentist to the practice at a time when stability among the team and patients of the practice is under the stress of ownership transition.

The challenges to this new working relationship are that the seller often has difficulty taking off his/her owner hat with all that ownership entails and putting on an associate hat as an employee of the practice. This is only made worse if the seller has a dominant personality and the buyer does not. Clearly defined roles, as well as repercussions for not working within those roles, is critical to addressing this common problem.

Another challenge is that the former owner does not buy in to the new owner's goals, expectations, and standards. This can result in conflict between the two sides, and dividing the team into two camps.

These challenges create another challenge: how to terminate the working relationship of the former owner. While that termination should be no different than any other employer-employee relationship, it is complicated by the long-term relationship that exists between the former owner and the patients and team.

Sale to a Dental Service Organization

The Dental Service Organization (aka Dental Support Organization - DSO) has become increasingly popular over the past couple of decades. These corporate-owned companies establish, purchase, or contract with dentist-owned practices to provide business support services which include Human Resources, Marketing & Branding, Recruiting, IT Services, Payroll, Capital & Financing, Tax Services, Accounting, Risk Management, and Practice Support. DSOs allow non-dentists, such as private equity groups, to invest in ownership of dental practices.

There is little wonder why they have grown as fast as they have. They take over the business of the practice, which many practice owners consider a burden, and they typically pay top price for dental practices they purchase. They usually pay one hundred percent or more of the practice annual average revenue, twenty to thirty percent greater than the average sale price when the purchase involves a non-DSO buyer.

In addition to paying a top purchase price and taking over the management responsibilities of the practice, DSOs also provide continuing education and mentoring for young dentists. Their larger size and buying power allow them to incorporate the latest technological advances, decrease overhead, and increase profitability.

A big disadvantage to the seller in a DSO purchase is giving up control over practice decisions. The previous owner is now an employee, and the conversion often isn't easy. The former owner doesn't have the same autonomy or security; they may be held to production quotas that are challenging; and the team may not embrace the new ownership and related policies, with ensuing turnover.

The typical terms of the DSO purchase have the seller working in the practice for at least three years for a certain number of days at a defined level of production. The seller must also participate in company-sponsored events such as team training and continuing education. The DSO typically pays the seller sixty to seventy-five percent of the sale price at the time of purchase and the remainder upon satisfying the purchase terms at a designated future date.

The GSO: Forming Your Own DSO-Like Business Structure

While there are some things to like about the DSO business structure, the biggest downside for most practice owners is the loss of ownership and the ramifications related to autonomy, income, and equity growth potential.

A Group Service Organization (GSO) is a new model that allows practice owner(s) to continue to own and grow their practice with additional providers and sometimes additional practices. Within a GSO, owners can maintain control over practice decisions, retain the ability to practice for as long as they want (as well as how and how much they want), and maintain or increase cash flow, while growing their equity value.

This involves a change in the business model. Privately owned dental practices exist as one entity - with no separation of the clinical or business management component. When the practice is sold, the entire practice entity is purchased, either in increments or in whole, as previously described. In a GSO, the business or management portion is separate from the clinical portion. The management portion is funded by revenue from the clinical portion. In the case of most DSOs, the percentage of collections taken from clinical revenue to fund the management ranges from seven to twelve percent.

In the GSO model, the practice owner(s) create a separate management LLC to fulfill the same responsibilities that a DSO performs, funded by revenue from the clinical entity in the seven to twelve percent range. The chosen percentage number within this range is based on existing profit margins, as well as the magnitude of the responsibilities the management portion will undertake.

As the practice owner grows the practice by adding associate providers, the practice owner may choose to work less, both of which have the potential to reduce the practice owner's cash flow. This is offset in the GSO business structure by two things:

1. The autonomy that the practice owner retains (as the majority owner of the clinical portion) with this transition model allows them to choose to perform more highly profitable procedures that can maintain or increase the practice owner's production even though working fewer hours/days in the practice.
2. The practice owner, as the sole or majority owner of the management portion, is now paid an additional seven to twelve percent of clinical-generated revenue.

Some of the associates may become partners, which will cause the practice owner's equity portion to be diluted. This is offset by the fact that the overall size of the clinical portion will grow from the added production (due to increased capacity), so while the percentage ownership in the clinical portion will be less, its value will be maintained or increased.

With the GSO transition model, the practice owner can participate in the practice and business for as long as they want, working the way they want, as frequently as they want. When they are working on the management side, they can also work remotely wherever they want. At some future date, when they are ready to sell some or all their clinical and management ownership portions, they can do so at either a pre-set or updated appraised value.

This transition model most closely aligns with the mantra of Sunrise Dental Solutions – Make More, Keep More, and Enjoy More, as well as the purpose for the owner of the prosperous dental practice – to achieve both financial and lifestyle freedom.

Throughout this book, we have referenced the important role that a practice coach and consultant plays in this purpose. Ambitious people are naturally attracted to individuals or organizations that can help them get to where they want to go. They realize that figuring it out themselves takes a lot of time and involves a lot of trial and error. Ambitious people are by nature impatient and want to get to where they want to go in as straight a line as possible. So, they associate themselves with others who know more than they do about achieving whatever it is that they are committed to. For this reason, I encourage the reader who desires to be a prosperous dental practice owner to associate with a coach and a network of other like-minded individuals.

THE KEY CONCEPT

The Key Concept of Learning from Others – Vernon Law said, "Experience is a hard teacher because she gives the test first, the lesson afterward." You can figure things out for yourself, which requires more time, effort, and money, or you can learn from the experience and wisdom of others who have done what you want to do. The choice between these two options should be easy, but most choose to make the wrong decision.

THE KEY CONCEPT

The Key Concept of Accountability – Accountability means being answerable for your actions and decisions. Being held accountable refers to the individual(s) whom you have chosen to answer to for doing what you agreed you would do. This individual can be yourself, another individual, or a group of individuals. The more respect you have for those who hold you accountable, the more likely you are to succeed in accomplishing your goals.

SUMMARY OF KEY POINTS FROM CHAPTER 4 - THE TRANSITION OPTIONS

1. Dentists should begin their career with a plan for how they want it to evolve, up to and including how they want their career to end.

2. Profit from a business comes not only in the form of cash flow, but also through equity. Successful practice owners are always looking for ways to increase the value of their equity in the business, even if that means decreasing their percentage of ownership.

3. What everyone who appreciates the importance of a financial vision – financial freedom – needs is their "number." That number is the amount of money they need upon retirement to support their chosen lifestyle until their anticipated time of death.

4. Continually growing the practice until its sale requires the practice owner to operate the practice at high levels, which includes updating technology, upgrading and refining systems, attending the finest continuing education available, marketing the practice, and investing in the attraction and retention of the best team possible.

5. The phrase "*Retire in Practice*" describes dentists who continue as owners while working less chairside, in some cases working only in a managerial role. This way they continue to participate in the cash flow and equity of the practice even if they end their clinical dentistry career.

6. Prior to the sale to an associate, the practice should have a successful associate relationship of one to five years. The definition of a successful working relationship with an associate is when the associate meets the expectations of the practice owner, and the practice owner meets those of the associate.

7. Associateships fail for two reasons: the inherent disadvantages of the associate arrangement, and the wrong person is chosen for the associate position.

8. The search for the right associate starts with the practice owner determining the characteristics of the right associate. By being as specific as possible about those characteristics, the practice owner can better advertise and screen for them, as well as recognize them when they appear.

9. Associates can be paid two basic ways – a fixed rate (salary or per diem) or commission. From the standpoint of less financial risk for the practice owner, as well as more motivation to produce more, commission wins out.

10. The ideal compensation percentage to pay an associate is the point at which the senior dentist takes home one dollar for every dollar the associate takes home from the dentistry the associate produces.

11. The associate needs to appreciate that his or her success is closely tied to their ability to work harmoniously with the team. One of the biggest mistakes a new associate makes is entering a new practice with the mindset that their dental degree means they are more important to the practice than a team member without a dental degree.

12. The team and the associate need to understand that when it comes to scheduling, the practice owner's schedule is the highest priority. The associate's production cannot come at the expense of the practice owner's production.
13. The practice owner must accept responsibility for mentoring the new associate. Like any endeavor, it must begin with a plan that includes clear-cut objectives, time-associated goals, regularly-scheduled meetings, feedback, and support.
14. A partner must be carefully selected and, in almost every instance, a partnership should be preceded by an associateship.
15. Forming a privately-owned DSO-like business structure, a GSO, allows the practice owner(s) to continue to own and grow their practice with additional providers, and sometimes additional practices, all while maintaining control over practice decisions, retaining the ability to practice for as long as they want and how and how much they want, maintaining or increasing cash flow, while growing their equity value.

Glossary

KEY CONCEPTS

Accountability – Accountability means being answerable for your actions and decisions. Being held accountable refers to the individual(s) whom you have chosen to answer to for doing what you agreed you would do. This individual can be yourself, another individual, or a group of individuals. The more respect you have for those who hold you accountable, the more likely you are to succeed in accomplishing your goals.

Accountability Versus Responsibility – Within a team, a designated individual should be assigned and accept primary accountability for the outcome of a key system. Accountability makes for a deeper commitment on the part of the designated individual, while allowing more efficient management of the assigned system. Responsibility in this context refers to sharing in the outcome of key systems.

Asking – In the New Testament Bible Jesus taught the message of asking: "Ask and it shall be given. Knock and the door will be opened to you." (Matthew 7:7,8). In fact, there are more than a hundred Bible verses with the message, "You have not because you ask not." The key is to ask. Asking is the first step in seeking knowledge (remember the acronym A-S-K – Always Seeking Knowledge), and knowledge is essential to influencing others.

Attraction – Based on the quote by Paul J. Meyer, the Law of Attraction is this: "Whatever you can vividly imagine, ardently desire, earnestly believe in, and expectantly act toward, with God's help, must inevitably come to pass. That which you are seeking, is seeking you."

Believability, Likeability, and Trust (BLT) – When faced with a decision about where to go and who to buy from for any product or service, people rely on trusted sources. They tend to trust those they like, and they often believe those they like. Therefore, if you want to be trusted and believed, first seek to be liked.

Build It and They Will Come – We usually attribute this famous quote to the film *Field of Dreams*, referring to building a baseball diamond in a cornfield where players of past eras would return. In the business world, it refers to creating capacity for growth. Savvy business owners don't just respond to demand, they create demand and remove all obstacles to the flow of new business.

Compensating for Quality (aka "You get what you pay for") – Henry Ford once said, "In industry, there is only one rule: achieve the highest possible quality of products at the lowest possible costs and pay the highest salaries."

Compounding Interest – Compound interest is considered one of the great miracles of all of human history and economics. Albert Einstein described it as the most powerful force in our society. When you allow money to accumulate at compound interest over a long enough period of time, it increases more than most people realize.

Controlling the Conversation – You dominate a conversation by talking; you control a conversation by asking questions.

Delegation – Any role that a team member can legally perform to the standards set by the practice owner should be delegated to that team member.

Emotional Decision-Making – While it's logical for people to make big decisions based on logic, that is the exception rather than the rule. Ask yourself, "What are the biggest decisions I've ever made?" Your answers would probably be marriage, purchasing a home, choosing a career path, and others. More than likely, these decisions were emotionally charged. You may have used logic to justify the emotional decision, but if you had done it the other way around, you likely would not have decided to move forward.

15X – In general, consumers need to experience a marketing message at least fifteen times before making a decision to act on that message.

Learning from Others – The Vernon Law says, "Experience is a hard teacher because she gives the test first, the lesson afterward." You can figure things out for yourself, which requires more time, effort, and money, or you can learn from the experience and wisdom of others who have done what you want to do. The choice between these two options should be easy, but most choose to make the wrong decision.

Leverage – By expanding a team member's role, efficiency and effectiveness are enhanced.

Like Likes Like – In high school chemistry class we learned this concept: Chemicals with similar structures when mixed together form a solution. The same applies when choosing people to work with. Choose those individuals who mix well with you, who in the most important ways see the world as you do.

Outcome Visualization – To your brain, visualizing success is as real as actually achieving success. Once your brain believes in the outcome, the outcome becomes more possible and, when practiced regularly, inevitable. Denis Waitley said, "When you visualize, then you materialize."

Persistence and Determination – Calvin Coolidge once said, "Nothing in this world can take the place of persistence. Talent will not; nothing is more common than unsuccessful men with talent. Genius will not; unrewarded genius is almost a proverb. Education will not; the world is full of educated derelicts. Persistence and determination alone are omnipotent."

Positive Affirmation – "Affirmations are proven methods of self-improvement because of their ability to rewire our brains. Much like exercise, they raise the level of feel-good hormones and push our brains to form new clusters of "positive thought" neurons. In the sequence of thought-speech-action, affirmations play an integral role by breaking patterns of negative thoughts, negative speech, and, in turn, negative actions." – Dr. Carmen Harra.

Rock, Sand, and Water – The rock, sand, and water metaphor has been applied to many aspects of life. The teaching exercise for the concept involves a jar and a combination of three components that can fill that jar – rocks, sand, and water. Rocks represent the most important things required to accomplish the purpose of filling the jar. Sand, while necessary, has less value. Water represents the least value of all. The basic premise is that in order to accomplish the most, and more importantly accomplish the most important first, rocks need to go in first, followed by sand, and lastly by water. In terms of a dental practice, the jar represents the schedule, rocks represent highly productive appointments, sand represents less productive appointments, and water represents appointments that have no production when it comes to dollar value. Given that the purpose of a schedule is to schedule to goal, then highly productive appointments (rocks) must go in first, followed by less productive ones.

Storytelling – Telling a story is an excellent way to make a point. People are drawn in to an account of someone like them who faced a similar challenge and overcame it. Every good story has a hero, a plot, and a point to be made. The point can precede the story or follow the story. Make a point, tell a story – tell a story, make a point.

Team Member Quality – Decide on a scale of 1-10, with 10 being the best, what quality of practice and business you want. Then realize that whatever number you've chosen, the quality of each team member on a similar scale cannot be less than the number you've chosen for your practice.

Trust but Verify – The business owner must trust that everyone in their employment will conduct themselves in a moral, ethical, and legal manner. This is critical given that these team members will be delegated important responsibilities involving the organization's success. A lack of trust with any individual must be resolved to the business owner's satisfaction as soon as possible. Even in the presence of this trust, the business owner must do their due diligence to confirm that trust is well-placed.

JOB DESCRIPTIONS (AKA TEAM MEMBER OBJECTIVES)

DENTAL ASSISTANT

<Team Member Name>

Design of the Position: The Dental Assistant will assist the doctor chairside to deliver quality, comfortable care in a stress-free environment. This will include readiness and cleanliness of the operatory and preparation of the patient for dental treatment. This team member needs to be able and willing to perform chairside assistance, capturing x-rays, recording information in patient electronic records, performing expanded duties if qualified, and opening/closing office.

ESSENTIAL PERFORMANCE AND RESPONSIBILITIES are as follows. Other duties may be appointed:

A. Preparation Responsibilities

- Turn on all cart, x-ray, intra-oral units, wall switches, ultrasonic, autoclave, etc., for the start of the day.
- Evaluate sterilization area for cleanliness and organization for the beginning of the day and throughout the day.
- Make sure all the treatment rooms are ready, stocked, and clean (certain rooms may apply to specific assistants).
- Seat patients and review with patient the treatment to be performed. Ask if there are any questions or concerns, and make the doctor aware of any.
- Be responsible for the appearance of the treatment rooms.

B. Assisting Responsibilities

- Assist the doctor at all times.
- Anticipate the doctor's needs at all times, preparing in advance for the next step.
- Capture digital x-rays, download, and display on the monitor for doctor to view.
- Take impressions, if qualified.
- Fabricate temporary crowns and bridges, if qualified.
- Assist doctor with administration of nitrous oxide and any other medications that need to be given during the appointment, if qualified.
- Perform all expanded duties, if qualified.
- Show an interest in and participate in all meetings.
- Be willing to participate in seminars and webinars that facilitate both professional and personal growth.
- Calm and reassure patients throughout dental procedure.
- Work safely and follow safety and office protocol.

C. Charting Responsibilities

- Make sure the patient's record is complete and all services for that day of treatment are recorded prior to dismissing the patient. Include the next appointment to be scheduled, the treatment to be provided, and the time units needed to perform the treatment.
- It is imperative that all chart notes are accurate for each procedure. If additional information is necessary, seek the proper person for advice.
- Complete all charts, routing slips, treatment cards, and lab slips before patient leaves the office.
- Make sure that patient records arrive at the front desk at the same time as the departing patient or, preferably, before.

D. Patient Care Responsibilities

- Welcome, seat, and dismiss patients cheerfully.
- Show care, concern, and respect for patient's well-being and comfort at all times.
- Ensure that the patient is comfortable. Request additional assistance if needed.
- Make sure that the patient is thoroughly suctioned out with no remaining debris present intra-orally.
- Ensure that the patient's face is clean and free of debris before exiting treatment room to the front desk; provide hand mirror and moist towel if needed.
- If patients wish to rinse their mouth, direct them to the sink, mouthwash, and cups.
- Give, and make sure that all patients are aware of, post-operative instructions for any procedure performed, for the rest of the day and for the time between visits. If additional assistance or direction is required, be responsible for asking the appropriate person(s).
- Review follow-up appointments with the patient and what they should do if any questions or concerns arise; make patient aware of how important it is to get needed treatment scheduled before it requires more extensive treatment.
- Escort patients to the business office and inform them who they will be seeing to discuss financial arrangements and to schedule future appointments.
- Guide patients to the business office and do a "2 on 1" transfer of power with the next team member, discussing treatment performed today, future treatment and appointments needed, any appropriate financial information from the doctor, etc.
- Reassure patients that all their needs will be taken care of.
- Contact patients at the end of the day to see how well they are doing.

E. Overall Practice Responsibilities

- Present a positive image of dental services to be rendered.
- Present a positive relationship with other team members and the doctor in front of patients.
- Be punctual to work, and during appointments with patient seating and dismissing.
- Use downtime constructively.
- Engage only in positive conversation regarding another team member.
- Maintain a clean, well-groomed professional manner.

- Do not allow personal phone use to interfere with work.
- Assist business office with the following if time permits: Greet patients as they enter office, answer phone, take messages, make appointments, make financial arrangements, confirm appointments.
- Perform light housekeeping such as vacuuming, removing trash, cleaning kitchen area and patient/employee bathrooms.
- Participate in seminars, meetings, etc.

F. Sterilization Responsibilities
- Follow OSHA guidelines for all procedures.
- Ensure that mask, gowns, gloves, and safety glasses are worn and accessible at all times during dental procedures, clean-up of the treatment rooms, and sterilizing instruments.
- Be responsible for the appearance and organization of the sterilization area.
- Be responsible for the sterilization of instruments and set-up of trays.
- Clean sinks in treatment areas and sterilization area.
- Empty trash, clean and disinfect treatment rooms and sterilization area.

G. Equipment Responsibilities (if appointed, assistants may have specific duties)
- Maintain and keep record of all handpieces and attachments.
- Screen curing light units for sufficient light intensity.
- Clean and/or change vacuum traps and suction units weekly and drain compressor.
- Be responsible for a maintenance plan for all equipment.

H. Laboratory Responsibilities (if appointed)
- Pour, mount, and trim study models and other lab procedures, if qualified.
- Make sure all lab cases are back for the next day.
- Be responsible for the lab area.
- Be responsible for lab equipment maintenance.
- Be responsible for communicating with laboratory.

I. Ordering Responsibilities (if appointed)
- Be responsible for ordering all clinical supplies.
- Keep track of back-ordered items and returned items.
- Look for best prices and discounts on all supplies.

CREDENTIALS and REQUIREMENTS: To perform this position successfully, an individual must be able to perform each duty within expectations. The terms listed below are representative of the knowledge, skill, and experience required in this role. Reasonable arrangements may be made to enable individuals with disabilities to perform the essential functions.

EDUCATION and/or EXPERIENCE: High school diploma or graduate degree and completion of accredited dental assistant program; 2 years general dentistry experience with some specialized experience preferred, or 4 years related experience and/or training; or combination of education and experience.

LANGUAGE SKILLS: Ability to read and interpret common business periodicals, professional journals, technical procedures, and governmental regulations. Ability to write reports such as detailed information in patient records and communicate with patient without interference or language barriers.

MATHEMATICAL SKILLS: Ability to add, subtract, multiply, and divide in all units of measure, using whole numbers, common fractions, and decimals.

LICENSES, CERTIFICATIONS, and REGISTRATION (may vary by state)

- State Registered or Certification from an accredited dental Assistant program
- X-ray Certification
- Cardio-Pulmonary Resuscitation (CPR) Certification
- Sedation Certification, if appropriate

REPORTS TO: Assistant Team Leader / Office Manager / Practice Owner

HOURS:

I have read and understand the Job Description/Team Member Objectives information presented to me so that I can perform my role to the highest standards of this practice.

______________________________ _______________

Assistant Signature Date

______________________________ _______________

Practice Owner / Office Manager Signature Date

REGISTERED DENTAL HYGIENIST

<Team Member Name>

Design of the Position: The Dental Hygienist is the chief preventive and periodontal treatment provider in the practice. This team member motivates, educates, and provides excellent treatment. It is also essential that this team member recognize early signs of periodontal disease so that prevention and early treatment of the disease averts its most serious consequences to the patient. Discovering areas of disease or structural breakdown along with complete documentation, both periodontally and restoratively, will facilitate the doctor's diagnosis and treatment recommendations.

ESSENTIAL PERFORMANCE AND RESPONSIBILITIES are as follows. Other duties may be appointed:

A. Preparation and Hygiene Responsibilities

- Welcome and seat patient cheerfully.
- Have treatment room properly set up and ready for the hygiene procedure.
- Show care and concern for patient's welfare and make comfortable at all times.
- Review and update patient's health history.
- Perform a head and neck/oral cancer exam.
- Capture digital radiographs and display on monitor for doctor to view and interpret.
- Chart patient's existing hard tissue restorations and note any areas of concern.
- Perform periodontal evaluation (probing depths, bleeding points, mobility, and recession) and communicate findings to patient and doctor.
- Chart patient's progress with home care; document non-compliance.
- Utilize technology (intra-oral camera, etc.) as appropriate.
- Discuss any unfinished, previously diagnosed, treatment.
- Perform oral prophylaxis, if appropriate.
- Administer fluoride treatment.
- Give anesthesia, if qualified, when asked for, or as hygiene treatment dictates.
- Perform root debridement therapy.
- Complete scheduled treatment.
- Educate and motivate the patient on proper oral hygiene and corrective and/or preventive measures.
- Observe patient for decay and restorative problems that will hamper periodontal treatment success.
- Present appropriate educational literature.
- Assist doctor in hygiene examination.
- Schedule patient for the appropriate re-care appointment, emphasizing the significance of continuing care.
- Use appropriate verbal skills to educate and motivate patients.
- While still in the treatment room, make sure patient's electronic record is complete and all services for the day's treatment are recorded, as well as the next continuing care or treatment visit, and time units required. Return patient records to

the business office and escort the patient to the appropriate team member for final processing, employing a "2 on 1" transfer of power.
- Contact any root debridement therapy patient that evening to see how well they are doing.
- Make patient hygiene appointments in treatment room prior to leaving, if appropriate.

B. Sterilization Responsibilities
- Assist the hygiene assistant in setting up and disinfecting treatment rooms and instrument trays in accordance with office policy and OSHA standards.
- Assist the hygiene assistant in sterilizing and disinfecting instruments and intra-oral devices in accordance with office policy and OSHA standards.
- Ensure that masks, gloves, gown, and safety glasses are worn and accessible at all times during dental procedures and cleanup of treatment rooms and instruments.

C. Equipment Responsibilities
- Clean and maintain the hygiene hand pieces.
- Sharpen hygiene instruments and see that instruments are ordered as needed, if appropriate.

D. Overall Practice Responsibilities
- Assist other team members when time permits.
- Participate in morning meeting and give information regarding new and existing patients for the day, any concerns, time issues, etc.
- Send a personal note to patients that deserve special attention.
- Present a positive image of dental services to be rendered.
- Present a positive relationship with other team members and the doctor in front of patients.
- Be punctual to work and with patient seating and dismissing.
- Use downtime constructively.
- Engage only in positive conversation regarding another team member.
- Maintain a clean, well-groomed professional manner.
- Do not allow personal phone use to interfere with work.
- Assist business office with the following if time permits: Greet patients as they enter office, answer phone, take messages, make appointments, make financial arrangements, confirm appointments.
- Perform light housekeeping such as vacuuming, removing trash, cleaning kitchen area and patient/employee bathrooms.
- Be able to calm and reassure patients facing uncomfortable or painful dental procedures.
- Be able to quickly record detailed information in a readable, legible, condensed form.
- Be able to work safely and follow established safety and office procedures.

CREDENTIALS and REQUIREMENTS: To perform this position successfully, an individual must be able to perform each duty within expectations. The terms listed below are representative of the knowledge and experience required of this role. Reasonable arrangements may be made to enable individuals with disabilities to perform the essential functions.

EDUCATION and/or EXPERIENCE: High school diploma or graduate equivalent degree and completion of accredited dental hygiene program; 1 year general dentistry experience or 2 years related experience and/or training; or equivalent combination of education and experience.

LANGUAGE SKILLS: Ability to read and interpret professional journals, technical procedures, and government regulations. Ability to write or type reports such as detailed information in patient records and communicate with patients without interference or language barriers.

MATHEMATICAL SKILLS: Ability to add, subtract, multiply, and divide in all units of measure, using whole numbers, common fractions, and decimals. Ability to compute rate, ratio, and percent.

LICENSES, CERTIFICATIONS, and REGISTRATION (may vary by state)

- State Registered Dental Hygiene License
- Cardio-Pulmonary Resuscitation (CPR) Certification
- Local Anesthesia Certification, if appropriate
- Sedation Certification, if appropriate
- Laser Certification, if appropriate

REPORTS TO: Hygiene Team Leader / Office Manager / Practice Owner

HOURS:

I have read and understand the Job Description/Team Member Objectives information presented to me so that I can perform my role to the highest standards of this practice.

______________________________ _______________

Hygienist Signature Date

______________________________ _______________

Practice Owner / Office Manager Signature Date

HYGIENE ASSISTANT

<Team Member Name>

Design of the Position: The Hygiene Assistant is responsible for seeing that the hygiene schedule runs smoothly and on time, by being one step ahead of the Hygienist. The Hygiene Assistant will take radiographs (when properly trained and certified), turn over hygiene operatories (break down and setup), stock hygiene rooms, record periodontal readings, sterilize instruments, make doctor aware of patient check time, and keep Hygienist aware of schedule changes at all times.

ESSENTIAL PERFORMANCE AND RESPONSIBILITIES are as follows. Other duties may be assigned:

A. Preparation and Assisting Responsibilities

- Record periodontal readings, treatment completed, and treatment that needs to be done for the hygienist.
- Print out financial arrangements and treatment plan.
- Review charts day before and inform hygienist of treatment needs and medical alerts.
- Take radiographs (FMX/BWX/PANO/CT SCAN) as needed.
- Quickly clean hygiene treatment rooms once the patient has been brought to the business office, so that the next patient can be seated as soon as possible.
- Communicate with hygiene scheduling coordinator and front desk about hygiene schedule changes and doctor-patient flow.
- Make sure all essential forms for the next day are completed before leaving the office.
- Assist the hygiene scheduling coordinator with scheduling, filling appointment times, and moving patients to make the schedule flow smoothly, as time permits.
- Assist the clinical assistants in cleaning of their operatories as needed to make schedule flow smoothly.
- Assist the scheduling and financial coordinator as time permits.
- Set up and clean treatment room and instrument trays in accordance with office procedures and OSHA requirements.
- Sterilize and disinfect instruments and intra-oral devices in accordance with OSHA requirements, office procedures, and industry standards.

B. Sterilization Responsibilities

- Follow OSHA guidelines for all procedures.
- Ensure that mask, gloves, safety glasses, and gown are worn at all times during dental procedures, clean-up of treatment rooms, and sterilizing instruments.
- Be responsible for the appearance and organization of the sterilization area.
- Be responsible for the sterilization of instruments and set-up of trays.
- Clean sinks in treatment areas and sterilization areas.
- Empty trash and clean and disinfect treatment rooms and sterilization area.

C. Overall Practice Responsibilities

- Greet arriving patients.
- Assist front desk with answering phones when needed.
- Perform light housekeeping, including such tasks as vacuuming, removing trash, cleaning kitchen area and patient/employee bathrooms.
- Present a positive image of dental services to be rendered.
- Present a positive relationship with other team members and doctor in front of patients.
- Be punctual to work and in carrying out responsibilities.
- Use downtime constructively.
- Make sure personal phone use does not interfere with work.
- Engage only in positive conversation regarding another team member.
- Maintain a clean, well-groomed professional manner.

CREDENTIALS and REQUIREMENTS: To perform this position successfully, an individual must be able to perform each duty within expectations. The terms listed below are representative of the knowledge, skill, and experience required in this role. Reasonable arrangements may be made to enable individuals with disabilities to perform the essential functions.

EDUCATION and/or EXPERIENCE: High school diploma or graduate equivalent degree. Two years general dentistry experience preferred.

LANGUAGE SKILLS: Ability to read and interpret common business periodicals, professional journals, technical procedures, and governmental regulations. Ability to write reports such as detailed information in patient charts and communicate with patients without interference or language barriers.

MATHEMATICAL SKILLS: Ability to add, subtract, multiply, and divide in all units of measure, using whole numbers, common fractions, and decimals.

LICENSES and CERTIFICATIONS

- X-ray Certification
- Cardio-Pulmonary Resuscitation (CPR) Certification

REPORTS TO: Hygiene Team Leader / Office Manager / Practice Owner

HOURS:

I have read and understand the Job Description/Team Member Objectives information presented to me so that I can perform my role to the highest standards of this practice.

______________________________ ________________

Hygiene Assistant Signature Date

______________________________ ________________

Practice Owner / Office Manager Signature Date

SCHEDULING COORDINATOR/HYGIENE

<Team Member Name>

Design of the Position: The Hygiene Scheduling Coordinator is responsible for successful scheduling of the Hygiene Department to goal on a daily basis. In order to accomplish this the Hygiene Scheduling Coordinator utilizes every source available, such as the "ASAP call" list, today's and the upcoming schedule, and the overdue for hygiene appointment list to schedule each hygienist to goal.

ESSENTIAL PERFORMANCE AND RESPONSIBILITIES are as follows. Other duties may be appointed:

A. Appointment Scheduling Responsibilities

- Make sure that the phone is answered before the third ring at all times, with a smile.
- Whenever a patient calls to schedule an appointment, pull up the patient's record in order to have all the information available to schedule the appointment efficiently.
- Pre-block the schedule according to procedures and time allotments, using "RDT (Root Debridement Therapy), SPT (Supportive Periodontal Therapy), & NPE (New Patient Exam)".
- Be responsible for keeping hygienist scheduled to goal.
- Make sure appointments are made for new patients within three days of their initial call.
- Attend the morning meeting and discuss the hygiene production numbers from the previous day and the current day, and opportunities for today and tomorrow. Ask others in the meeting for ideas to assist with scheduling.
- Keep a record of patients who don't schedule hygiene appointments prior to leaving the office.
- Form an "ASAP call" list for any appointment that can be moved forward.
- Confirm appointments according to office policy.
- Manage late patients/no shows/last-minute cancellations, using correct verbal skills.
- At the end of each business day, provide each hygienist with a copy of the schedule with patients' telephone numbers to call that evening to see how well they are doing.
- Schedule all hygiene appointments.

B. Emergencies Responsibilities

- True emergencies should always be seen as soon as possible.

C. Financial Management Responsibilities

- Collect over-the-counter payments to meet daily and monthly collection goals.
- Accurately post appointment procedures and print insurance claim forms for patients as needed.
- Notify the financial coordinator of any patients with unsettled balances that want to schedule treatment.
- Cover for the financial or scheduling coordinator during breaks and lunch periods.

D. Continuing and Re-care Responsibilities

- Be accountable for keeping a continuing care system and follow up appointments.
- Appoint next hygiene visit at time of current visit.
- Perform regular chart audits to reactivate patients who are overdue for preventive maintenance, or periodontal care.
- Be responsible for the re-care system.

E. Office Procedures Responsibilities

- Arrange financial consultations with financial coordinator for any recommended restorative treatment, using a "2 on 1" transfer of power.
- Be accountable for keeping the hygienist scheduled to goal; make adjustments as necessary during the day to assure that goals are reached.
- Record chart notations for important items, pre-medication, medical alerts, and any other notification that will help in treating patients.
- Keep all patients' records up to date.
- Confirm that requested x-rays have been received.
- Help direct patient flow for the hygienist and hygiene assistant.
- As changes in the schedule occur during the workday, note the changes on the daily posted schedules.
- Ensure that all the essential forms for the next workday are ready before closing the office.
- Keep the hygienist informed and current on all aspects of the office, patient status, recommendations, scheduling, etc.
- Assist the financial coordinator as time permits.
- Concentrate on the current patient, whether in person or on the phone. This person is always the first priority. Patients on the phone should not be put on hold while another call is answered or another patient is waiting. The phone system will take messages while the current patient's needs are being addressed.

F. Overall Practice Responsibilities

- Greet and dismiss patients cheerfully.
- Present a positive image of dental services to be rendered.
- Present a positive relationship with other team members and the doctor in front of patients.
- Be punctual to work, with patient checkout, and with schedule.
- Uses downtime constructively.
- Engage only in positive conversation regarding another team member.
- Maintain a clean, well-groomed professional manner.
- Do not allow personal phone use to interfere with work.
- Assist other front desk personnel with the following if time permits: make and confirm doctor appointments, make financial arrangements.
- Perform light housekeeping such as vacuuming, removing trash, cleaning kitchen area and patient/employee bathrooms.

CREDENTIALS and REQUIREMENTS: To perform this position successfully, an individual must be able to perform each duty within expectations. The terms listed below are representative of the knowledge, skill, and experience required in this role. Reasonable arrangements may be made to enable individuals with disabilities to perform the essential functions.

EDUCATION and/or EXPERIENCE: High school diploma or graduate equivalent degree and 6 months data entry experience; 6 months to 1 year experience in basic use of computers; 6 months experience with dental insurance billing helpful; or equivalent combination of education and experience.

LANGUAGE SKILLS: Ability to read and interpret standardized forms, insurance and/or computer procedures, and governmental regulations. Ability to write letters and memos in response to patient and/or insurance company inquiries. Ability to communicate with patients, team members, visitors, maintenance personnel, and insurance personnel without interference or language barriers. Sufficient understanding of dental terminology and procedures to communicate with dental and medical professionals, team members, and insurance personnel.

MATHEMATICAL SKILLS: Ability to add, subtract, multiply, and divide in all units of measure, using whole numbers, common fractions, and decimals.

LICENSES and CERTIFICATIONS

- Cardio-Pulmonary Resuscitation (CPR) Certification

REPORTS TO: Hygiene & Business Office Team Leader / Office Manager / Practice Owner

HOURS:

I have read and understand the Team Member Objectives information presented to me so that I can perform my role to the highest standards of this practice.

______________________________ _______________

Scheduling Coordinator/Hygiene Signature | Date

______________________________ _______________

Practice Owner / Office Manager Signature | Date

SCHEDULING COORDINATOR/RESTORATIVE

<Team Member Name>

Design of the Position: The Restorative Scheduling Coordinator is responsible for successful scheduling of the doctor(s) to goal on a daily basis. The Restorative Scheduling Coordinator uses every resource available to accomplish that objective: reviewing the "ASAP-call" list, checking upcoming weeks of the schedule to move patients forward, getting new patients in sooner, reviewing the unscheduled patient list, informing the entire team of the opportunities, and performing more treatment on patients currently in today's schedule (if permitted).

ESSENTIAL PERFORMANCE AND RESPONSIBILITIES are as follows. Other duties may be appointed:

A. Appointment Scheduling Responsibilities

- Make sure that the phone is answered before the third ring at all times, with a smile.
- Whenever a patient calls to schedule an appointment, pull the patient's chart, so that all information needed to schedule the appointment efficiently is available.
- In order to consistently schedule to goal, pre-block the schedule according to procedures and time allotments, using the "rock, sand and, water" principle.
- Schedule treatment by room availability.
- Ensure that new patient appointments are scheduled within three days of their initial call.
- Attend the morning meeting and discuss the production numbers from the previous and the current day, and opportunities that are available the current day and following day. Solicit assistance from everyone on the team with the schedule.
- Keep a record of patients who don't schedule treatment prior to leaving the office to use as a source when trying to fill the schedule.
- Form an "ASAP call" list for any appointment that can be moved forward.
- Confirm restorative appointments according to office policy (left messages are not considered confirmed).
- Manage late patients/no shows/last-minute cancellations, using correct verbal skills.
- Post the daily schedule in designated areas and make sure each doctor has a copy.
- At the end of each business day, provide the doctor with a copy of the schedule with the patients' telephone numbers to call that evening to see how well they are doing.

B. Emergencies Responsibilities

- True emergencies should always be seen as soon as possible.

C. Financial Management Responsibilities

- Collect over-the-counter payments to meet daily and monthly collection goals.
- Accurately post appointment procedures and print/submit insurance claim forms for patients as needed.
- Notify the financial coordinator of any patients with unsettled balances that want to schedule treatment.
- Cover for any business office personnel during breaks and lunch periods.

D. Marketing Responsibilities

- Participate with the marketing team to coordinate all practice marketing systems.
- Share positive and negative information received from patients to improve "5 Star Service" in the practice.
- Complete the Telephone Information Slip on all new patients and emergency patients.
- Encourage all new patients to schedule a comprehensive examination.
- Encourage acceptance of needed treatment and encourage patients to schedule immediately because treatment prolonged will only be more extensive and expensive.
- Trace referral source of all new patients and prepare a month-end report by computer or manually.

E. Continuing Care and Re-care Responsibilities

- Be responsible for working on the continuing care system and follow-up appointments.
- Appoint next hygiene visit at time of current visit.
- Perform regular chart audits to reactivate patients who haven't been in during the last 12 months.

F. Office Procedures Responsibilities

- Schedule all restorative appointments, keeping an "ASAP call" list for short notice fill-ins.
- Arrange financial consultations with financial coordinator for any recommended restorative treatment, using a "2 on 1" transfer of power.
- Be accountable for keeping the doctors scheduled to their goals. Make adjustments as necessary during the day to assure that goals are reached.
- Keep all patient records up to date.
- Help direct patient flow for the doctors and assistants.
- As changes in the schedule occur during the day, note the changes on the daily posted schedules in the sterilization area or other designated areas.
- Make sure that all the essential forms for the next day are ready before closing the office.
- Keep the doctor(s) informed and current on all aspects of the office, patient

status, recommendations, scheduling, etc.
- Assist the financial coordinator and any other member of the team as time permits.
- Assist the current patient, whether in person or on the phone. That patient is your first priority. Do not put your phone patient on hold while you answer another call or deal with another patient who is waiting.

G. Overall Practice Responsibilities
- Welcome and dismiss patients cheerfully.
- Present a positive image of dental services to be rendered.
- Present a positive relationship with other team members and your doctor in front of patients.
- Be punctual to work, and with patient scheduling and check-out.
- Use downtime constructively.
- Engage only in positive conversation regarding another team member.
- Maintain a clean, well-groomed professional manner.
- Do not allow personal phone use to interfere with work.
- Assist front desk with the following if time permits: Greet patients as they enter office, answer phone, take messages, make and confirm appointments, make financial arrangements.
- Perform light housekeeping such as vacuuming, removing trash, cleaning kitchen area and patient/employee bathrooms.
- Show interest and be willing to participate in meetings, seminars, etc.

CREDENTIALS and REQUIREMENTS: To perform this position successfully, an individual must be able to perform each duty within expectations. The terms listed below are representative of the knowledge, skill, and experience required in this role. Reasonable arrangements may be made to enable individuals with disabilities to perform the essential functions.

EDUCATION and/or EXPERIENCE: High school diploma or graduate equivalent degree and 6 months data entry experience; experience in basic use of computers.

Experience in basic use of computers; 6 months experience with dental insurance billing helpful; or equivalent combination of education and experience.

LANGUAGE SKILLS: Ability to read and interpret standardized forms, insurance and/or computer procedures, and governmental regulations. Ability to write reports and memos in response to insurance inquiries. Ability to communicate with patients, team members, visitors, maintenance personnel, and insurance personnel without interference or language barriers. Sufficient understanding of dental terminology and procedures to communicate with dental and medical professionals.

MATHEMATICAL SKILLS: Ability to add, subtract, multiply, and divide in all units of measure, using whole numbers, common fractions, and decimals.

LICENSES and CERTIFICATIONS

- Cardio-Pulmonary Resuscitation (CPR) Certification
- Valid Driver's License

REPORTS TO: Business Office Team Leader / Office Manager / Practice Owner

HOURS:

I have read and understand the Team Member Objectives information presented to me so that I can perform my role to the highest standards of this practice.

____________________________________ __________________

Scheduling Coordinator/Restorative Signature Date

____________________________________ __________________

Practice Owner / Office Manager Signature Date

FINANCIAL COORDINATOR

<Team Member Name>

Design of the Position: The Financial Coordinator position includes many important aspects; sound financial arrangements and collecting money are the financial foundation of the business. The Financial Coordinator has the responsibility to make thorough financial arrangements with patients, collect money in advance and at time of treatment, collect outstanding accounts, file insurance claims properly, and perform follow-up. With the financial goals of the business in mind, these tasks need to be performed at a high level for the best interest of the patient and the practice.

ESSENTIAL PERFORMANCE AND RESPONSIBILITIES are as follows. Other duties may be appointed:

A. Financial Arrangements Responsibilities

- Make specific and thorough financial arrangements with all patients, who have agreed to the treatment recommended, according to the financial policy of the office.
- Be accountable for requesting and collecting money over the counter.
- Ensure that patients receive a copy of any written financial arrangement prior to exiting the office.
- Be accountable for the distribution and explanation of weekly and monthly computer data regarding collections, accounts receivable, and adjustments.
- Be accountable for the safekeeping and accounting of all cash, check, and credit card transactions.
- Be accountable for entries and messages into the computer regarding financial arrangements and insurance information.
- Balance cash on hand each day.
- Make sure that the bank deposit records match the day sheet total.
- Compare accounts payable invoices to bills, if appointed.
- Subtract the In-the-Mail (ITM) amount tallied from the deposit to determine the Over-the-Counter (OTC) rate for the day. Give this OTC amount to the person responsible for entering the Monthly Assessment Reports and daily team bonus records.

B. Collection Control Responsibilities

- Ensure that all fees for dental care planned or provided are collected on or before the day of treatment.
- Properly estimate any patient's estimated portion of payment due after insurance if the practice accepts assignment from the insurance company.
- Ensure that at least 60% of all collections are received over the counter (in the office).
- Ensure that the accounts receivable monthly production ratio is no more than .6X average monthly production.
- Oversee and keep current all collection issues. Make sure that all agreements not kept are addressed and resolved with the patient.

- Run an aged monthly receivables report (30-60-90 days) and be prepared to review with the doctor, office manager, and scheduling coordinator on a monthly basis.
- Use a collection tracking system so that any team member can see the current status and arrangements for all patients regarding treatment and their account.
- Forward uncollectible accounts to collection agency, when necessary and with the practice owner's permission.
- Ensure that each patient record has today's treatment and fee posted prior to the appointment, and that there is no outstanding balance on the patient's account.
- Provide receipts to patients before they leave the office.
- Write off any accounts that cannot be collected, when necessary and with practice owner's permission.
- Represent doctor in small claims court, if necessary and/or appointed.
- Post all insurance checks received in the mail to correct accounts; deposit checks on the day they are received.
- Post daily charges and receipts to practice accounting software.
- Prepare aged receivables report 30-60-90 days with most recent payment activity, if requested by doctor.

C. Insurance Control Responsibilities

- Preserve, monitor and follow up with practice insurance systems.
- Keep the master insurance file current.
- Estimate patient portion of treatment needed, verify insurance coverage, ask patient to sign, and give patient a copy.
- Be responsible for handling all insurance claims received and sent.
- Correspond with insurance companies regarding claims and contact insurance adjusters when necessary.
- Send overpayments to patients when necessary or credit their account.
- Follow up on claims not paid within 45 days, or according to office policy.
- Make sure that the patient understands and agrees that insurance coverage is an agreement between the patient and the insurance company; the full amount is ultimately the responsibility of the patient.

D. Marketing Responsibilities

- Promote acceptance of recommended treatment by making good financial arrangements and using correct dental terminology.
- Present a positive image of dental services rendered and work with patients to find an ultimate, suitable solution.
- Highlight the benefits of treatment in terms of what motivates patients to proceed with treatment.
- Have the ability to put patients at ease, reaffirm their decision to proceed, and prevent buyer's remorse.
- Respond to account inquiries from office team, patients, and insurance companies when needed.

E. Overall Practice Responsibilities

- Inform the doctor and team when a scheduled patient has arrived, as needed.
- Complete and input telephone information on all new patients and emergency patients.
- Encourage new patients to schedule a comprehensive exam.
- Schedule next treatment, if applicable.
- Dissuade patients from canceling and rescheduling their appointments by using suitable verbiage per office protocol.
- When making financial arrangements, be sure to include any previous outstanding balance to the total amount arranged.
- Make sure that the front desk is covered at all times; cover the scheduling coordinator position during breaks and lunch.
- Keep patient records up to date.
- Provide the doctor with a copy of the day sheet daily, showing procedures billed, patient payments, and a breakdown of OTC and ITM collections.
- Check records daily to be prepared to approach any patient with an overdue balance.
- Make sure that all necessary forms for the next day are ready before closing the office.
- Organize and maintain file systems for quick retrieval of information.
- Keep the practice owner informed and current on all aspects of the office, patient status, recommendations, delinquent accounts, etc.
- Be responsible for keeping desk area organized and clean.
- Have financial arrangement forms and supplies in neat and orderly fashion so retrieval is quick.
- Enter and maintain fee schedules in computer system.
- Run and maintain computer back-up media for office computer system.
- Work with computer technician during system upgrades, troubleshooting, and general system maintenance.
- Ensure appointment dates are on patient recall notices.
- Answer telephone within three rings, take messages, and communicate with insurance representatives.
- Download, send electronically, or print x-rays that need to be sent to insurance company.
- Be able to communicate clearly regarding accounting information.
- Be able to quickly write thorough information in a legible, condensed form.
- Be punctual to work, with financial arrangements, and in dismissing patients.
- Be able to work safely and follow established safety and office protocols.
- Have good memory skills.
- Present a positive relationship with other team members and doctor in front of patients.
- Use downtime constructively.
- Engage only in positive conversation regarding another team member.
- Maintain a clean, well-groomed professional manner.

- Do not allow personal phone use to interfere with work.
- Assist the rest of the business office with their duties, when time permits.
- Perform light housekeeping such as vacuuming, removing trash, cleaning kitchen area and patient/employee bathrooms.
- Show interest in and be willing to participate in meetings, seminars, and presentations.

CREDENTIALS and REQUIREMENTS: To perform this position successfully, an individual must be able to perform each duty within expectations. The terms listed below are representative of the knowledge, skill, and experience required in this role. Reasonable arrangements may be made to enable individuals with disabilities to perform the essential functions.

EDUCATION and/or EXPERIENCE: High school diploma or graduate equivalent degree and 6 months data entry experience; 6 months to 1 year experience in basic use of computers; 6 months experience with dental insurance billing helpful; or equivalent combination of education and experience.

LANGUAGE SKILLS: Ability to read and interpret standardized forms, insurance and/or computer procedures, and governmental regulations. Ability to write letters and memos in response to patient and/or insurance company inquiries. Adequate understanding of English language to respond to questions from patients and insurance companies regarding accounts, and from computer technicians regarding the computer system. Adequate experience using dental terminology and procedures to communicate with team, insurance company personnel, and medical and dental professionals.

MATHEMATICAL SKILLS: Capability to add, subtract, multiply, and divide in all units of measure, using whole numbers, common fractions, and decimals. Capability to compute rate, ratio, and percent.

LICENSES and CERTIFICATIONS

- Cardio-Pulmonary Resuscitation (CPR) Certification

REPORTS TO: Business Office Team Leader / Office Manager / Practice Owner

HOURS:

I have read and understand the Team Member Objectives information presented to me so that I can perform my role to the highest standards of this practice.

______________________________ _______________

Financial Coordinator Signature Date

______________________________ _______________

Practice Owner / Office Manager Signature Date

RECEPTIONIST

<Team Member Name>

Design of the Position: The Receptionist greets all patients pleasantly and with a smile. Whenever possible, the receptionist is the first team member to answer the phone. The Receptionist informs the team when the patient has arrived and makes sure that all team members have the correct information for that patient in the system.

ESSENTIAL FUNCTIONS AND RESPONSIBILITIES are as follows. Other duties may be appointed:

A. Preparation Responsibilities

- Welcome patients when arriving as if you have been expecting them (using their name).
- Enter all new patients' information into their electronic record.
- Call and get breakdown of insurance benefits from insurance companies.
- Answer phone calls by the third ring.
- Make sure that all necessary forms for the next day are ready before closing the office.
- Make sure that the front desk is covered at all times; cover any business office staff positions during breaks and lunch.
- Order all business office supplies, if applicable.
- Make sure that the reception area is neat and orderly throughout the day and before leaving the office.

B. Marketing Responsibilities

- Complete the Telephone Information Slip and enter information electronically on all new patients and emergency patients.
- Track referral sources of new patients on the computer or manually and prepare a month-end report.
- Track names of patients who left the practice and their reason for leaving. Ask patients to help you with valuable feedback on their reasons for leaving. Let them know, "If for any reason you are not happy where you are going, we'd be happy to welcome you back."
- Be responsible for monitoring need for, and distribution of, patient communications, including new patient welcome packets and sedation patient packets (if applicable).
- Keep the new patient control sheet current.

C. Overall Practice Responsibilities

- Maintain a neat and orderly appearance of the front desk area.
- Create and assemble new patient records and check for completeness.
- Welcome and dismiss patients cheerfully.
- Present a positive image of dental services to be rendered.
- Present a positive relationship with other team members and the doctor in front of patients.
- Be punctual to work, with checking patients in and out, and putting new patient information into computer.

- Use downtime constructively.
- Engage only in positive conversation regarding another team member.
- Maintain a clean, well-groomed professional manner.
- Do not allow personal phone use to interfere with work.
- Assist other team members of the business office when needed.
- Be able to schedule patients to goal for each provider.
- Be able to accept payment per the office protocol.
- Be able to call and confirm patients for scheduling.
- Perform light housekeeping such as vacuuming, removing trash, cleaning kitchen area and patient/employee bathrooms.
- Show interest in and be willing to participate in meetings, seminars, and presentations.

CREDENTIALS and REQURIMENTS: To perform this position successfully, an individual must be able to perform each duty within expectations. The terms listed below are representative of the knowledge, skill, and experience required in this role. Reasonable arrangements may be made to enable individuals with disabilities to perform the essential functions.

EDUCATION and/or EXPERIENCE: High school diploma or graduate equivalent degree and 6 months data entry experience; 6 months to 1 year experience in basic use of computer.

LANGUAGE SKILLS: Ability to read and interpret standardized forms, insurance, computer procedures, and governmental forms. Ability to write letters or emails using dental terminology correctly. Ability to communicate with patients, team members, visitors, maintenance personnel, and insurance personnel without interference or language barriers.

Sufficient understanding of dental terminology and procedures to communicate with dental and medical professionals.

MATHEMATICAL SKILLS: Ability to add, subtract, multiply, and divide in all units of measure, using whole numbers, common fractions, and decimals.

LICENSES, CERTIFICATIONS, and REGISTRATION

- Cardio-Pulmonary Resuscitation (CPR) Certification

REPORTS TO: Business Office Team Leader / Office Manager / Practice Owner

HOURS:

I have read and understand the Team Member Objectives information presented to me so that I can perform my role to the highest standards of this practice.

______________________________ ________________

Receptionist Signature Date

______________________________ ________________

Practice Owner / Office Manager Signature Date

DENTAL/LAB ASSISTANT

<Team Member Name>

Design of the Position: The Dental/Lab Assistant will assist the doctor chairside to deliver quality, comfortable care in a stress-free environment. This will include readiness and cleanliness of the operatory and preparation of patient for dental treatment. This team member needs to be able and willing to perform chairside assistance, capturing x-rays, recording information in patient charts, performing expanded duties if qualified, and opening/closing the office. In addition to dental assisting, this team member will have full accountability over the lab including the flow of the lab, communication with doctors and outside labs, and making sure all lab cases are at the office in a timely manner.

ESSENTIAL PERFORMANCE AND RESPONSIBILTIES are as follows. Other duties may be appointed:

A. Lab Responsibilities

- Pour-up impressions as they are received in the lab in a timely manner.
- Manually fabricate bite-guards, study models, bleach trays, custom trays, and other lab procedures and have ready before the due date.
- Use 3D printer to create implant guides, bite-guards, custom trays, study models, temporary crowns and bridges, and other lab procedures and have ready before due date.
- Make sure that outside laboratories receive and return cases on time.
- Make sure that all models and opposing models are mounted appropriately with bite registrations or by lab recommendations.
- Stock and clean the lab daily.
- Be responsible for the organization of model closet and keep it up to date.
- Mix impression material and assist as needed.
- Record and file all lab slips daily in the appropriate location.
- Clean out impression trays and facebows daily so that they are available.
- Put all models away and make sure that they are filed accurately and neatly.
- Maintain lab equipment and keep in good condition.
- Change plaster trap as needed.
- Inform doctor about cases that are due to go out that day or the next day that need attention.
- Call and communicate with all outside laboratory technicians on a regular basis.
- Maintain quality control over all impressions and models submitted to in-house and outside lab.
- Have a check-in system and out-going cases system in place so anyone can go into lab and help if downtime occurs.

B. Preparation Responsibilities

- Turn on all cart, x-ray, intra-oral units, wall switches, ultrasonic, autoclave, and other equipment for the start of the day.
- Evaluate sterilization area for cleanliness and organization at start of day and throughout the day.

- Make sure all the treatment rooms are ready, stocked and clean (certain rooms may apply to specific assistants).
- Seat patients and review with them the treatment that is going to be performed. Ask if there are any questions or concerns, and make sure doctor is made aware of any.
- Be responsible for the appearance of the treatment rooms.

C. Assisting Responsibilities

- Assist the doctor at all times.
- Anticipate the doctor's needs at all times, looking forward to the next step.
- Capture digital x-rays, download, and display for the doctor.
- Take impressions, if qualified.
- Fabricate temporary crowns and bridges, if qualified.
- Assist doctor with administration of nitrous oxide and any other medications that need to be given during appointment time, if qualified.
- Perform all expanded duties, if qualified.
- Show an interest in and participate in meetings.
- Be willing to participate in seminars and presentations that facilitate professional and personal growth.
- Be able to calm and reassure patients throughout dental procedures.
- Be able to work safely and follow safety and office protocol.

D. Charting Responsibilities

- Chart all existing restorations and treatment to be performed; record the date, service rendered, and fee, if suitable.
- Make sure the patient's record is complete and all services for that day of treatment are recorded prior to dismissing the patient. Include the next appointment to be scheduled, the treatment to be provided, and the time units needed to perform the treatment.
- Ensure that all chart notes are comprehensive and accurate for each procedure. If additional information is necessary, be responsible for seeking the proper person for advice.
- Complete all routing and lab slips before patient leaves the treatment room.
- Ensure that all paperwork arrives at the front desk at the same time as the departing patient or, preferably, before.

E. Patient Care Responsibilities

- Welcome, seat, and dismiss patients cheerfully.
- Show care, concern, and respect for patients' well-being and comfort at all times.
- Make sure that the patient is thoroughly suctioned out with no remaining debris present intra-orally.
- Ensure that the patient's face is clean and free of debris before exiting treatment room to the front desk; provide hand mirror and moist towel if needed.
- If patients wishes to rinse their mouth, direct them to the sink, mouthwash, and cups.

- Give post-operative instructions for any procedure performed, and ensure patient understands the instructions for the rest of the day and for the time between visits.
- Review follow-up appointments, what to do if questions or concerns arise, and how important it is to get needed treatment scheduled before it causes more extensive and expensive care.
- Escort the patient to the front desk and do a "2 on 1" transfer of power with the next team member, discussing treatment performed today, future treatment and appointments needed, appropriate financial arrangements, etc. Reassure patient that all their needs will be taken care of and that you will see them soon.
- Contact patients at the end of the day to see how well they are doing.

F. Sterilization Responsibilities

- Follow OSHA guidelines for all procedures.
- Ensure that mask, gloves, gown, and safety glasses are worn and accessible at all times during dental procedures, clean-up of treatment rooms, and sterilizing instruments.
- Be responsible for the appearance and organization of the sterilization area.
- Be responsible for the sterilization of instruments and set-up of trays.
- Clean sinks in treatment areas and sterilization area.
- Remove trash, clean and disinfect treatment rooms and sterilization area.

G. Overall Practice Responsibilities

- Greet, seat, and dismiss patients cheerfully.
- Present a positive image of dental services to be rendered.
- Present a positive relationship with other team members and doctor in front of patients.
- Be punctual to work and with patient seating and dismissal.
- Use downtime constructively.
- Engage only in positive conversation regarding another team member.
- Maintain a clean, well-groomed professional manner.
- Do not allow personal phone use to interfere with work.
- Assist business office with the following if time permits: Greet patients as they enter office, answer phone, take messages, make and confirm appointments, make financial arrangements.
- Perform light housekeeping such as vacuuming, removing trash, cleaning kitchen area and patient/employee bathrooms.

H. Equipment Responsibilities (if appointed, assistants may have specific duties)

- Maintain and keep record of all handpieces, attachments and maintenance.
- Monitor curing light units for sufficient light intensity.
- Clean and/or change vacuum traps and suction units every week.
- Be responsible for a maintenance plan for all equipment.

I. **Ordering Responsibilities.**
   - Be responsible for ordering all clinical supplies.
   - Keep track of back-ordered items and returned items.
   - Search for best prices and discounts on all supplies.

CREDENTIALS and REQUIREMENTS: To perform this position successfully, an individual must be able to perform each duty within expectations. The terms listed below are representative of the knowledge, skill, and experience required in this role. Reasonable arrangements may be made to enable individuals with disabilities to perform the essential functions.

EDUCATION and/or EXPERIENCE: High school diploma or graduate equivalent degree and completion of accredited dental assistant program; 2 years general dentistry experience with some specialized experience preferred, or 4 years related experience and/or training; or combination of education and experience.

LANGUAGE SKILLS: Ability to read and interpret general business periodicals, professional journals, technical procedures, and governmental regulations. Ability to write reports such as detailed information in patient records, and communicate with patients without interference or language barriers.

MATHEMATICAL SKILLS: Ability to add, subtract, multiply, and divide in all units of measure, using whole numbers, common fractions, and decimals.

LICENSES, CERTIFICATIONS, and REGISTRATION (may vary by state)
- State Registered or Certification from an accredited dental assistant program
- X-ray Certification
- Cardio-Pulmonary Resuscitation (CPR) Certification
- Sedation Certification, if appropriate.

REPORTS TO: Assistant Team Leader / Office Manager / Practice Owner

HOURS:

I have read and understand the Team Member Objectives information presented to me so that I can perform my role to the highest standards of this practice.

______________________________ ______________

Assistant's Signature Date

______________________________ ______________

Practice Owner / Office Manager Signature Date

PATIENT CARE SPECIALIST

<Team Member Name>

Design of the Position: The Patient Care Specialist (PCS) is the first team member in personal contact with the new patient and acts as liaison between patient and doctor. The PCS sets a tone of comfort and concern toward the new patient through easy conversation and a non-threatening attitude. The PCS is to discover exactly what the patient wants to accomplish at the appointment and in the future. The PCS is to complete radiographs, hard tissue, soft tissue, temporomandibular, and periodontal exams (may vary due to team member responsible for this position and state laws), as well as any intra-oral pictures needed. The PCS will discuss the findings, being careful not to diagnose (the doctor will make the ultimate determination about clinical findings, their interpretation, and recommended treatment), in an educational manner and careful not to intimidate or overwhelm the patient. Excellent patient education and motivation is as important as providing treatment. The PCS is to help phase treatment according to patient's budget and explain financial arrangements for the treatment. When the new patient exam is complete the PCS is to escort the patient to the financial coordinator's desk to schedule the first appointment and/or apply for financing. The PCS is responsible to follow up on the new patient if no appointment was scheduled that day and to present the doctor with a spreadsheet of information regarding new patients scheduled and not scheduled.

ESSENTIAL PERFORMANCE AND RESPONSIBILITIES are as follows. Other duties may be appointed:

A. Preparation and Appointment Responsibilities

- Welcome and seat patient cheerfully.
- Have treatment room set up and ready for new patient exam.
- Show care and concern for patient welfare and comfort at all times.
- Perform a head and neck/oral cancer exam.
- Capture digital x-rays, intraoral scan, CBCT, and display for doctor to view.
- Chart patient existing hard tissue restorations and note any areas of concern.
- Perform periodontal evaluation (probing depths, bleeding points, mobility, and recession) and communicate findings to patient and doctor.
- Document patient home care.
- Utilize technology (intra-oral camera, patient education software, etc.) as appropriate.
- Discuss and educate patient on any potential needed treatment.
- Perform oral prophylaxis, if appropriate.
- Administer fluoride treatment.
- Estimate patient insurance benefits and explain them.
- Review and update patient medical history.
- Phase treatment to fit patient budget.

- Follow up with patients who have not scheduled and make appointment within two weeks.
- Complete sedation paperwork and vitals for appropriate patient (may not apply to all offices).
- Communicate with doctors through new patient monitoring spreadsheet.

B. Hygiene Responsibilities

- Give anesthesia, if qualified, when asked for, or as hygiene treatment dictates.
- Perform root debridement therapy, if appropriate.
- Perform laser treatment, if appropriate.
- Call any root debridement patient that evening to see how well they are doing.
- Request "completion of treatment" letters from the scheduling coordinator when finishing periodontal treatment phase.
- Send personal notes to patients that deserve special treatment.
- Complete scheduled treatment for that day.
- Educate the patient on proper oral hygiene and corrective and/or preventive measures.
- Present appropriate literature to patients.
- Quote treatment fees to patients, upon request.
- Assist and chart for the doctor examination.
- Inform the scheduling coordinator of the appropriate re-care appointment for the patient, emphasizing the importance of continuing care at the appropriate treatment interval.
- Use appropriate verbal skills to educate and motivate patients.
- While still in the treatment room, make sure patient's records are complete and all services for the day's treatment are recorded in the appropriate areas, as well as the next continuing care or treatment visit with time units.
- Return paperwork to the front desk and escort the patient to appropriate team member for final processing, employing a "2 on 1" transfer of power.

C. Sterilization Responsibilities

- Assist the hygiene assistant in setting up and disinfecting treatment rooms and instrument trays in accordance with office policy and OSHA standards.
- Assist the hygiene assistant in sterilizing and disinfecting instruments and intra-oral devices in accordance with office policy and OSHA standards.
- Ensure that masks, gloves, gown, and safety glasses are worn and accessible at all times during dental procedures and cleanup of treatment rooms and instruments.

D. Overall Practice Responsibilities

- Assist other team members when time permits.
- Participate in morning meeting and provide information regarding new patients for the day, along with any comments about the patient.
- Call new patients to confirm two to three days prior to appointment, according to office policy.

- Send a personal note card to every new patient within one week of NPE.
- Greet, seat, and dismiss patients cheerfully.
- Present a positive image of dental services to be rendered.
- Present a positive relationship with other team members and doctor in front of patients.
- Be punctual to work and with patient seating and dismissing.
- Use downtime constructively.
- Engage only in positive conversation regarding another team member.
- Maintain a clean, well-groomed professional manner.
- Do not allow personal phone use to interfere with work.
- Assist business office with the following if time permits: Greet patients as they enter office, answer phone, take messages, make and confirm appointments, and make financial arrangements.
- Perform light housekeeping such as vacuuming, removing trash, cleaning kitchen area and patient/employee bathrooms.
- Be able to calm and reassure patients facing uncomfortable or painful dental procedures.
- Be able to quickly write and type detailed information in a readable, legible, condensed form.
- Be able to work safely and follow established safety and office procedures.

E. Equipment Responsibilities

- Clean and maintain handpieces.
- Sharpen hygiene instruments.

CREDENTIALS and REQUIREMENTS: To perform this position successfully, an individual must be able to perform each duty within expectations. The terms listed below are representative of the knowledge, skill, and experience required in this role. Reasonable arrangements may be made to enable individuals with disabilities to perform the essential functions.

EDUCATION and/or EXPERIENCE: High school diploma or graduate equivalent degree and completion of accredited dental hygiene program; 1-year general dentistry experience, or two years related experience and/or training; or equivalent combination of education and experience.

LANGUAGE SKILLS: Ability to read and interpret professional journals, technical procedures, and government regulations. Ability to write reports, such as detailed information in patient charts, and communicate with patients without interference or language barriers.

MATHEMATICAL SKILLS: Ability to add, subtract, multiply, and divide in all units of measure, using whole numbers, common fractions, and decimals.

LICENSES, CERTIFICATIONS, and REGISTRATION (may vary by state)

- State Registered Dental Hygiene License
- Cardio-Pulmonary Resuscitation (CPR) Certification
- Local Anesthesia Certification, if appropriate.
- Sedation Certification, if appropriate.
- Laser Treatment Certification, if appropriate.

REPORTS TO: Hygiene Team Leader / Office Manager / Practice Owner

HOURS:

I have read and understand the Team Member Objectives information presented to me so that I can perform my role to the highest standards of this practice.

______________________________ ______________

PCS Signature Date

______________________________ ______________

Practice Owner / Office Manager Signature Date

TEAM LEADER

<Team Member Name>

Design of the Position: The Team Leader is accountable for the success of the department they oversee. The Team Leader is the designated individual that the practice owner can seek out for answers or concerns regarding that person's team, and for a solution as well. The Team Leader interviews and recommends hiring and terminating team members. They are responsible for appropriate disciplinary action of their team, both verbal and in writing, including explanation of improvements needed as well as the consequences of not improving. They keep their team up to date on office policy changes, upcoming seminars, and any other information that the team needs to be aware of. They are the liaison between their team, the office manager (if applicable), and the practice owner.

ESSENTIAL PERFORMANCE RESPONSIBILITIES are as follows:

A. Be accountable for the team.

- Interview, hire and recommend termination of team members.
- Discipline with verbal warning and/or written warning, as required, and inform about consequences when improvements have not been made.
- Be accountable to the office manager and the practice owner.
- Conduct a monthly meeting which addresses challenges within the team and fosters communication between team and management.
- Meet privately with the doctor once a month and report any necessary information that the practice owner needs to know.
- Conduct a SWOT (strength, weakness, opportunity, and threat) analysis of the team twice a year or more often as needed.
- Be aware of the team member objectives and responsibilities of each team member and ensure that team members are fulfilling their job descriptions. If there are shortfalls, find solutions to improve that team member or make changes.
- Handle team member requests, such as a CE course or new equipment. Requests should be researched by the team member. If the team leader approves the request, team leader brings it to the doctor/team leader meeting.

B. Overall team leader responsibilities.

- Support the team.
- Support the doctor(s)/owner.
- Be available to team members for requests, challenges, and issues.
- Be a problem solver.
- Discipline as needed, both verbally and in writing, and request termination of team member's employment, if necessary.
- Handle conflicts among team members or teams.

- Report to the office manager and/or doctor/owner as needed.
- Motivate team members.
- Give 89 day and annual reviews to team members.
- Take responsibility for team problems and assure the doctor/owner that such a problem will not happen again.
- Set goals for the team and the office.
- Arrange and facilitate a monthly meeting with the department.
- Attend a monthly meeting with office manager and other team leaders.
- Attend a monthly meeting with practice owner/team leaders/associate dentists/ office manager.
- Train new team members.

CREDENTIALS and REQUIREMENTS: To perform this position successfully, an individual must be able to perform each duty within expectations. The terms listed below are representative of the knowledge, skill, and experience required in this role. Reasonable arrangements may be made to enable individuals with disabilities to perform the essential functions.

EDUCATION and/or EXPERIENCE: High school diploma or graduate equivalent degree and completion of accredited dental hygiene or dental assisting program for hygiene department and assistant department team leaders respectively. 1-year general dentistry experience, or two years related experience and/or training; or equivalent combination of education and experience.

LANGUAGE SKILLS: Ability to read and interpret professional journals, technical procedures, and government regulations. Ability to write reports, such as detailed information in patient charts, and communicate with patients without interference or language barriers.

MATHEMATICAL SKILLS: Ability to add, subtract, multiply, and divide in all units of measure, using whole numbers, common fractions, and decimals.

LICENSES, CERTIFICATIONS, and REGISTRATION (may vary by state)

- State Registered Dental Hygiene License (Hygiene Team Leader)
- Cardio-Pulmonary Resuscitation (CPR) Certification
- State Registered or Accredited Dental Assisting Certification (Dental Assistant Team Leader)
- Local anesthesia Certification, if appropriate.

REPORTS TO: Office Manager / Practice Owner

HOURS:

I have read and understand the Team Member Objectives information presented to me so that I can perform my role to the highest standards of this practice.

______________________________ ____________________

Team Leader Signature Date

______________________________ ____________________

Office Manager Signature Date

______________________________ ____________________

Practice Owner Signature Date

OFFICE MANAGER

<Team Member Name>

Design of the Position: The Office Manager operates as an executive assistant to the practice owner(s). Many of the practice owner's daily operations responsibilities may be assigned to the Office Manager. The Office Manager works under the advisement of the practice owner to coordinate activities of clerical and clinical personnel, including work schedules and hiring and terminating team members. The Office Manager upholds and supports all accounting systems, scheduling systems, dental management systems, human resources and payroll, answers telephones, and greets patients and other visitors.

ESSENTIAL PERFORMANCE AND RESPONSIBILITIES are as follows. Other duties may be appointed:

A. Managerial Responsibilities

- Be accountable for understanding all office operation systems in order to oversee them and assist at any time.
- Oversee patient satisfaction within the practice, including monitoring, and addressing complaints.
- Accountable for all internal marketing systems, and responsible for all external marketing systems in the practice.
- Arrange employee work schedules in cooperation with team leaders.
- Examine and organize office protocols and procedures such as payroll, flow of correspondence, and other business office services.
- Evaluate office production in cooperation with team leaders to revise procedures to improve workflow efficiency.
- Open and distribute mail.
- Compute and record monthly bonuses and 401(k) contributions.
- Prepare procedures for systematic preservation, protection, retrieval, transfer, and disposal of records.
- Prepare agenda and conduct team leader meetings.
- Record minutes of team meetings, print and distribute minutes to team members.
- Maintain office personnel records including vacation, sick leave, wages, bonuses, absence records, performance reviews, terminations, and transfers in accordance with applicable laws and regulations.
- Conduct reference checks and schedule appropriate pre-employment tests for job candidates.
- Plan and conduct new employee orientation to foster positive attitude toward practice goals.
- Ensure that all team members read and understand office policies as outlined in the Office Policy Manual.
- Schedule routine meetings with team leaders, team members, and doctor(s).
- Assist with preparation and facilitate team leader evaluations.

- Handle all employee relations issues such as policy interpretation, team morale, and benefits.
- Compile daily, weekly, monthly, quarterly, and year-end reports such as cash receipts, expenditures, and other items pertinent to operation of business.
- Be responsible for distribution and interpretation of weekly and monthly computer reports.
- Produce production reports for the office and for each provider.
- Produce office collections report, both in-the-mail (ITM) and over-the counter (OTC).
- Produce report on number of new patients and their referral sources.
- Handle team member requests.
- Participate in morning meetings.
- Schedule flights, arrange transportation, and make hotel reservations for seminars for doctor(s) and all team members.
- Maintain the Message on Hold System.
- Send thank-you letters to patients for referrals.
- Send sympathy and get-well cards to patients.
- Prepare paperwork for monthly and quarterly taxes.
- Maintain the bonus system.
- Control payroll on a biweekly basis.

B. Overall practice responsibilities

- Welcome patients and visitors when needed.
- Schedule appointments, make financial arrangements, and answer the telephone when needed.
- Coordinate patient flow.
- Update team member objectives as needed.
- Collect numbers for 401(k) census.
- Tally time hours for payroll purposes.
- Arrange and facilitate monthly meeting with team leaders, monthly meeting with doctor(s) and team leaders, and monthly meeting with doctor/owner.
- Present positive image of dental services to be rendered.
- Be punctual to work and with duties surrounding position.
- Use downtime constructively.
- Engage only in positive conversation regarding other team members.
- Maintain a clean, well-groomed professional manner.
- Do not allow personal phone use to interfere with work.
- Be capable of calming patients facing uncomfortable or painful dental procedures.
- Work safely and follow established safety and office protocols.
- Be capable of resolving personnel issues and arbitrating team member conflict with and without assistance from the practice owner.
- Present a positive relationship with doctor and team members in front of patients.

SUPERVISORY RESPONSIBILITIES: Direct the entire team and accomplish management responsibilities in agreement with the practice's policies and applicable laws. Responsibilities include interviewing, hiring, and terminating team members in conjunction with the team leaders. Train business office employees: plan, assign and direct work; assess performance; reward and discipline team members; address complaints and resolve issues.

CREDENTIALS and REQUIRMENTS: To perform this position successfully, an individual must be able to perform each duty within expectations. The terms listed below are representative of the knowledge, skill, and experience required of the individual. Reasonable arrangements may be made to enable individuals with disabilities to perform the essential functions.

EDUCATION and/or EXPERIENCE: Associate degree or 2 years of college, or equivalent from a 2-year college in business administration or accounting; 3 years dental management experience including experience in personnel/human resources and 1 to 2 years data entry, word processing and general computer experience.

LANGUAGE SKILLS: Ability to read, evaluate, and interpret general business periodicals, professional journals, technical procedures, and governmental regulations. Ability to produce reports, business correspondence, and procedure manuals according to office protocol. Ability to communicate with patients, team members, visitors, maintenance personnel, and insurance personnel without interference or language limitations. Sufficient understanding of dental terminology and procedures to communicate with dental and medical professionals.

MATHEMATICAL SKILLS: Ability to add, subtract, multiply, and divide in all units of measure, using whole numbers, common fractions, and decimals. Ability to compute rate, ratio, and percent.

LICENSES and CERTIFICATIONS

- Cardio-Pulmonary Resuscitation (CPR) Certification

REPORTS TO: Practice Owner

HOURS:

I have read and understand the Team Member Objectives information presented to me so that I can perform my role to the highest standards of this practice.

______________________________ ______________

Office Manager Signature Date

______________________________ ______________

Practice Owner Signature Date

CHIEF OPERATING OFFICER

<Team Member Name>

Design of the Position: The Chief Operating Officer (COO) acts as an executive supervisor in a large group or multi-facility practice. Many day-to-day operations duties may be transferred to the COO who works under the direction of the practice owner(s). The COO is the liaison between the practice owner(s) and each location and their team leaders, and if applicable, office managers. The COO coordinates the activities of all personnel in the organization including work scheduling and staffing, maintaining all accounting systems including general accounting, dental management systems, and payroll.

ESSENTIAL FUNCTIONS AND RESPONSIBILITIES are as follows. Other duties may be assigned:

- Be responsible for understanding ALL office operation systems in order to oversee them.
- Oversee internal marketing and customer satisfaction.
- Prepare employee work schedules in cooperation with team leaders.
- Analyze and organize office operations and procedures such as preparation of payrolls, flow of correspondence, and other clerical services.
- Evaluate office production in cooperation with team leaders to revise procedures or devise new methods of improving workflow efficiency.
- Open and distribute mail.
- Compute and record bonuses.
- Formulate procedures for systematic retention, protection, retrieval, transfer, and disposal of records.
- Prepare agenda and conduct team leader/office manager meetings.
- Record minutes of team meetings; print and distribute to staff members.
- Maintain office personnel records including paid time off, wages, bonuses, absence, performance reviews, terminations, and transfers in accordance with applicable laws and regulations.
- Conduct reference checks and schedule appropriate pre-employment tests for job candidates.
- Plan and conduct new employee orientation to foster positive attitude toward practice goals.
- Ensure that all team members read and understand office policies as outlined in the Office Policy Manual.
- Schedule routine meetings with team and doctor(s).
- Assist with preparation and facilitate team leader evaluations.
- Handle all employee relations issues such as policy interpretation, staff morale, conflict resolution, and benefits.

- Compile daily, weekly, monthly, quarterly, and year-end reports such as cash receipts, expenditures, and other items pertinent to operation of business.
- Be responsible for distribution and interpretation of weekly and monthly computer reports.
- Produce production reports for the office and for each provider.
- Produce office collections report, both in-the-mail (ITM) and over-the counter (OTC).
- Produce report on number of new patients and their referral sources.
- Handle team member requests.
- Participate in morning meetings.
- Schedule flights, arrange transportation, make hotel reservations for seminars.
- Prepare data for monthly and quarterly taxes.
- Be responsible for payroll.
- Maintain practice budget.
- Be responsible for overhead containment.
- Participate with practice owner in strategic planning and business development.
- Schedule and facilitate monthly meetings with team leaders, doctors and team leaders, and the monthly meeting of the entire team.

SECONDARY FUNCTIONS AND RESPONSIBILITIES:

- Greet patients and visitors.
- Schedule appointments and make financial arrangements with patients.
- Answer the telephone and take messages.
- Coordinate patient flow.
- Update job descriptions as needed.

SUPERVISORY RESPONSIBILITIES: Directly supervise dental team employees in accordance with the organization's policies and applicable laws. Responsibilities include interviewing and hiring all employees and training front office employees; planning, assigning, and directing work; appraising performance; rewarding and disciplining employees; addressing complaints and resolving problems.

QUALIFICATIONS AND REQUIREMENTS: To perform this job successfully, an individual must be able to perform each essential duty satisfactorily. The requirements listed below are representative of the knowledge, skill, and/or ability required. Reasonable accommodations may be made to enable qualified individuals with disabilities to perform the essential functions.

EDUCATION and/or EXPERIENCE: Minimum of 2 years of college or an associate degree (AA) or equivalent from 2-year college in business administration or accounting; 3 years dental management experience including experience in personnel/human resources and 1 to 2 years data entry, word processing and general computer experience; or 5 to 7 years related experience and/or training; or equivalent combination of education and experience.

LANGUAGE SKILLS: Ability to read, analyze, and interpret general business periodicals, professional journals, technical procedures, and governmental regulations. Ability to write reports, business correspondence, and procedure manuals. Sufficient command of English language to reassure patients and effectively present information and respond to questions from patients, employees, and the general public. Sufficient command of dental terminology and procedures to communicate with dental and medical professionals.

MATHEMATICAL SKILLS: Ability to add, subtract, multiply, and divide in all units of measure, using whole numbers, common fractions, and decimals. Ability to compute rate, ratio, and percent.

OTHER SKILLS and ABILITIES

- Ability to calm and reassure patients facing uncomfortable or painful dental procedures.
- Ability to work safely and follow established safety and office procedures.
- Ability to resolve personnel issues and mediate staff difficulties with and without assistance from the practice owner.

REPORTS TO: Practice Owner(s)

HOURS:

I have read and understand the Team Member Objectives information presented to me so that I can perform my role to the highest standards of this practice.

____________________________ ________________

Chief Operating Officer Signature Date

____________________________ ________________

Practice Owner Signature Date

ASSOCIATE DENTIST

<Team Member Name>

Design of the Position: Under direct supervision or working independently, the Associate Dentist diagnoses and treats dental conditions. The Associate Dentist designs treatment options for patients with other support personnel and prepares, presents, and administers treatment plans. In addition, this position requires great communication skills, leadership qualities, and an entrepreneurial spirit.

ESSENTIAL FUNCTIONS:

- Examine patients to diagnosis oral disease and recommend solutions as well as elective treatment.
- Provide treatment in accordance with standards of care, to include but not limited to:
  - Extraoral exams
  - Intraoral exams
  - Interpretation of digital radiographs including periapical, bitewing, 2D panoramic, 3D panoramic, and CBCT
  - Preventive treatment, including sealants, fluoride, and any other prophylactic dental treatment
  - Removal of tooth decay and filling with the appropriate restorative material
  - Administering local anesthetics
  - Administering sedative agents if qualified
  - Repair of fractured teeth with the appropriate restoration
  - Tooth extractions – non-surgical and surgical
  - Model preparation
  - All dental laboratory procedures the office performs
  - Prosthetic replacement of missing teeth including complete dentures, partial dentures, fixed crown and bridge, implant-retained overdentures, and fixed detachable dentures
  - Dental implant placement
  - Write prescriptions for appropriate medications including analgesic, antibiotic, anti-inflammatory, muscle relaxant, anti-emetic, and sedative.
  - Endodontic treatment except for those procedures more appropriate for endodontic referral such as retreatments
  - Pediatric dentistry
  - Laser dentistry including gingival troughing prior to impressions or scans, crown lengthening, biopsies, and tissue removal
  - Cosmetic dental procedures including bleaching, chairside labial composite veneers, porcelain veneers and crowns, Botox and dermal fillers (if qualified)
  - Treat temporomandibular dysfunction using orthotic appliances, muscle relaxants, trigger point injections, and Botox (if qualified)

  - Periodontal treatment to prevent, treat, and restore supportive structures
  - Surgical treatment including incision, flap reflection and management, suturing, sinus lifts and grafts, socket preservation grafts, ridge augmentation grafting, and alveoloplasty
  - Draw blood, start IVs, and administer sedative (oral and IV), analgesics and anti-emetic drugs intravenously, if trained and certified
  - Refer patient to specialists whenever it is in the patient's best interest
  - Manage asepsis and infection, using and maintaining hazard control protocols as established by OSHA and practice standards
- Represent the practice in a professional, pleasant, and cooperative manner.
- Maintain regular, consistent and punctual attendance in accordance with assigned schedule and time-off policies.
- Comfortably and efficiently handle multiple deadlines and task assignments.
- Work both independently and cooperatively in team settings.
- Travel when required to participate in continuing education.
- Other duties and tasks, as assigned and periodically required.

SUCCESS FACTORS:

- Maintain the highest level of confidentiality to HIPAA standards.
- Adhere to strict safety guidelines and procedures of OSHA and office standards.
- Be comfortable maintaining a professional demeanor and attitude while working around body fluids and odors that may be unpleasant.
- Be detail oriented in order to work efficiently in small spaces and maintain patient comfort and satisfaction.
- Meet all assigned production goals without sacrificing patient comfort or satisfaction.
- Be flexible and understand that job duties may change from time to time, requiring assistance in other areas of the office or lab.
- Excel in forward thinking in order to anticipate the needs of patients, as well as guiding office personnel during exams and treatments.
- Demonstrate active listening: giving full attention to what other people are saying, taking time to understand the points being made, asking questions as appropriate, and not interrupting at inappropriate times.
- Demonstrate good reading comprehension: understanding written sentences and paragraphs in work related documents.
- Demonstrate excellent communication skills: talking to others to convey information effectively, provide patient education, and respond to patient questions simply and effectively.
- Perform routine maintenance on dental equipment to maintain and adjust, as necessary.
- Be committed to the vision and goals of the practice, including production standards and goals.

SUPERVISORY RESPONSIBILITIES: Directly supervise dental team members in accordance with the organization's policies and applicable laws. Responsibilities include interviewing, hiring and training employees; planning, assigning, and directing work; appraising performance; rewarding and disciplining (as assigned by the practice owner); addressing complaints and resolving problems.

QUALIFICATIONS AND REQUIREMENTS: To perform this job successfully, an individual must be able to perform each essential duty satisfactorily. The requirements listed herein are representative of the knowledge, skill, and/or ability required. Reasonable accommodations may be made to enable qualified individuals with disabilities to perform the essential functions.

EDUCATION and/or EXPERIENCE: Minimum of 4 years of undergraduate and university degree. Graduation from a college of dentistry within the United States, and a certificate to practice dentistry in the state of the practice. Minimum of 2 years of experience as a practicing dentist.

LANGUAGE SKILLS: Ability to read, analyze, and interpret general business periodicals, professional journals, technical procedures, and governmental regulations. Ability to write reports, business correspondence, and procedure manuals. Sufficient command of English language to reassure patients, effectively present information, and respond to questions from patients, employees, and the general public. Sufficient command of dental terminology and procedures to communicate with dental and medical professionals.

MATHEMATICAL SKILLS: Ability to add, subtract, multiply, and divide in all units of measure, using whole numbers, common fractions, and decimals. Ability to compute rate, ratio, and percent.

REPORTS TO: Practice Owner

HOURS:

I have read and understand the Team Member Objectives information presented to me so that I can perform my role to the highest standards of this practice.

______________________________ __________________

Associate Dentist Signature Date

______________________________ __________________

Practice Owner Signature Date

SUNRISE DENTAL SOLUTIONS MONTHLY ASSESSMENT REPORT (MAR) EXAMPLE

Coach: Tony Feck

SDS
SUNRISE DENTAL SOLUTIONS

Monthly Assessment Report

Dr. [redacted]

December 2020

Table Of Contents

SUNRISE DENTAL SOLUTIONS Dr. [redacted] December 2020 Page 2

PRACTICE PRODUCTIVITY

Provider Days Worked

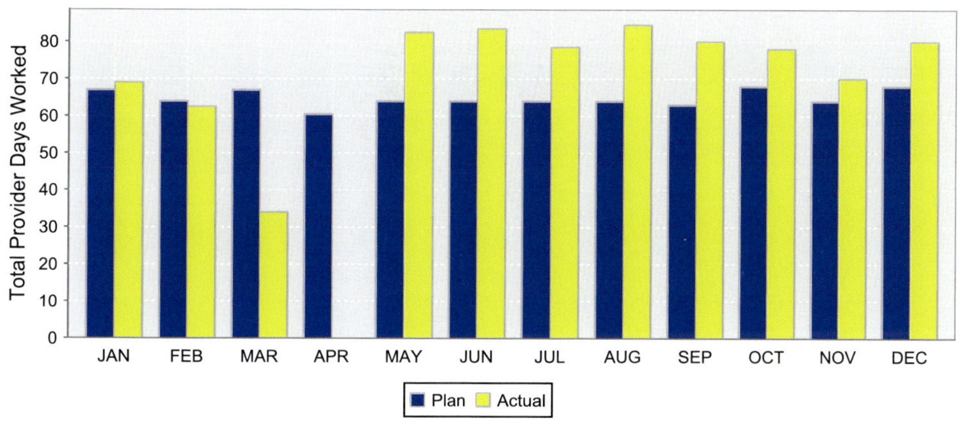

Dr. [redacted]

Days Worked December	16.0
+/- No./Plan for Month	(1.0)
Loss/Gain in Production	($9,489)

Days Worked YTD	158.0
+/- No./Plan for Year	(36.0)
Loss/Gain in Production	($341,605)

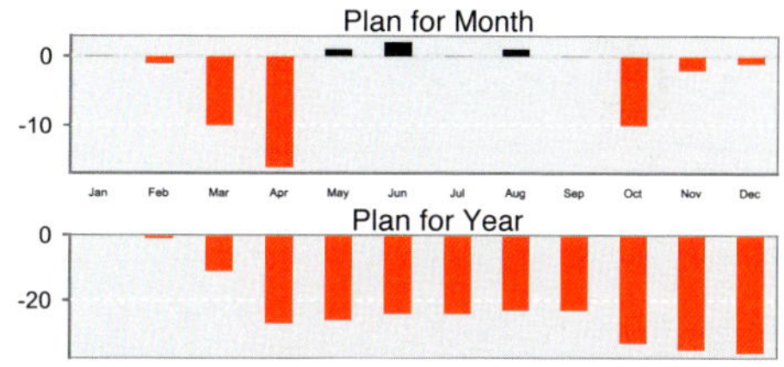

Dr. [redacted]

Days Worked December	16.0
+/- No./Plan for Month	(1.0)
Loss/Gain in Production	($7,558)

Days Worked YTD	176.5
+/- No./Plan for Year	(16.0)
Loss/Gain in Production	($120,931)

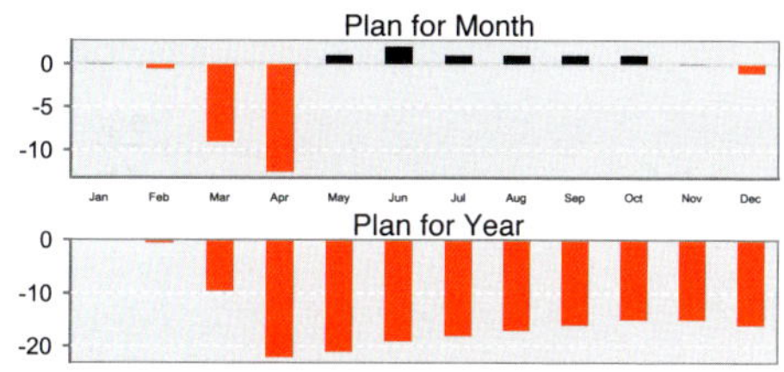

SUNRISE DENTAL SOLUTIONS Dr. [redacted] December 2020 Page 2A

PRACTICE PRODUCTIVITY

Provider Days Worked

Hygienist: [redacted]

Days Worked December	9.0
+/- No./Plan for Month	(8.0)
Loss/Gain in Production	($9,216)

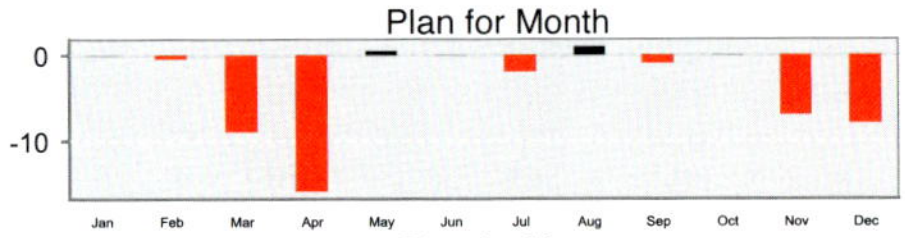

Days Worked YTD	153.0
+/- No./Plan for Year	(42.0)
Loss/Gain in Production	($48,385)

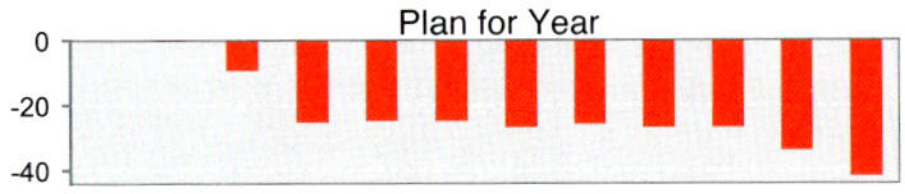

Hygienist: [redacted]

Days Worked December	7.0
+/- No./Plan for Month	(10.0)
Loss/Gain in Production	($11,365)

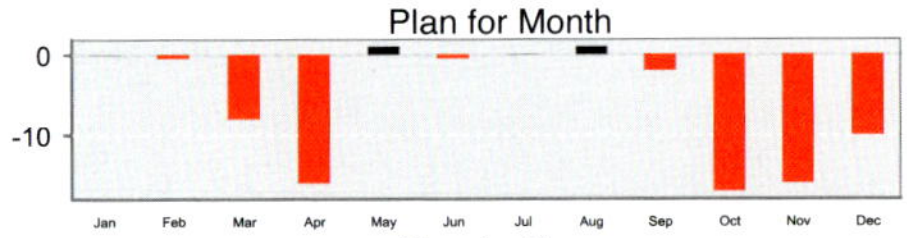

Days Worked YTD	128.0
+/- No./Plan for Year	(68.0)
Loss/Gain in Production	($77,280)

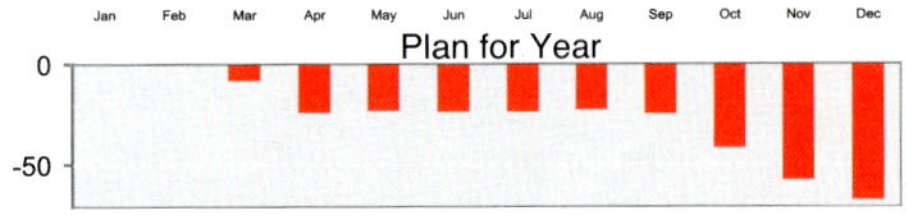

Hygienist: [redacted]

Days Worked December	0.0
+/- No./Plan for Month	0.0
Loss/Gain in Production	$0

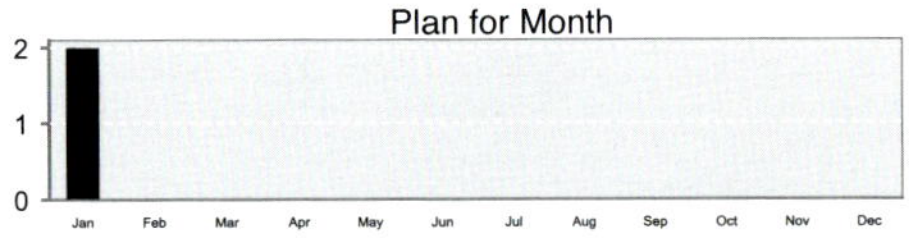

Days Worked YTD	2.0
+/- No./Plan for Year	2.0
Loss/Gain in Production	$0

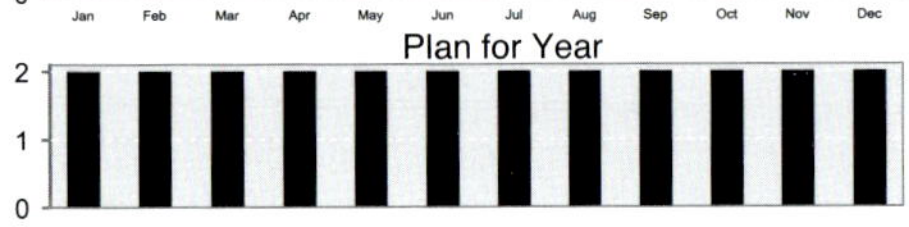

SUNRISE DENTAL SOLUTIONS Dr. [redacted] December 2020 Page 3

PRACTICE PRODUCTIVITY

Office Production

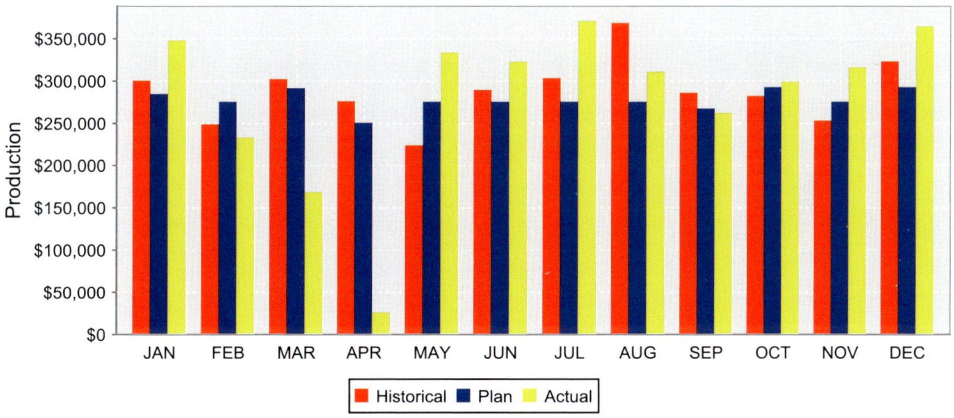

Month	Actual	Planned	$ Difference	% Difference	Average Production/Day	Historical	$ Difference	% Difference
January	347,274	284,400	62,874	22%	20,428	300,073	47,200	16%
February	232,664	275,200	(42,536)	(15%)	15,011	248,626	(15,963)	(6%)
March	167,915	291,300	(123,385)	(42%)	15,265	301,912	(133,997)	(44%)
April	25,575	250,350	(224,775)	(90%)	0	275,841	(250,265)	(91%)
May	332,998	275,200	57,798	21%	19,588	223,826	109,172	49%
June	322,235	275,200	47,035	17%	17,902	289,187	33,047	11%
July	370,338	275,200	95,138	35%	21,785	303,053	67,286	22%
August	310,224	275,200	35,024	13%	18,248	368,168	(57,944)	(16%)
September	261,869	267,200	(5,331)	(2%)	15,404	285,754	(23,885)	(8%)
October	298,668	292,400	6,268	2%	16,593	282,085	16,583	6%
November	315,745	275,200	40,545	15%	19,734	252,928	62,817	25%
December	364,029	292,400	71,629	24%	22,752	322,836	41,193	13%
YTD Totals	3,349,535	3,329,250	20,285	1%	----------	3,454,290	(104,755)	(3%)
YTD Average	279,128	277,438	1,690	1%	18,660	287,857	(8,730)	(3%)

Date of Last Record Production Month - July, 2020
Amount of Last Record Production Month - $370,338.16

Dental

Date of Last Fee Increase - December, 2009
Percent of Last Fee Increase - 10.95%

Hygiene

Date of Last Fee Increase - November, 2014
Percent of Last Fee Increase - 3.00%

SUNRISE DENTAL SOLUTIONS Dr. [redacted] December 2020 Page 4

PRACTICE PRODUCTIVITY

Departmental Production - Doctors

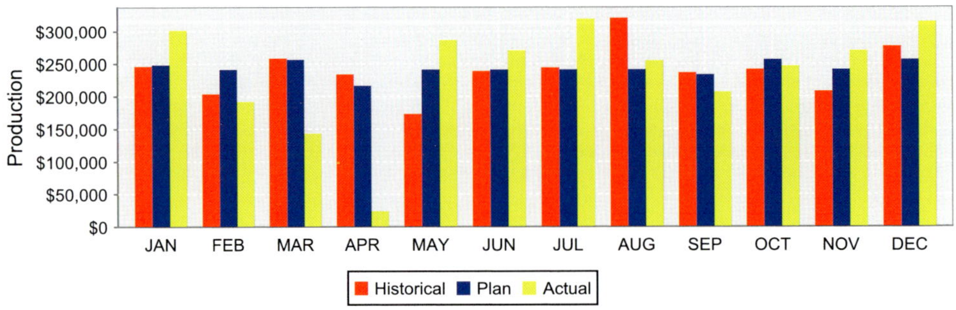

Month	Actual	Planned	$ Difference	% Difference	Average Production/Day	Historical	$ Difference	% Difference
January	302,100	248,700	53,400	21%	9,155	246,319	55,781	23%
February	192,207	241,600	(49,393)	(20%)	6,302	204,113	(11,906)	(6%)
March	143,628	256,700	(113,072)	(44%)	9,575	258,687	(115,058)	(44%)
April	24,220	216,750	(192,530)	(89%)	0	234,186	(209,966)	(90%)
May	286,604	241,600	45,004	19%	8,430	173,589	113,015	65%
June	270,739	241,600	29,139	12%	7,521	239,260	31,479	13%
July	319,463	241,600	77,863	32%	9,681	244,621	74,842	31%
August	254,987	241,600	13,387	6%	7,500	320,978	(65,991)	(21%)
September	207,086	233,600	(26,514)	(11%)	6,471	236,847	(29,761)	(13%)
October	246,837	256,700	(9,863)	(4%)	9,873	241,843	4,994	2%
November	270,338	241,600	28,738	12%	9,011	208,215	62,123	30%
December	315,076	256,700	58,376	23%	9,846	277,131	37,944	14%
YTD Totals	2,833,286	2,918,750	(85,464)	(3%)	----------	2,885,790	(52,504)	(2%)
YTD Average	236,107	243,229	(7,122)	(3%)	8,470	240,483	(4,375)	(2%)

December Average Production/Day

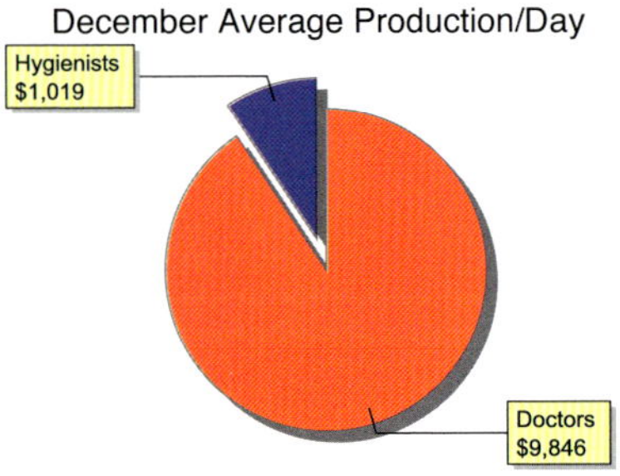

YTD Production by Department

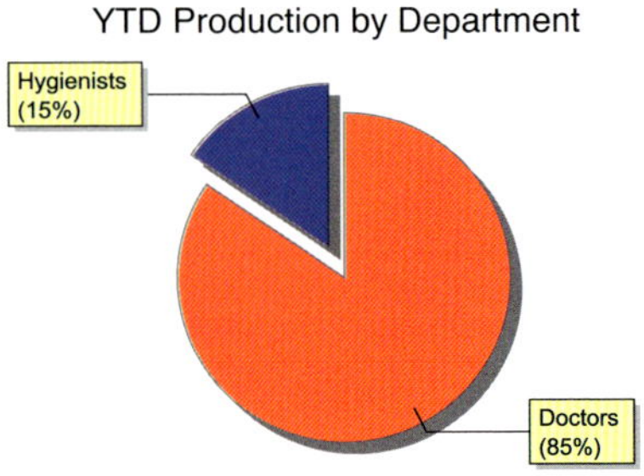

Date of Last Record Production Month - August, 2019
Amount of Last Record Production Month - $320,978.19

SUNRISE DENTAL SOLUTIONS Dr. [redacted] December 2020 Page 4A

PRACTICE PRODUCTIVITY

Departmental Production - Hygienists

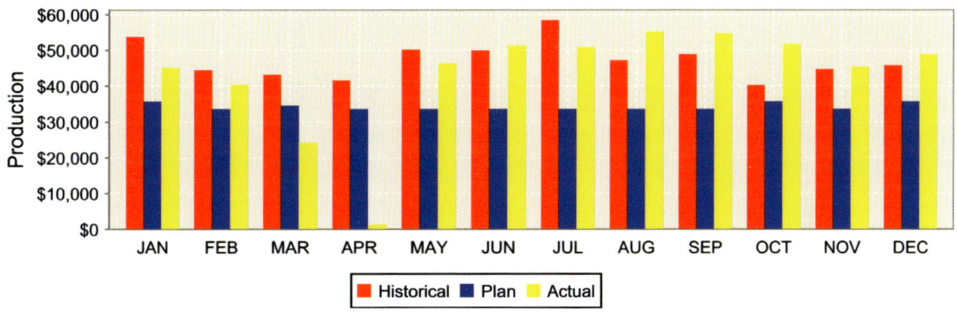

Month	Actual	Planned	$ Difference	% Difference	Average Production/Day	Historical	$ Difference	% Difference
January	45,173	35,700	9,473	27%	1,255	53,754	(8,581)	(16%)
February	40,456	33,600	6,856	20%	1,264	44,514	(4,057)	(9%)
March	24,287	34,600	(10,313)	(30%)	1,278	43,226	(18,939)	(44%)
April	1,355	33,600	(32,245)	(96%)	0	41,654	(40,299)	(97%)
May	46,394	33,600	12,794	38%	957	50,237	(3,843)	(8%)
June	51,496	33,600	17,896	53%	1,084	49,927	1,569	3%
July	50,875	33,600	17,275	51%	1,118	58,432	(7,557)	(13%)
August	55,237	33,600	21,637	64%	1,094	47,190	8,047	17%
September	54,783	33,600	21,183	63%	1,141	48,907	5,876	12%
October	51,831	35,700	16,131	45%	978	40,242	11,589	29%
November	45,407	33,600	11,807	35%	1,135	44,713	694	2%
December	48,954	35,700	13,254	37%	1,020	45,705	3,249	7%
YTD Totals	516,249	410,500	105,749	26%	----------	568,499	(52,251)	(9%)
YTD Average	43,021	34,208	8,812	26%	1,103	47,375	(4,354)	(9%)

December Average Production/Day

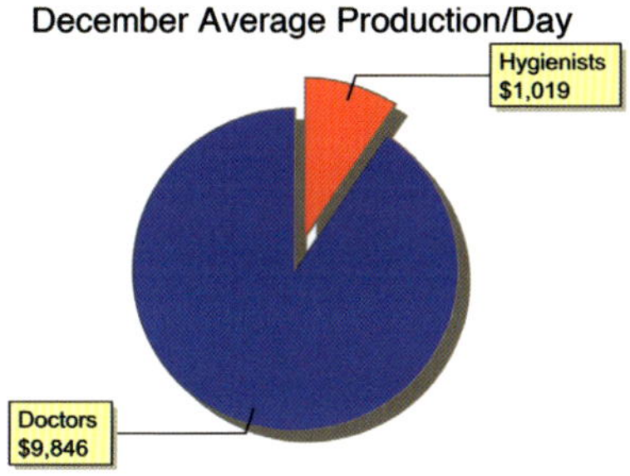

YTD Production by Department

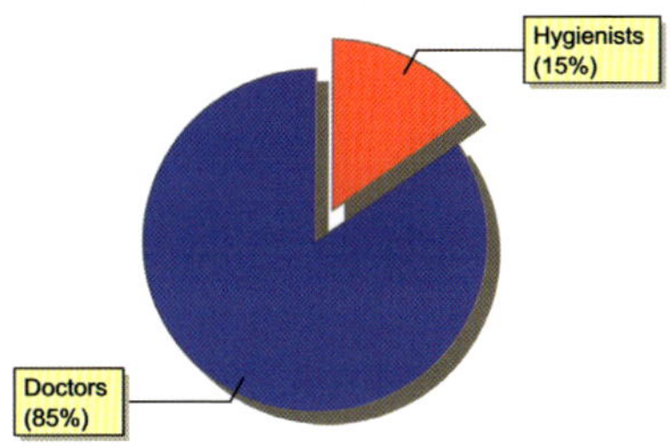

Date of Last Record Production Month - March, 2017
Amount of Last Record Production Month - $66,413.04

SUNRISE DENTAL SOLUTIONS Dr. [redacted] December 2020 Page 5

PRACTICE PRODUCTIVITY

Individual Provider Production - Dr. [redacted]

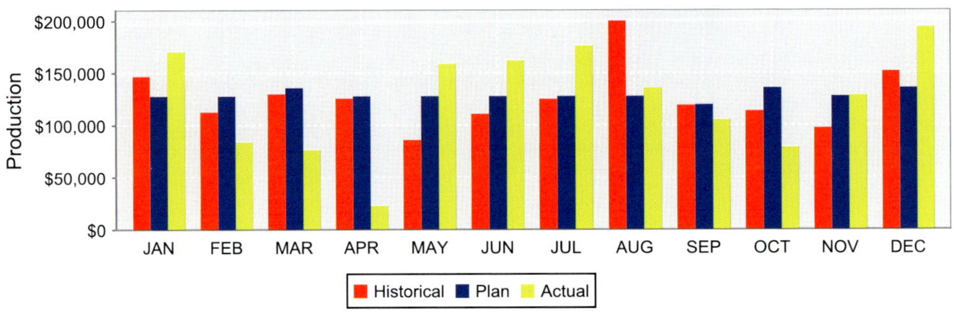

Month	Actual	Planned	$ Difference	% Difference	Average Production/Day	Historical	$ Difference	% Difference
January	170,844	128,000	42,844	33%	10,678	147,100	23,744	16%
February	84,503	128,000	(43,497)	(34%)	5,634	112,943	(28,440)	(25%)
March	77,016	136,000	(58,984)	(43%)	11,002	130,201	(53,185)	(41%)
April	23,338	128,000	(104,662)	(82%)	0	125,910	(102,572)	(81%)
May	159,273	128,000	31,273	24%	9,369	86,254	73,018	85%
June	162,495	128,000	34,495	27%	9,027	111,207	51,288	46%
July	176,473	128,000	48,473	38%	11,030	125,366	51,108	41%
August	136,127	128,000	8,127	6%	8,007	200,326	(64,199)	(32%)
September	105,971	120,000	(14,029)	(12%)	7,065	119,528	(13,557)	(11%)
October	79,488	136,000	(56,512)	(42%)	11,355	114,104	(34,616)	(30%)
November	129,190	128,000	1,190	1%	9,228	97,798	31,392	32%
December	194,547	136,000	58,547	43%	12,159	151,925	42,622	28%
YTD Totals	1,499,265	1,552,000	(52,735)	(3%)	----------	1,522,662	(23,397)	(2%)
YTD Average	124,939	129,333	(4,395)	(3%)	9,489	126,888	(1,950)	(2%)

Provider % of Total Practice

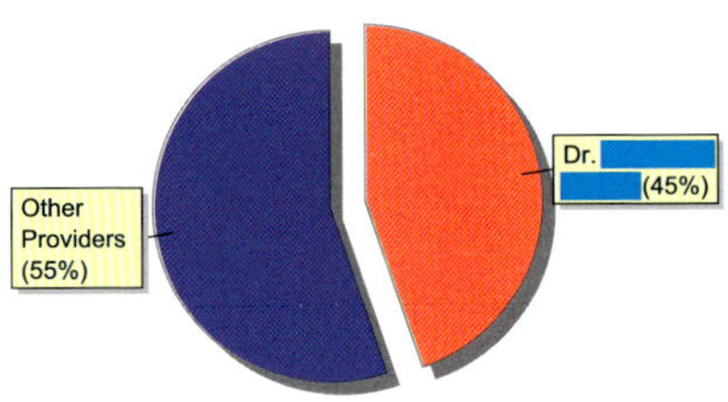

Date of Last Record Production Month - February, 2018
Amount of Last Record Production Month - $212,111.45

SUNRISE DENTAL SOLUTIONS Dr. [redacted] December 2020 Page 5A

PRACTICE PRODUCTIVITY

Individual Provider Production - Dr. [redacted]

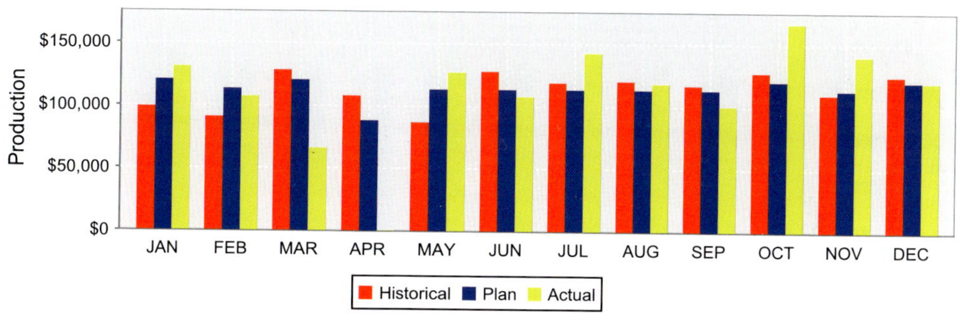

Month	Actual	Planned	$ Difference	% Difference	Average Production/Day	Historical	$ Difference	% Difference
January	131,256	120,700	10,556	9%	7,721	99,220	32,036	32%
February	107,704	113,600	(5,896)	(5%)	6,949	91,170	16,535	18%
March	66,612	120,700	(54,088)	(45%)	8,327	128,486	(61,873)	(48%)
April	882	88,750	(87,868)	(99%)	0	108,276	(107,395)	(99%)
May	127,332	113,600	13,732	12%	7,490	87,335	39,997	46%
June	108,245	113,600	(5,355)	(5%)	6,014	128,054	(19,809)	(15%)
July	142,990	113,600	29,390	26%	8,411	119,255	23,734	20%
August	118,860	113,600	5,260	5%	6,992	120,653	(1,792)	(1%)
September	101,115	113,600	(12,485)	(11%)	5,948	117,319	(16,204)	(14%)
October	167,349	120,700	46,649	39%	9,297	127,739	39,610	31%
November	141,148	113,600	27,548	24%	8,822	110,417	30,731	28%
December	120,528	120,700	(172)	(0%)	7,533	125,206	(4,678)	(4%)
YTD Totals	1,334,021	1,366,750	(32,729)	(2%)	----------	1,363,129	(29,108)	(2%)
YTD Average	111,168	113,896	(2,727)	(2%)	7,558	113,594	(2,426)	(2%)

Provider % of Total Practice

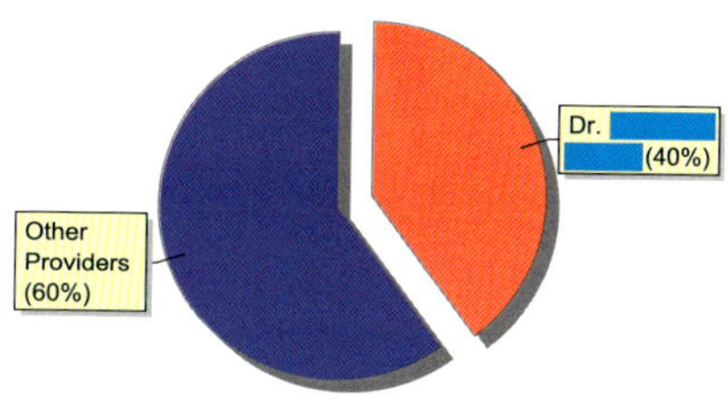

Date of Last Record Production Month - October, 2020
Amount of Last Record Production Month - $167,349.20

SUNRISE DENTAL SOLUTIONS Dr. [redacted] December 2020 Page 6

PRACTICE FINANCIALS

Monthly Collections

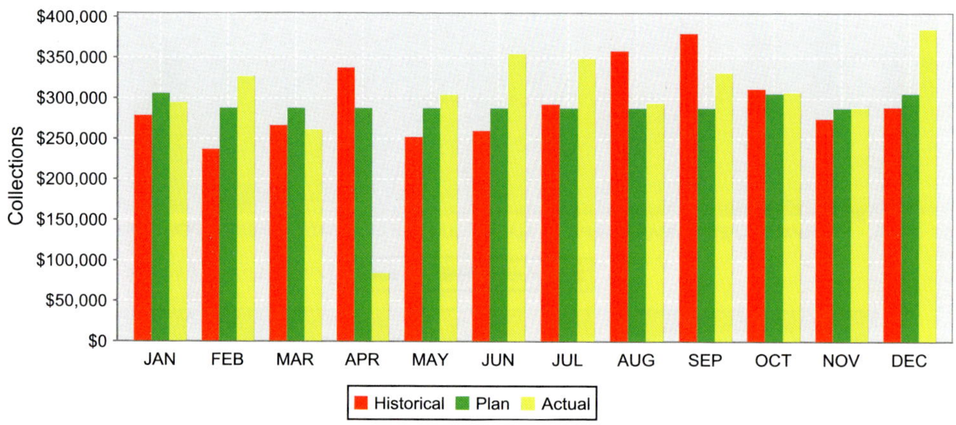

Month	Actual	Planned	$ Difference	% Difference	Average Collections/Day	Historical	$ Difference	% Difference
January	294,970	306,000	(11,030)	(4%)	17,351	278,837	16,133	6%
February	327,214	288,000	39,214	14%	21,111	237,385	89,829	38%
March	261,802	288,000	(26,198)	(9%)	23,800	266,602	(4,801)	(2%)
April	84,808	288,000	(203,192)	(71%)	0	337,623	(252,816)	(75%)
May	304,899	288,000	16,899	6%	17,935	252,435	52,464	21%
June	354,982	288,000	66,982	23%	19,721	260,275	94,707	36%
July	349,453	288,000	61,453	21%	20,556	292,805	56,648	19%
August	294,644	288,000	6,644	2%	17,332	358,434	(63,789)	(18%)
September	331,960	288,000	43,960	15%	19,527	379,936	(47,975)	(13%)
October	307,786	306,000	1,786	1%	17,099	311,798	(4,012)	(1%)
November	289,144	288,000	1,144	0%	18,071	274,987	14,157	5%
December	385,829	306,000	79,829	26%	24,114	289,262	96,567	33%
YTD Totals	3,587,491	3,510,000	77,491	2%	----------	3,540,380	47,111	1%
YTD Average	298,958	292,500	6,458	2%	19,986	295,032	3,926	1%

Date of Last Record Collections Month - December, 2020
Amount of Last Record Collections Month - $385,829.25

SUNRISE DENTAL SOLUTIONS Dr. [redacted] December 2020 Page 7

PRACTICE FINANCIALS

Collections as % of Production

Collections as % of Production

Month	Percentage
January	85%
February	141%
March	156%
April	332%
May	92%
June	110%
July	94%
August	95%
September	127%
October	103%
November	92%
December	106%
Average YTD	107%
Historical	102%
Planned	107%

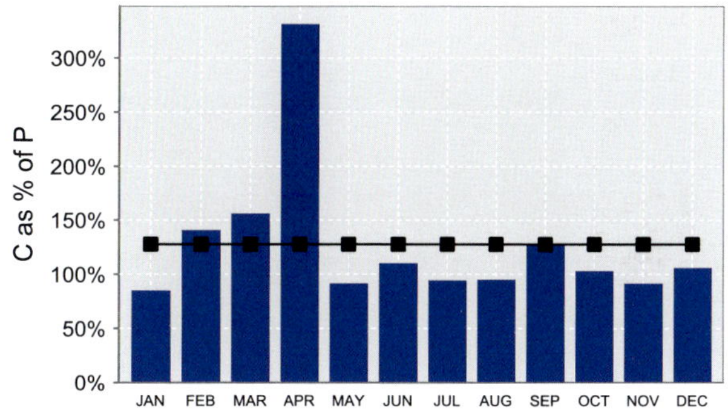

Accounts Receivable Trend

1.	Previous Month AR:	229,305	
2.	Current Month Production:	364,029	
3.	Current Month Collections:	385,829	
4.	Expected AR:	207,505	(1+2-3)
5.	Actual AR:	217,275	
6.	Difference:	9,770	(4-5)
7.	Net Change in AR:	(12,030)	(1-5)

Accounts Receivable Trend Key

Expected A/R
- calculated by SDS without accounting for any type of adjustments

Actual A/R
- reporter by client (after any month end adjustments for courtesies, insurance write-off, bad debt etc.)

Difference
- if a negative number (red), it reflects some amount of adjustments. If (big red), examine reasons for this, refer to page 11!
- if black, then collections exceeded production due to pre-payments or good collections

Net Change in A/R
- if (red) then client A/R descreased from last month and the outstanding money is coming in. (Good!)
- if black, then client A/R has increased from last month and outstanding money is accumulating. (NOT good!)

Over-The-Counter vs
In-The-Mail Collections

Month	$ OTC	%	$ ITM	%
January	222,170	75%	72,799	25%
February	146,632	45%	180,582	55%
March	158,392	61%	103,410	39%
April	36,021	42%	48,786	58%
May	245,814	81%	59,084	19%
June	241,853	68%	113,129	32%
July	266,500	76%	82,954	24%
August	188,554	64%	106,091	36%
September	238,307	72%	93,653	28%
October	227,646	74%	80,141	26%
November	201,023	70%	88,121	30%
December	287,812	75%	98,017	25%
Average YTD	205,060	69%	93,897	31%
Total YTD	2,460,724	69%	1,126,767	31%

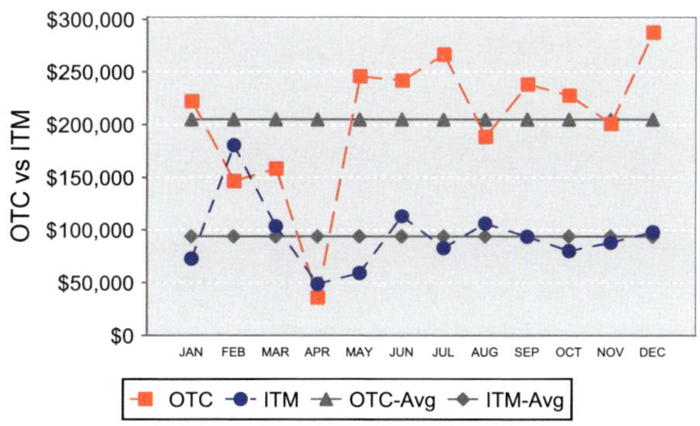

SUNRISE DENTAL SOLUTIONS Dr. [redacted] December 2020 Page 8

PRACTICE FINANCIALS

Accounts Receivable

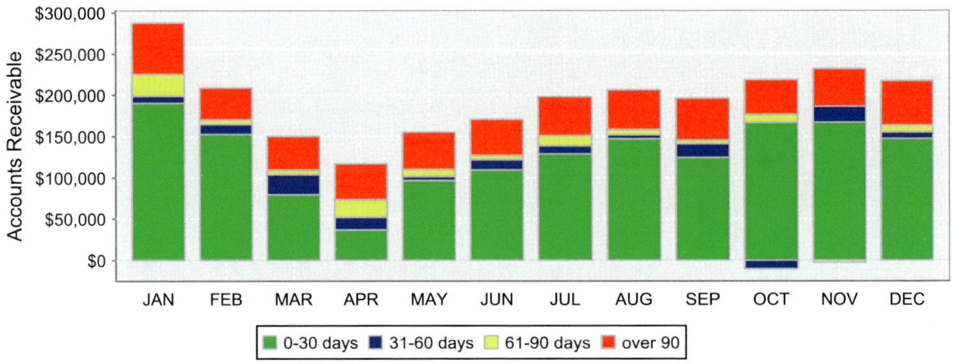

Month	0-30 days	31-60 days	61-90 days	90+ days	% Overdue	Total
January	190,214	8,542	26,063	62,843	34%	287,663
February	152,614	12,084	5,255	38,847	27%	208,800
March	79,768	24,106	5,392	40,963	47%	150,228
April	36,688	15,183	21,684	43,392	69%	116,948
May	96,755	4,754	8,236	45,474	38%	155,220
June	109,591	12,287	4,878	43,790	36%	170,546
July	128,927	9,645	12,313	47,253	35%	198,137
August	147,159	4,682	6,136	48,243	29%	206,220
September	124,562	16,461	4,403	50,729	36%	196,155
October	166,803	(10,384)	9,521	42,177	20%	208,118
November	166,980	19,228	(2,535)	45,632	27%	229,305
December	147,428	7,641	8,196	54,009	32%	217,275
Average	128,957	10,353	9,128	46,946	34%	195,384

AR/Monthly Production Ratio

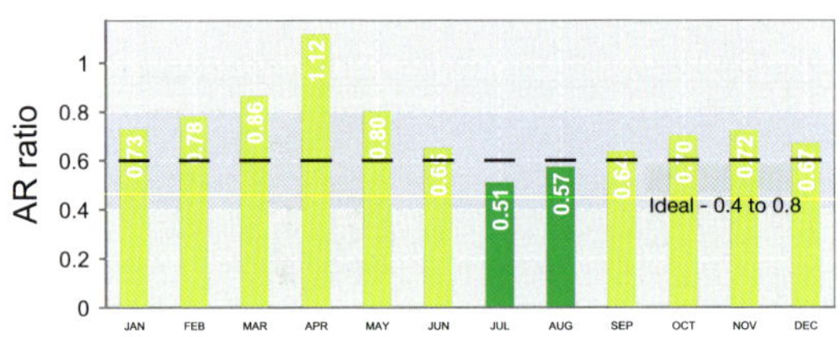

December % of AR by aging

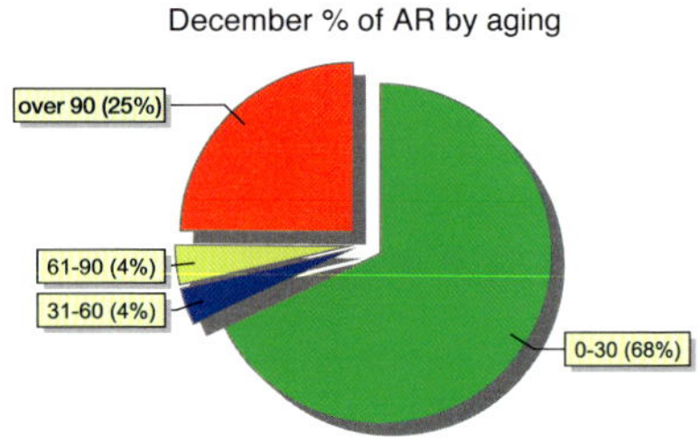

SUNRISE DENTAL SOLUTIONS Dr. [redacted] December 2020 Page 9

PRACTICE GROWTH

New Patients by Month

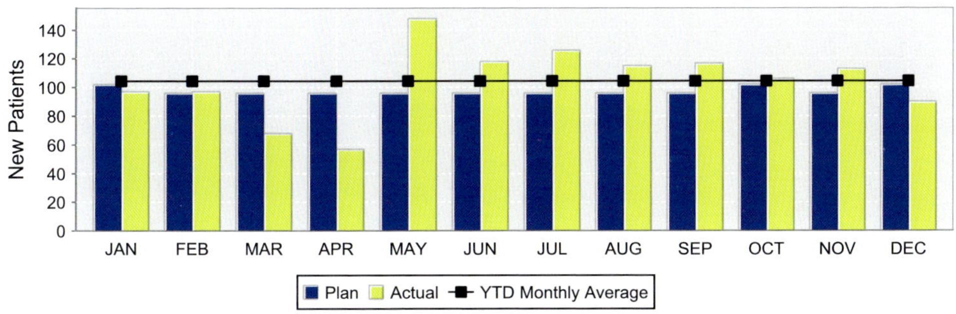

Sources of New Patient and YTD Totals

Referral Type	JAN	FEB	MAR	APR	MAY	JUN	JUL	AUG	SEP	OCT	NOV	DEC	YTD Total	Monthly Average	December %	YTD %	Gross Production
Website/Internet	18.0	18.0	31.0	0.0	39.0	29.0	42.0	36.0	26.0	33.0	38.0	31.0	341.00	28.42	34%	27%	$701,618
Radio	13.0	13.0	12.0	0.0	36.0	29.0	25.0	16.0	19.0	24.0	25.0	20.0	232.00	19.33	22%	19%	$477,347
Referral-Patient	35.0	35.0	17.0	0.0	7.0	23.0	20.0	13.0	22.0	18.0	17.0	18.0	225.00	18.75	20%	18%	$462,944
Signage/Walk-In	15.0	15.0	6.0	0.0	55.0	29.0	33.0	36.0	43.0	16.0	11.0	11.0	270.00	22.50	12%	22%	$555,533
Referral-Insurance	5.0	5.0	2.0	0.0	3.0	6.0	1.0	5.0	5.0	7.0	10.0	6.0	55.00	4.58	7%	4%	$113,164
Billboard	3.0	3.0	0.0	0.0	0.0	1.0	1.0	3.0	0.0	3.0	4.0	3.0	21.00	1.75	3%	2%	$43,208
Newspaper	3.0	3.0	0.0	0.0	2.0	0.0	0.0	4.0	2.0	0.0	5.0	1.0	20.00	1.67	1%	2%	$41,151
TV	0.0	0.0	0.0	0.0	3.0	0.0	0.0	1.0	0.0	2.0	1.0	0.0	7.00	0.58	0%	1%	$14,403
Word of Mouth	3.0	3.0	0.0	0.0	0.0	0.0	0.0	0.0	0.0	0.0	0.0	0.0	6.00	0.50	0%	0%	$12,345
Teledentistry	0.0	0.0	0.0	57.0	0.0	0.0	0.0	0.0	0.0	0.0	0.0	0.0	57.00	4.75	0%	5%	$117,279
Yellow Pages	2.0	2.0	0.0	0.0	3.0	1.0	3.0	0.0	0.0	2.0	0.0	0.0	13.00	1.08	0%	1%	$26,748
Viva Cards	0.0	0.0	0.0	0.0	0.0	0.0	1.0	1.0	0.0	1.0	2.0	0.0	5.00	0.42	0%	0%	$10,288
Totals	97.0	97.0	68.0	57.0	148.	118.	126.	115.	117.	106.	113.	90.0	1252.00	104.33	100%	100%	$2,576,028

December Referrals

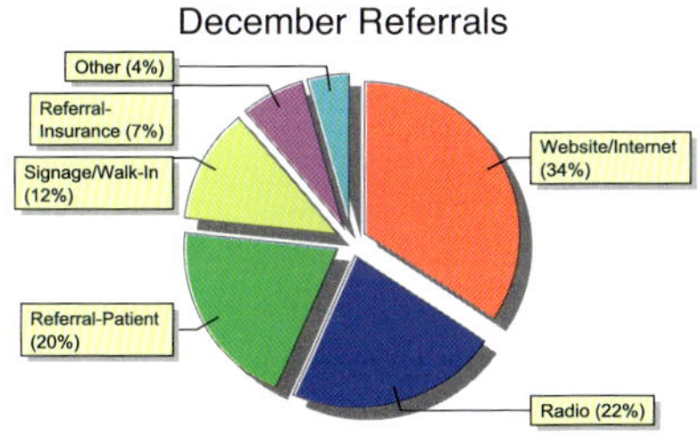

YTD Referrals

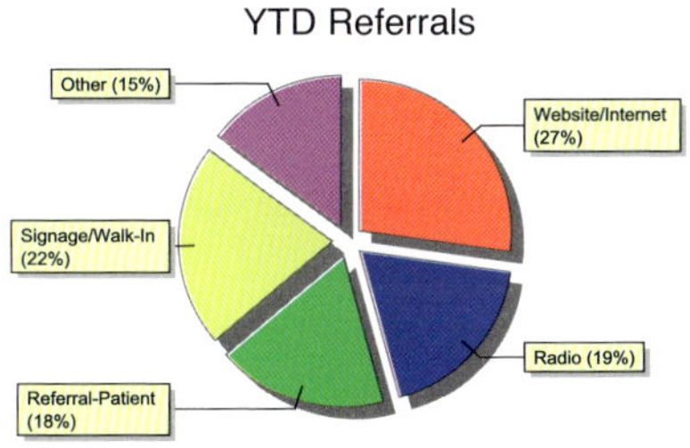

SUNRISE DENTAL SOLUTIONS Dr. [redacted] December 2020 Page 10

PRACTICE GROWTH

Value/ROI for New Patients

Value of New Patients as of - February 2015

	Gross Production	Difference from Previous Value	**Profit**
Dental	$1,865.40	$366.01	$418.52
Hygiene	$192.13	-$91.29	$43.11
Total	$2,057.53	$274.72	$461.63

	Feb-15 Dr. [redacted]		
Dental	$1,865.40		
Hygiene	$192.13		
Total	$2,057.53		

ROI of Marketing

Using Approximated Numbers

Source	Production Source	$ Spent Source	# of New Patients/Source	ROI/NP	ROI Ratio	ROI Rank/MO.
Website/Internet	63,783	5,385	31	1,884	11.844	4
Radio	41,151	4,306	20	1,842	9.557	5
Referral-Patient	37,036	0	18	2,058		2
Signage/Walk-In	22,633	0	11	2,058		3
Referral-Insurance	12,345	0	6	2,058		1
Billboard	6,173	1,295	3	1,626	4.766	7
Newspaper	2,058	238	1	1,820	8.663	6
TV	0	0	0	0		8
Teledentistry	0	0	0	0		9
Viva Cards	0	0	0	0		10
Others (combined)	2,058	0	1	2,058		0
YTD Totals	187,235	11,224	91	1,934		----------

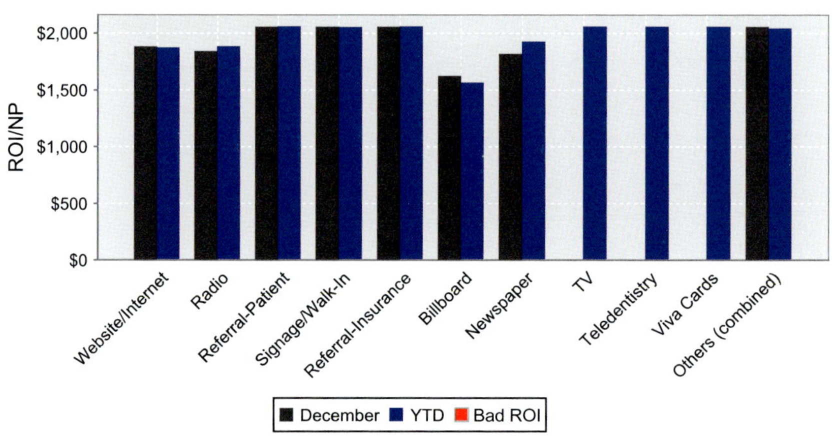

SUNRISE DENTAL SOLUTIONS Dr. [redacted] December 2020 Page 11

PRACTICE PROFITABILITY

Write-Offs

Month	PPO	EmpDent	Charitable	BadDebts	CPF	Barter	Senior	Misc	subTotal	RefOvPmt	MarkOffer	OutFinanc	SmileCard	PayToday	subTotal	TOTAL
January	1,120	0	693	411	2,289	140	0	0	4,653	872	0	8,816	0	0	9,687	$14,341
February	3,086	2,290	502	1,037	3,265	1,499	0	0	11,679	25,835	0	2,944	0	822	29,601	$41,280
March	126	6,236	1,326	6,387	8,755	0	0	8	22,837	3,742	0	3,219	0	133	7,093	$29,930
April	2,906	1,290	0	0	0	10,807	0	0	15,002	9,219	0	854	0	0	10,072	$25,074
May	2,108	919	0	998	7,006	352	0	0	11,382	4,404	0	1,276	0	446	6,126	$17,509
June	3,842	203	7,126	-344	6,012	164	0	0	17,002	8,147	25	6,279	0	0	14,451	$31,453
July	4,278	297	342	-142	1,316	3,977	0	5,900	15,969	10,100	550	9,246	0	792	20,688	$36,657
August	2,175	3,479	5,500	678	1,106	1,116	0	0	14,053	15,335	50	5,586	0	555	21,526	$35,580
September	3,093	16,407	0	-982	-281	0	0	0	18,237	21,591	581	2,256	0	0	24,428	$42,665
October	2,577	646	289	0	2,450	848	0	0	6,811	866	100	4,012	0	468	5,446	$12,257
November	3,187	16,407	0	17	1,630	0	0	0	21,242	3,101	581	4,280	0	0	7,962	$29,204
December	1,232	615	3,332	19,624	18,123	2,850	0	1,276	47,051	21,154	0	4,989	0	120	26,263	$73,314
Totals	$29,729	$48,789	$19,110	$27,684	$51,670	$21,753	$0	$7,184	$205,919	$124,366	$1,887	$53,756	$0	$3,336	$183,345	$389,263
YTD %	8%	13%	5%	7%	13%	6%	0%	2%	53%	32%	0%	14%	0%	1%	47%	----------
% of Prod	1%	1%	1%	1%	2%	1%	0%	0%	----------	4%	0%	2%	0%	0%	----------	----------
Rank	5	4	8	6	3	7	12	9	----------	1	11	2	13	10	----------	----------

December Write-Offs

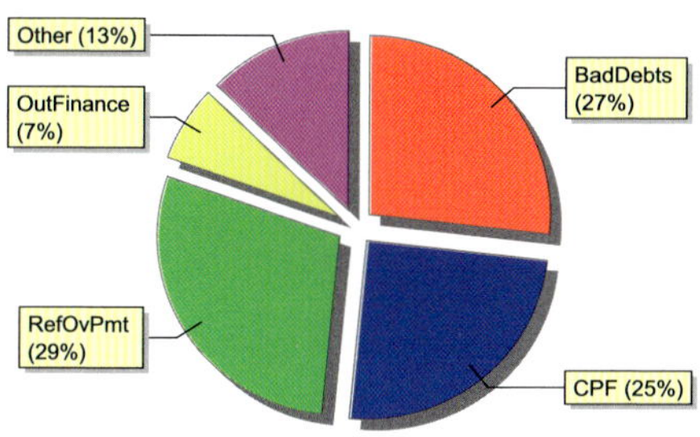

YTD Write-Offs

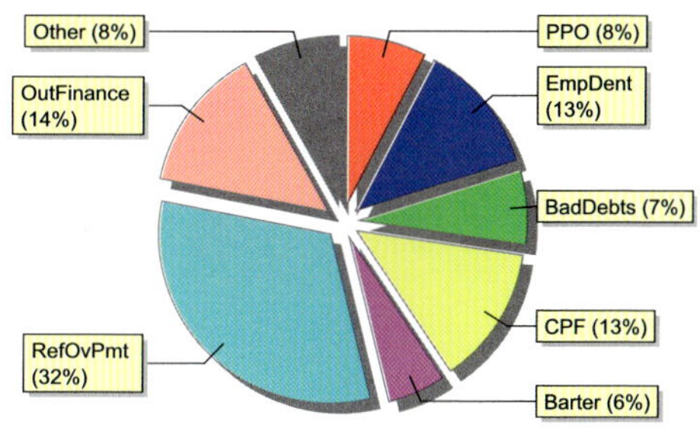

Misc - any source of write-offs not included in existing categories
PPO - Preferred Provider Organization, dentist is under contract to provide member patients with a reduced fee
EmpDent - employee dentistry benefits
Charitable - pre-arranged charity dental services
BadDebts - patients who don't ever pay for services
CPF - close personal friends, families and professional friends of the doctor/practice
Barter - dental services exchanged for services or products
Senior - senior citizen discount
RefOvPmt - refund of monies paid due to overpayment, including miscalculated insurance estimates
MarkOffer - special pricing related to marketing offers for discounts (mail brochures, newspaper, etc.)
OutFinance - adjustments made for outside financing services (Wells Fargo, Dental Fee Plan, etc.)
SmileCard - discounts similar to MarkOffer but tracked separately
PayToday - courtesy allowance offered to patients who pay in advance of treatment

SUNRISE DENTAL SOLUTIONS Dr. [redacted] December 2020 Page 12

PRACTICE PROFITABILITY

Expenses

Fixed Expenses

Category	This Month	% Expenses	% Collections	YTD	% YTD Expenses	AVG SDS 2019	% YTD Collections
Business Insurance	1,812	0.57%	0.47%	37,198	1.34%	1.26%	1.04%
Dues	3,909	1.22%	1.01%	18,853	0.68%	0.56%	0.53%
Equipment Lease	0	0.00%	0.00%	0	0.00%	0.88%	0.00%
Fixed Miscellaneous	0	0.00%	0.00%	9,873	0.35%	1.48%	0.28%
Janitorial	800	0.25%	0.21%	10,400	0.37%	0.54%	0.29%
Loan Payments	1,919	0.60%	0.50%	120,331	4.32%	4.16%	3.35%
Phone	774	0.24%	0.20%	21,088	0.76%	0.48%	0.59%
Rent	13,500	4.21%	3.50%	162,000	5.82%	4.85%	4.52%
Service Contracts	0	0.00%	0.00%	0	0.00%	1.06%	0.00%
Taxes	7,005	2.18%	1.82%	120,102	4.32%	2.37%	3.35%
Utilities	1,637	0.51%	0.42%	20,290	0.73%	0.63%	0.57%
SubTotals	31,357	9.78%	8.13%	520,135	18.69%	18.29%	14.50%

Variable Expenses

Category	This Month	% Expenses	% Collections	YTD	% YTD Expenses	AVG SDS 2019	% YTD Collections
Advertising	19,219	5.99%	4.98%	181,499	6.52%	4.12%	5.06%
Bank Charges	1,602	0.50%	0.42%	28,138	1.01%	1.31%	0.78%
Business Supplies	3,814	1.19%	0.99%	40,524	1.46%	0.99%	1.13%
Charitable Contributions	0	0.00%	0.00%	0	0.00%	0.38%	0.00%
Clinical Supplies	25,293	7.89%	6.56%	206,360	7.42%	8.14%	5.75%
Continuing Education Doctors	0	0.00%	0.00%	10,959	0.39%	1.02%	0.31%
Continuing Education Team	500	0.16%	0.13%	9,055	0.33%	0.90%	0.25%
Employee Benefits	10,902	3.40%	2.83%	87,966	3.16%	2.55%	2.45%
Equipment Purchase	27,369	8.54%	7.09%	108,668	3.91%	3.30%	3.03%
Equipment Service	683	0.21%	0.18%	13,708	0.49%	0.86%	0.38%
Gross Associate(s) Salaries/Wages	0	0.00%	0.00%	0	0.00%	11.02%	0.00%
Gross Salaries/Wages	127,148	39.66%	32.95%	1,011,703	36.36%	29.18%	28.20%
Laboratory Fees	32,303	10.07%	8.37%	242,528	8.72%	8.26%	6.76%
Legal/Professional	7,342	2.29%	1.90%	98,269	3.53%	2.57%	2.74%
Office Improvement	2,279	0.71%	0.59%	71,021	2.55%	1.42%	1.98%
Postage	170	0.05%	0.04%	3,964	0.14%	0.16%	0.11%
Refunds	21,154	6.60%	5.48%	115,962	4.17%	2.26%	3.23%
Travel/Entertainment	9,491	2.96%	2.46%	32,136	1.15%	1.08%	0.90%
Variable Miscellaneous	0	0.00%	0.00%	0	0.00%	2.20%	0.00%
SubTotals	289,268	90.22%	74.97%	2,262,460	81.31%	81.71%	63.07%
Expense Totals	320,625	100%	83%	2,782,595	100%	100%	78%

December Expenses

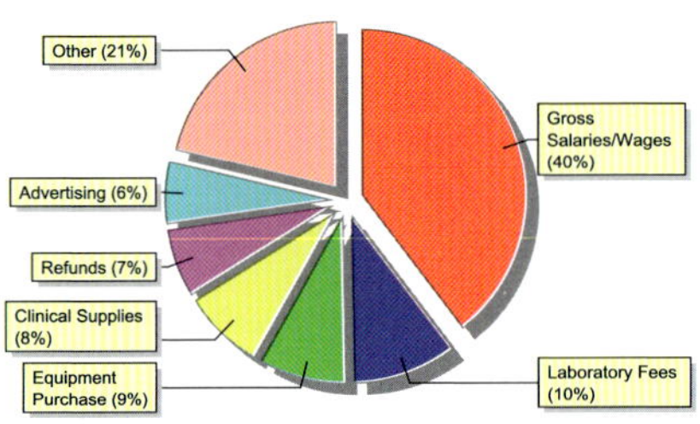

YTD Expenses

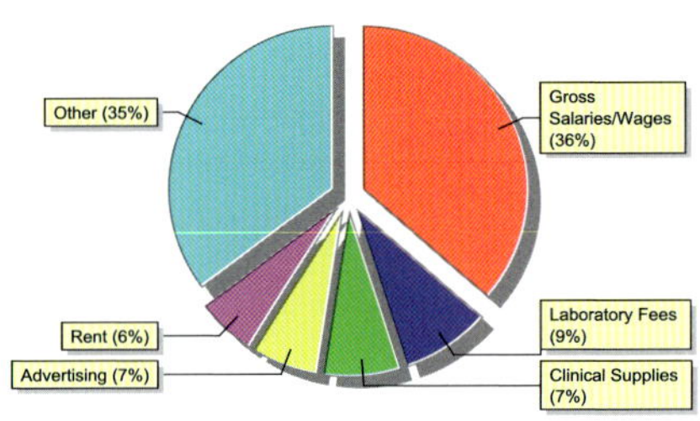

SUNRISE DENTAL SOLUTIONS Dr. [redacted] December 2020 Page 13

PRACTICE PROFITABILITY

Overhead

Practice Overhead

Month	% Month	% YTD
January	80.85%	80.85%
February	67.91%	74.05%
March	72.43%	73.57%
April	134.20%	78.87%
May	63.21%	75.13%
June	59.09%	71.63%
July	81.88%	73.44%
August	91.78%	75.82%
September	89.02%	77.50%
October	65.21%	76.20%
November	83.88%	76.90%
December	83.10%	77.56%
Average	77.56%	77.56%

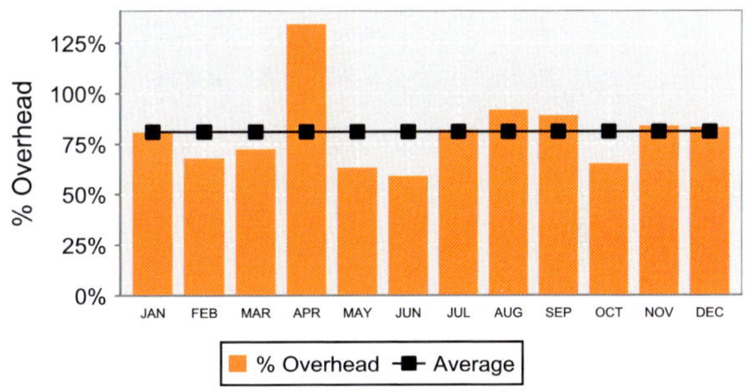

Practice Profitability

Month	Net Income
January	56,483
February	105,004
March	72,189
April	(29,007)
May	112,157
June	145,211
July	63,312
August	24,213
September	36,445
October	107,089
November	46,596
December	65,204
Total	804,896
Average	67,075

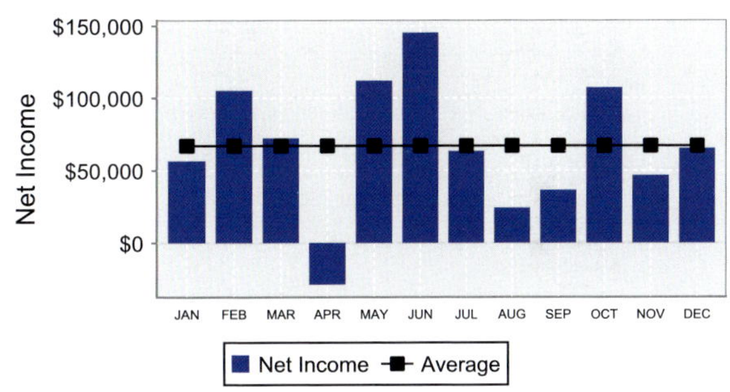

Production/Collections

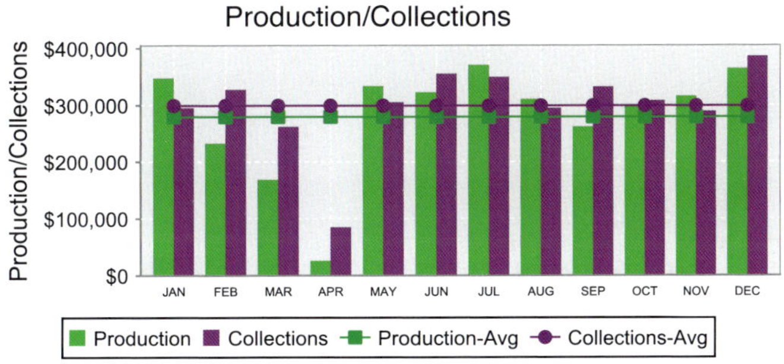

"Preferred Provider" Allowance Vs. Practice Fees Analysis

Practice Name | Date: MM/YR

Overhead %

Proc. Code	Procedure	Practice Fee	Delta Dental Premier	Cigna PPO	PPO #3 Fee	PPO #4 Fee	PPO #5 Fee	PPO #6 Fee	PPO #7 Fee	PPO #8 Fee	PPO #9 Fee	PPO #10 Fee
120	Periodic Oral Exam	$ -	$ -	$ -								
150	Comprehensive Oral Exam	$ -	$ -	$ -								
274	Bitewings 4 Films	$ -	$ -	$ -								
1110	Prophylaxis Adult	$ -	$ -	$ -								
2332	Resin 3 Surface Anterior	$ -	$ -	$ -								
2392	2 Surface Posterior Composite	$ -	$ -	$ -								
2740	Crown Porcelain/Ceramic	$ -	$ -	$ -								
2950	Crown Build-Up Including Pins	$ -	$ -	$ -								
3310	Root Canal-Anterior	$ -	$ -	$ -								
5110	Denture Complete Upper	$ -	$ -	$ -								
7140	Simple Extraction	$ -	$ -	$ -								
7210	Surgical Extraction	$ -	$ -	$ -								
2952	Post and Core Buildup	$ -	$ -	$ -								
1351	Sealant	$ -	$ -	$ -								

Proc. Code	Procedure	Practice Fee	Delta Dental Premier $ Diff.	Cigna PPO $ Diff.	PPO #3 $ Diff.	PPO #4 $ Diff.	PPO #5 $ Diff.	PPO #6 $ Diff.	PPO #7 $ Diff.	PPO #8 $ Diff.	PPO #9 $ Diff.	PPO #10 $ Diff.
120	Periodic Oral Exam	$ -	$ -	$ -	$ -	$ -	$ -	$ -	$ -	$ -	$ -	$ -
150	Comprehensive Oral Exam	$ -	$ -	$ -	$ -	$ -	$ -	$ -	$ -	$ -	$ -	$ -
274	Bitewings 4 Films	$ -	$ -	$ -	$ -	$ -	$ -	$ -	$ -	$ -	$ -	$ -
1110	Prophylaxis Adult	$ -	$ -	$ -	$ -	$ -	$ -	$ -	$ -	$ -	$ -	$ -
2332	Resin 3 Surface Anterior	$ -	$ -	$ -	$ -	$ -	$ -	$ -	$ -	$ -	$ -	$ -
2392	2 Surface Posterior Composite	$ -	$ -	$ -	$ -	$ -	$ -	$ -	$ -	$ -	$ -	$ -
2740	Crown Porcelain/Ceramic	$ -	$ -	$ -	$ -	$ -	$ -	$ -	$ -	$ -	$ -	$ -
2950	Crown Build-Up Including Pins	$ -	$ -	$ -	$ -	$ -	$ -	$ -	$ -	$ -	$ -	$ -
3310	Root Canal-Anterior	$ -	$ -	$ -	$ -	$ -	$ -	$ -	$ -	$ -	$ -	$ -
5110	Denture Complete Upper	$ -	$ -	$ -	$ -	$ -	$ -	$ -	$ -	$ -	$ -	$ -
7140	Simple Extraction	$ -	$ -	$ -	$ -	$ -	$ -	$ -	$ -	$ -	$ -	$ -
7210	Surgical Extraction	$ -	$ -	$ -	$ -	$ -	$ -	$ -	$ -	$ -	$ -	$ -
2952	Post and Core Buildup	$ -	$ -	$ -	$ -	$ -	$ -	$ -	$ -	$ -	$ -	$ -
1351	Sealant	$ -	$ -	$ -	$ -	$ -	$ -	$ -	$ -	$ -	$ -	$ -

Proc. Code	Procedure	Practice Fee	Delta Dental Premier % Diff.	Cigna PPO % Diff.	PPO #3 % Diff.	PPO #4 % Diff.	PPO #5 % Diff.	PPO #6 % Diff.	PPO #7 % Diff.	PPO #8 % Diff.	PPO #9 % Diff.	PPO #10 % Diff.
120	Periodic Oral Exam	$ -	#DIV/0!	#DIV/0!	#DIV/0!	#DIV/0!	#DIV/0!	#DIV/0!	#DIV/0!	#DIV/0!	#DIV/0!	#DIV/0!
150	Comprehensive Oral Exam	$ -	#DIV/0!	#DIV/0!	#DIV/0!	#DIV/0!	#DIV/0!	#DIV/0!	#DIV/0!	#DIV/0!	#DIV/0!	#DIV/0!
274	Bitewings 4 Films	$ -	#DIV/0!	#DIV/0!	#DIV/0!	#DIV/0!	#DIV/0!	#DIV/0!	#DIV/0!	#DIV/0!	#DIV/0!	#DIV/0!
1110	Prophylaxis Adult	$ -	#DIV/0!	#DIV/0!	#DIV/0!	#DIV/0!	#DIV/0!	#DIV/0!	#DIV/0!	#DIV/0!	#DIV/0!	#DIV/0!
2332	Resin 3 Surface Anterior	$ -	#DIV/0!	#DIV/0!	#DIV/0!	#DIV/0!	#DIV/0!	#DIV/0!	#DIV/0!	#DIV/0!	#DIV/0!	#DIV/0!
2392	2 Surface Posterior Composite	$ -	#DIV/0!	#DIV/0!	#DIV/0!	#DIV/0!	#DIV/0!	#DIV/0!	#DIV/0!	#DIV/0!	#DIV/0!	#DIV/0!
2740	Crown Porcelain/Ceramic	$ -	#DIV/0!	#DIV/0!	#DIV/0!	#DIV/0!	#DIV/0!	#DIV/0!	#DIV/0!	#DIV/0!	#DIV/0!	#DIV/0!
2950	Crown Build-Up Including Pins	$ -	#DIV/0!	#DIV/0!	#DIV/0!	#DIV/0!	#DIV/0!	#DIV/0!	#DIV/0!	#DIV/0!	#DIV/0!	#DIV/0!
3310	Root Canal-Anterior	$ -	#DIV/0!	#DIV/0!	#DIV/0!	#DIV/0!	#DIV/0!	#DIV/0!	#DIV/0!	#DIV/0!	#DIV/0!	#DIV/0!
5110	Denture Complete Upper	$ -	#DIV/0!	#DIV/0!	#DIV/0!	#DIV/0!	#DIV/0!	#DIV/0!	#DIV/0!	#DIV/0!	#DIV/0!	#DIV/0!
7140	Simple Extraction	$ -	#DIV/0!	#DIV/0!	#DIV/0!	#DIV/0!	#DIV/0!	#DIV/0!	#DIV/0!	#DIV/0!	#DIV/0!	#DIV/0!
7210	Surgical Extraction	$ -	#DIV/0!	#DIV/0!	#DIV/0!	#DIV/0!	#DIV/0!	#DIV/0!	#DIV/0!	#DIV/0!	#DIV/0!	#DIV/0!
2952	Post and Core Buildup	$ -	#DIV/0!	#DIV/0!	#DIV/0!	#DIV/0!	#DIV/0!	#DIV/0!	#DIV/0!	#DIV/0!	#DIV/0!	#DIV/0!
1351	Sealant	$ -	#DIV/0!	#DIV/0!	#DIV/0!	#DIV/0!	#DIV/0!	#DIV/0!	#DIV/0!	#DIV/0!	#DIV/0!	#DIV/0!

Key

Key	Name of PPO
PPO #1	
PPO #2	
PPO #3	
PPO #4	
PPO #5	
PPO #6	
PPO #7	
PPO #8	
PPO #9	
PPO #10	

Rank - Best to Worst

PPO #1
PPO #2
PPO #3
PPO #4
PPO #5
PPO #6
PPO #7
PPO #8
PPO #9
PPO #10

Sunrise Team Achievement Rewards Program - Profit Available For Bonuses Per Practice Production Worksheet

Doctor Name

Collection Rate 96 **Overhead %** 50 **Desired Annual Owner Draw** $ 800,000.00

Calculating the Amount of Money Available to Pay Bonuses out of Profit after Owner's Draw at Various Levels of Production			Determining the Amount of Money Available to Pay out of Profit at Three Different Levels - 100% of Available Profit after Owner's Draw, as well as 90% and 80% Levels					
Annual Production	Profit	Profit After Draw	Annual Bonus $ Avail. 100%	Bonus $ Avail/Mo.	Annual Bonus $ Avail. 90%	Bonus $ Avail/Mo.	Annual Bonus $ Avail. 80%	Bonus $ Avail. Mo.
$ 1,200,000.00	$ 552,000.00	$ (248,000.00)	$ (248,000.00)	$ (20,666.67)	$ (223,200.00)	$ (18,600.00)	$ (198,400.00)	$ (16,533.33)
$ 1,250,000.00	$ 575,000.00	$ (225,000.00)	$ (225,000.00)	$ (18,750.00)	$ (202,500.00)	$ (16,875.00)	$ (180,000.00)	$ (15,000.00)
$ 1,300,000.00	$ 598,000.00	$ (202,000.00)	$ (202,000.00)	$ (16,833.33)	$ (181,800.00)	$ (15,150.00)	$ (161,600.00)	$ (13,466.67)
$ 1,350,000.00	$ 621,000.00	$ (179,000.00)	$ (179,000.00)	$ (14,916.67)	$ (161,100.00)	$ (13,425.00)	$ (143,200.00)	$ (11,933.33)
$ 1,400,000.00	$ 644,000.00	$ (156,000.00)	$ (156,000.00)	$ (13,000.00)	$ (140,400.00)	$ (11,700.00)	$ (124,800.00)	$ (10,400.00)
$ 1,450,000.00	$ 667,000.00	$ (133,000.00)	$ (133,000.00)	$ (11,083.33)	$ (119,700.00)	$ (9,975.00)	$ (106,400.00)	$ (8,866.67)
$ 1,500,000.00	$ 690,000.00	$ (110,000.00)	$ (110,000.00)	$ (9,166.67)	$ (99,000.00)	$ (8,250.00)	$ (88,000.00)	$ (7,333.33)
$ 1,550,000.00	$ 713,000.00	$ (87,000.00)	$ (87,000.00)	$ (7,250.00)	$ (78,300.00)	$ (6,525.00)	$ (69,600.00)	$ (5,800.00)
$ 1,600,000.00	$ 736,000.00	$ (64,000.00)	$ (64,000.00)	$ (5,333.33)	$ (57,600.00)	$ (4,800.00)	$ (51,200.00)	$ (4,266.67)
$ 1,650,000.00	$ 759,000.00	$ (41,000.00)	$ (41,000.00)	$ (3,416.67)	$ (36,900.00)	$ (3,075.00)	$ (32,800.00)	$ (2,733.33)
$ 1,700,000.00	$ 782,000.00	$ (18,000.00)	$ (18,000.00)	$ (1,500.00)	$ (16,200.00)	$ (1,350.00)	$ (14,400.00)	$ (1,200.00)
$ 1,750,000.00	$ 805,000.00	$ 5,000.00	$ 5,000.00	$ 416.67	$ 4,500.00	$ 375.00	$ 4,000.00	$ 333.33
$ 1,800,000.00	$ 828,000.00	$ 28,000.00	$ 28,000.00	$ 2,333.33	$ 25,200.00	$ 2,100.00	$ 22,400.00	$ 1,866.67
$ 1,850,000.00	$ 851,000.00	$ 51,000.00	$ 51,000.00	$ 4,250.00	$ 45,900.00	$ 3,825.00	$ 40,800.00	$ 3,400.00
$ 1,900,000.00	$ 874,000.00	$ 74,000.00	$ 74,000.00	$ 6,166.67	$ 66,600.00	$ 5,550.00	$ 59,200.00	$ 4,933.33
$ 1,950,000.00	$ 897,000.00	$ 97,000.00	$ 97,000.00	$ 8,083.33	$ 87,300.00	$ 7,275.00	$ 77,600.00	$ 6,466.67
$ 2,000,000.00	$ 920,000.00	$ 120,000.00	$ 120,000.00	$ 10,000.00	$ 108,000.00	$ 9,000.00	$ 96,000.00	$ 8,000.00
$ 2,050,000.00	$ 943,000.00	$ 143,000.00	$ 143,000.00	$ 11,916.67	$ 128,700.00	$ 10,725.00	$ 114,400.00	$ 9,533.33
$ 2,100,000.00	$ 966,000.00	$ 166,000.00	$ 166,000.00	$ 13,833.33	$ 149,400.00	$ 12,450.00	$ 132,800.00	$ 11,066.67
$ 2,150,000.00	$ 989,000.00	$ 189,000.00	$ 189,000.00	$ 15,750.00	$ 170,100.00	$ 14,175.00	$ 151,200.00	$ 12,600.00
$ 2,200,000.00	$ 1,012,000.00	$ 212,000.00	$ 212,000.00	$ 17,666.67	$ 190,800.00	$ 15,900.00	$ 169,600.00	$ 14,133.33
$ 2,250,000.00	$ 1,035,000.00	$ 235,000.00	$ 235,000.00	$ 19,583.33	$ 211,500.00	$ 17,625.00	$ 188,000.00	$ 15,666.67
$ 2,300,000.00	$ 1,058,000.00	$ 258,000.00	$ 258,000.00	$ 21,500.00	$ 232,200.00	$ 19,350.00	$ 206,400.00	$ 17,200.00
$ 2,350,000.00	$ 1,081,000.00	$ 281,000.00	$ 281,000.00	$ 23,416.67	$ 252,900.00	$ 21,075.00	$ 224,800.00	$ 18,733.33
$ 2,400,000.00	$ 1,104,000.00	$ 304,000.00	$ 304,000.00	$ 25,333.33	$ 273,600.00	$ 22,800.00	$ 243,200.00	$ 20,266.67

SDS Profit-Sharing Rewards Program

Practice Name

Month/Year

Day, Daily Reward & Totals

Prod. Goal Levels & Team Members	Daily Goal	Daily Reward	1 - Act. Daily Amt.	1- Reward	2 - Act. Daily Amt.	2-Reward	3 - Act. Daily Amt.	3-Reward	4 - Act. Daily Amt.	4-Reward	5 - Act. Daily Amt.	5-Reward	6 - Act. Daily Amt.	6-Reward	Total Daily Amt.	Total Monthly Reward	Team Member
Doctor 1	$ -		$ -	$ -	$ -	$ -	$ -	$ -	$ -	$ -	$ -	$ -	$ -	$ -	$ -		
		$ -		$ -		$ -		$ -		$ -		$ -		$ -		$ -	
		$ -		$ -		$ -		$ -		$ -		$ -		$ -		$ -	
		$ -		$ -		$ -		$ -		$ -		$ -		$ -		$ -	
		$ -		$ -		$ -		$ -		$ -		$ -		$ -		$ -	
		$ -		$ -		$ -		$ -		$ -		$ -		$ -		$ -	
			1 - Act. Daily Amt.	1- Reward	2 - Act. Daily Amt.	2-Reward	3 - Act. Daily Amt.	3-Reward	4 - Act. Daily Amt.	4-Reward	5 - Act. Daily Amt.	5-Reward	6 - Act. Daily Amt.	6-Reward	Total Daily Amt.	Total Monthly Reward	Team Member
Doctor 2	$ -		$ -	$ -	$ -	$ -	$ -	$ -	$ -	$ -	$ -	$ -	$ -	$ -	$ -		
		$ -		$ -		$ -		$ -		$ -		$ -		$ -		$ -	
		$ -		$ -		$ -		$ -		$ -		$ -		$ -		$ -	
		$ -		$ -		$ -		$ -		$ -		$ -		$ -		$ -	
		$ -		$ -		$ -		$ -		$ -		$ -		$ -		$ -	
		$ -		$ -		$ -		$ -		$ -		$ -		$ -		$ -	
			1 - Act. Daily Amt.	1- Reward	2 - Act. Daily Amt.	2-Reward	3 - Act. Daily Amt.	3-Reward	4 - Act. Daily Amt.	4-Reward	5 - Act. Daily Amt.	5-Reward	6 - Act. Daily Amt.	6-Reward	Total Daily Amt.	Total Monthly Reward	Team Member
Doctor 3	$ -		$ -	$ -	$ -	$ -	$ -	$ -	$ -	$ -	$ -	$ -	$ -	$ -	$ -		
		$ -		$ -		$ -		$ -		$ -		$ -		$ -		$ -	
		$ -		$ -		$ -		$ -		$ -		$ -		$ -		$ -	
		$ -		$ -		$ -		$ -		$ -		$ -		$ -		$ -	
		$ -		$ -		$ -		$ -		$ -		$ -		$ -		$ -	
		$ -		$ -		$ -		$ -		$ -		$ -		$ -		$ -	
			1 - Act. Daily Amt.	1- Reward	2 - Act. Daily Amt.	2-Reward	3 - Act. Daily Amt.	3-Reward	4 - Act. Daily Amt.	4-Reward	5 - Act. Daily Amt.	5-Reward	6 - Act. Daily Amt.	6-Reward	Total Daily Amt.	Total Monthly Reward	Team Member
Hygiene 1	$ -		$ -	$ -	$ -	$ -	$ -	$ -	$ -	$ -	$ -	$ -	$ -	$ -	$ -		
		$ -		$ -		$ -		$ -		$ -		$ -		$ -		$ -	
		$ -		$ -		$ -		$ -		$ -		$ -		$ -		$ -	
		$ -		$ -		$ -		$ -		$ -		$ -		$ -		$ -	
			1 - Act. Daily Amt.	1- Reward	2 - Act. Daily Amt.	2-Reward	3 - Act. Daily Amt.	3-Reward	4 - Act. Daily Amt.	4-Reward	5 - Act. Daily Amt.	5-Reward	6 - Act. Daily Amt.	6-Reward	Total Daily Amt.	Total Monthly Reward	Team Member
Hygiene 2	$ -		$ -	$ -	$ -	$ -	$ -	$ -	$ -	$ -	$ -	$ -	$ -	$ -	$ -		
		$ -		$ -		$ -		$ -		$ -		$ -		$ -		$ -	
		$ -		$ -		$ -		$ -		$ -		$ -		$ -		$ -	
		$ -		$ -		$ -		$ -		$ -		$ -		$ -		$ -	
			1 - Act. Daily Amt.	1- Reward	2 - Act. Daily Amt.	2-Reward	3 - Act. Daily Amt.	3-Reward	4 - Act. Daily Amt.	4-Reward	5 - Act. Daily Amt.	5-Reward	6 - Act. Daily Amt.	6-Reward	Total Daily Amt.	Total Monthly Reward	Team Member
Hygiene 3	$ -		$ -	$ -	$ -	$ -	$ -	$ -	$ -	$ -	$ -	$ -	$ -	$ -	$ -		
		$ -		$ -		$ -		$ -		$ -		$ -		$ -		$ -	
		$ -		$ -		$ -		$ -		$ -		$ -		$ -		$ -	
		$ -		$ -		$ -		$ -		$ -		$ -		$ -		$ -	

SENIOR DOCTOR'S NET TAKE-HOME/DAY BEFORE TAX*

PREPARED FOR

SUNRISE DENTAL SOLUTIONS

ASSOCIATE ASSUMPTIONS:

No. of Days Worked/mo.: 16 | Collections% 81% | Lab Fees 5% | Assist. Cost/day $ 130 | Practice Profit % after Associate Comp. 0,25

Compensation Percentage / Prod. Rate/Day	1000	1100	1200	1300	1400	1500	1600	1700	1800	1900	2000	2100	2200	2300	2400	2500	2600	2700	2800	2900	3000
25%	197	213	230	246	263	279	296	312	328	345	361	378	394	411	427	443	460	476	493	509	526
26%	195	211	227	244	260	276	292	308	325	341	357	373	390	406	422	438	455	471	487	503	520
27%	193	209	225	241	257	273	289	305	321	337	353	369	385	401	417	433	449	465	481	497	513
28%	191	207	222	238	254	270	286	302	317	333	349	365	381	397	412	428	444	460	476	492	507
29%	189	204	220	236	251	267	283	298	314	329	345	361	376	392	408	423	439	454	470	486	501
30%	187	202	218	233	248	264	279	295	310	326	341	356	372	387	403	418	434	449	464	480	495
31%	185	200	215	230	246	261	276	291	307	322	337	352	367	383	398	413	428	444	459	474	489
32%	183	198	213	228	243	258	273	288	303	318	333	348	363	378	393	408	423	438	453	468	483
33%	181	195	210	225	240	255	270	284	299	314	329	344	358	373	388	403	418	433	447	462	477
34%	179	193	208	222	237	252	266	281	296	310	325	339	354	369	383	398	412	427	442	456	471
35%	177	191	205	220	234	249	263	278	292	306	321	335	350	364	378	393	407	422	436	450	465
36%	175	189	203	217	231	246	260	274	288	302	317	331	345	359	374	388	402	416	430	445	459
37%	173	187	201	215	229	243	257	271	285	299	313	327	341	355	369	383	397	411	425	439	453
38%	171	184	198	212	226	240	253	267	281	295	309	322	336	350	364	378	391	405	419	433	447
39%	169	182	196	209	223	237	250	264	277	291	305	318	332	345	359	373	386	400	413	427	441
40%	167	180	193	207	220	234	247	260	274	287	301	314	327	341	354	368	381	394	408	421	435
41%	164	178	191	204	217	230	244	257	270	283	296	310	323	336	349	362	376	389	402	415	428
42%	162	175	188	201	214	227	240	253	266	279	292	305	318	331	344	357	370	383	396	409	422
43%	160	173	186	199	212	224	237	250	263	276	288	301	314	327	340	352	365	378	391	403	416
44%	158	171	184	196	209	221	234	247	259	272	284	297	309	322	335	347	360	372	385	398	410
45%	156	169	181	194	206	218	231	243	255	268	280	293	305	317	330	342	355	367	379	392	404
46%	154	167	179	191	203	215	227	240	252	264	276	288	301	313	325	337	349	361	374	386	398
47%	152	164	176	188	200	212	224	236	248	260	272	284	296	308	320	332	344	356	368	380	392
48%	150	162	174	186	197	209	221	233	245	256	268	280	292	303	315	327	339	351	362	374	386
49%	148	160	171	183	195	206	218	229	241	252	264	276	287	299	310	322	334	345	357	368	380
50%	146	158	169	180	192	203	215	226	237	249	260	271	283	294	306	317	328	340	351	362	374
51%	144	155	167	178	189	200	211	222	234	245	256	267	278	289	301	312	323	334	345	357	368
52%	142	153	164	175	186	197	208	219	230	241	252	263	274	285	296	307	318	329	340	351	362
53%	140	151	162	172	183	194	205	216	226	237	248	259	269	280	291	302	312	323	334	345	356
54%	138	149	159	170	180	191	202	212	223	233	244	254	265	275	286	297	307	318	328	339	349
55%	136	146	157	167	178	188	198	209	219	229	240	250	260	271	281	292	302	312	323	333	343
56%	134	144	154	165	175	185	195	205	215	226	236	246	256	266	276	287	297	307	317	327	337
57%	132	142	152	162	172	182	192	202	212	222	232	242	252	262	271	281	291	301	311	321	331
58%	130	140	150	159	169	179	189	198	208	218	228	237	247	257	267	276	286	296	306	315	325
59%	128	138	147	157	166	176	185	195	204	214	224	233	243	252	262	271	281	290	300	310	319
60%	126	135	145	154	163	173	182	191	201	210	220	229	238	248	257	266	276	285	294	304	313
61%	124	133	142	151	161	170	179	188	197	206	215	225	234	243	252	261	270	279	289	298	307
62%	122	131	140	149	158	167	176	185	194	202	211	220	229	238	247	256	265	274	283	292	301
63%	120	129	137	146	155	164	172	181	190	199	207	216	225	234	242	251	260	269	277	286	295
64%	118	126	135	144	152	161	169	178	186	195	203	212	220	229	237	246	255	263	272	280	289
65%	116	124	133	141	149	158	166	174	183	191	199	208	216	224	233	241	249	258	266	274	283

*Based on associate compensation of percentage of collections off of their production minus their lab fees and assistant costs

ASSOCIATE NET TAKE-HOME/DAY BEFORE TAX* **PREPARED FOR**

SUNRISE DENTAL SOLUTIONS

ASSUMPTIONS:
No. of Days Worked/mo.: 16 | Collections% 81% | Lab Fees 0% | Assist. Cost/day $ -

	Prod. Rate/Day	1000	1100	1200	1300	1400	1500	1600	1700	1800	1900	2000	2100	2200	2300	2400	2500	2600	2700	2800	2900	3000
Compensation	25%	203	223	243	263	284	304	324	344	365	385	405	425	446	466	486	506	527	547	567	587	608
Percentage	26%	211	232	253	274	295	316	337	358	379	400	421	442	463	484	505	527	548	569	590	611	632
	27%	219	241	262	284	306	328	350	372	394	416	437	459	481	503	525	547	569	590	612	634	656
	28%	227	249	272	295	318	340	363	386	408	431	454	476	499	522	544	567	590	612	635	658	680
	29%	235	258	282	305	329	352	376	399	423	446	470	493	517	540	564	587	611	634	658	681	705
	30%	243	267	292	316	340	365	389	413	437	462	486	510	535	559	583	608	632	656	680	705	729
	31%	251	276	301	326	352	377	402	427	452	477	502	527	552	578	603	628	653	678	703	728	753
	32%	259	285	311	337	363	389	415	441	467	492	518	544	570	596	622	648	674	700	726	752	778
	33%	267	294	321	347	374	401	428	454	481	508	535	561	588	615	642	668	695	722	748	775	802
	34%	275	303	330	358	386	413	441	468	496	523	551	578	606	633	661	689	716	744	771	799	826
	35%	284	312	340	369	397	425	454	482	510	539	567	595	624	652	680	709	737	765	794	822	851
	36%	292	321	350	379	408	437	467	496	525	554	583	612	642	671	700	729	758	787	816	846	875
	37%	300	330	360	390	420	450	480	509	539	569	599	629	659	689	719	749	779	809	839	869	899
	38%	308	339	369	400	431	462	492	523	554	585	616	646	677	708	739	770	800	831	862	893	923
	39%	316	347	379	411	442	474	505	537	569	600	632	663	695	727	758	790	821	853	885	916	948
	40%	324	356	389	421	454	486	518	551	583	616	648	680	713	745	778	810	842	875	907	940	972
	41%	332	365	399	432	465	498	531	565	598	631	664	697	731	764	797	830	863	897	930	963	996
	42%	340	374	408	442	476	510	544	578	612	646	680	714	748	782	816	851	885	919	953	987	1021
	43%	348	383	418	453	488	522	557	592	627	662	697	731	766	801	836	871	906	940	975	1010	1045
	44%	356	392	428	463	499	535	570	606	642	677	713	748	784	820	855	891	927	962	998	1034	1069
	45%	365	401	437	474	510	547	583	620	656	693	729	765	802	838	875	911	948	984	1021	1057	1094
	46%	373	410	447	484	522	559	596	633	671	708	745	782	820	857	894	932	969	1006	1043	1081	1118
	47%	381	419	457	495	533	571	609	647	685	723	761	799	838	876	914	952	990	1028	1066	1104	1142
	48%	389	428	467	505	544	583	622	661	700	739	778	816	855	894	933	972	1011	1050	1089	1128	1166
	49%	397	437	476	516	556	595	635	675	714	754	794	833	873	913	953	992	1032	1072	1111	1151	1191
	50%	405	446	486	527	567	608	648	689	729	770	810	851	891	932	972	1013	1053	1094	1134	1175	1215
	51%	413	454	496	537	578	620	661	702	744	785	826	868	909	950	991	1033	1074	1115	1157	1198	1239
	52%	421	463	505	548	590	632	674	716	758	800	842	885	927	969	1011	1053	1095	1137	1179	1221	1264
	53%	429	472	515	558	601	644	687	730	773	816	859	902	944	987	1030	1073	1116	1159	1202	1245	1288
	54%	437	481	525	569	612	656	700	744	787	831	875	919	962	1006	1050	1094	1137	1181	1225	1268	1312
	55%	446	490	535	579	624	668	713	757	802	846	891	936	980	1025	1069	1114	1158	1203	1247	1292	1337
	56%	454	499	544	590	635	680	726	771	816	862	907	953	998	1043	1089	1134	1179	1225	1270	1315	1361
	57%	462	508	554	600	646	693	739	785	831	877	923	970	1016	1062	1108	1154	1200	1247	1293	1339	1385
	58%	470	517	564	611	658	705	752	799	846	893	940	987	1034	1081	1128	1175	1221	1268	1315	1362	1409
	59%	478	526	573	621	669	717	765	812	860	908	956	1004	1051	1099	1147	1195	1243	1290	1338	1386	1434
	60%	486	535	583	632	680	729	778	826	875	923	972	1021	1069	1118	1166	1215	1264	1312	1361	1409	1458
	61%	494	544	593	642	692	741	791	840	889	939	988	1038	1087	1136	1186	1235	1285	1334	1383	1433	1482
	62%	502	552	603	653	703	753	804	854	904	954	1004	1055	1105	1155	1205	1256	1306	1356	1406	1456	1507
	63%	510	561	612	663	714	765	816	868	919	970	1021	1072	1123	1174	1225	1276	1327	1378	1429	1480	1531
	64%	518	570	622	674	726	778	829	881	933	985	1037	1089	1140	1192	1244	1296	1348	1400	1452	1503	1555
	65%	527	579	632	684	737	790	842	895	948	1000	1053	1106	1158	1211	1264	1316	1369	1422	1474	1527	1580

*Based on associate compensation of percentage of collections off of their production minus their lab fees and assistant costs

ASSOCIATESHIP AGREEMENT

This Employment Agreement is made by and between ____________________, an individual with a mailing address of ________________________________, [Your City & State Here] ____________ (hereinafter referred to as "Practice Owner") and ______________________, an individual with an address of __________________ ________________________ (hereinafter referred to as "Employee").

RECITALS:
First, that [Your Name] is a dentist, duly licensed to practice as such in the State of [Your State], and is currently engaged in the practice of general dentistry, operating at ____________________________ under the name of ____________ (the "Practice").

Second, that Employee is a general dentist, duly licensed to practice as such in the State of [Your State].

Third, that [Your Name] and Employee desire that Employee work as an employee-dentist in the Practice on the terms and subject to the conditions set forth in this Agreement.

AGREEMENTS:
In consideration of the foregoing recitals, the agreements and covenants set forth in this Agreement, and the mutual benefits to be derived therefrom, the receipt and adequacy of which are hereby acknowledged, [Your Name] and Employee, intending to be legally bound, hereby agree as follows:

1. **EMPLOYMENT AND TERM**: [Your Name] hereby employs Employee, and Employee accepts employment by, and agrees to serve, [Your Name], for a term beginning ________________, unless sooner terminated as provided in this Agreement (the "Initial Term"). The Initial Term of this Agreement shall be automatically renewed for successive annual terms, commencing ________________, unless either party notifies the other to the contrary not less than thirty (30) days prior to the end of the then current term (the "Term").
2. **DUTIES OF EMPLOYEE**: Throughout the Term of this Agreement, Employee shall:
   - Perform general dentistry services (including, without limitation, all professional dentistry and hygiene services customarily performed by general dentists in the State of [Your State]) to all patients of the Practice with due care and at a professional standard consistent with that prevalent in the community, and always pursuant to the terms and in accordance with the conditions set forth in this Agreement;
   - Devote all of [his or her] professional time and energy exclusively to the practice of general dentistry for the Practice;
   - Work during reasonable and customary business hours established by [Your Name] at [Your Name's] office or offices. The parties shall reasonably cooperate to determine Employee's work schedule, but [Your Name] shall ultimately have absolute discretion in determining when and how much Employee shall work;

- Use [his/her] best efforts, skill and ability to promote the Practice and its interests, and participate in all quality assurance and accreditation efforts.

3. **COMPENSATION**: As full compensation for the services to be provided by Employee pursuant to this Agreement, Employee shall be paid as follows:
   - **Percentage of Collections**: Employee shall be paid _______ percent (_%) of the Adjusted Production generated by the dental services personally rendered by Employee when those funds are actually received ("Employee's Percentage"). For purposes of this Agreement, "Adjusted Production" shall mean the associate's production reduced by discounts, reduced fees, insurance and other write-offs, laboratory remakes, and uncollectable accounts generated directly by dental services rendered personally by Employee. Employee shall be paid Employee's Percentage every _________. Any payments made on a particular account by a patient or carrier shall be allocated first to the oldest outstanding portion of any such account regardless of whether the service provided that generated that portion of the account was rendered by [Your Name] or Employee or any other employee of [Your Name]. Notwithstanding the foregoing, during the first __ (_) months of the Initial Term of this Agreement, Employee shall be paid the greater of (i) _________ dollars ($___) in net wages for every two-week period, or (ii) the Employee's Percentage.
   - **Payroll Matters**: All payments of compensation made by [Your Name] to Employee pursuant to this Section 2 shall be subject to required payroll deductions and contributions for tax withholdings, Social Security, unemployment, etc.

4. **ITEMS TO BE PROVIDED BY OWNER**: During the continuance of this Agreement, [Your Name] will provide, at no cost to Employee, the following benefits:
   - **Malpractice Liability Insurance Coverage** – In such form, with such insurer, and in such amount as [Your Name] shall determine, in [his/her] sole discretion; provided that such form and coverages shall be the same as that purchased by [Your Name] [himself/herself];
   - **Clinic Attire**
   - **Unpaid Vacation** – Made available to Employee, up to fifteen (15) days during any twelve (12) month period, subject to reasonable scheduling with [Your Name];
   - **Unpaid Sick Days** – Made available to Employee, up to six (6) days during any twelve (12) month period, for those days during which Employee is unable to work due to personal illness;
   - **Instrumentation & Equipment** – Appropriate dental and hygiene equipment and instrumentation;
   - **Staff Support** – Support from one or more dental assistant(s) as reasonably necessary, as well as access to Owner's hygienist(s) for the appointment of patients for necessary hygiene services, as well as support of the business office staff;
   - **Supplies** – Dental and hygiene supplies as reasonably needed, including stationery and business cards;

- **Continuing Education** – The cost of continuing education courses up to a maximum of $3,000 (or greater at Owner's discretion) which Owner specifically requests that Employee attend provided that Employee shall reimburse Owner for the total cost of such courses if Employee terminates this Agreement for any reason during the initial one (1) year term;
- **Health Insurance** – Health insurance under any plan selected by Owner in Owner's sole discretion at comparable allowances as provided to other employees of [Your Name].

Without limitation, Owner shall not either directly, or indirectly in the form of reimbursement, provide Employee with or pay for private disability insurance, automobile expenses, automobile insurance, or life insurance.

5. **ALLOCATION AND SCHEDULING OF PATIENTS**: Subject to the approval of [Your Name]'s patients, [Your Name] shall determine which of [Your Name]'s patients are treated by Employee.

6. **TERMINATION**: Notwithstanding anything to the contrary set forth in this Agreement, [Your Name] may immediately, without notice, discharge Employee as an employee in any of the following events:
   - Employee's right to practice dentistry in the State of [Your State] is suspended, revoked, or canceled;
   - Employee conducts [himself/herself] in an unprofessional, unethical, immoral, or fraudulent manner, or is cited for unprofessional or unethical conduct by any board, society, or group having any privilege or right to pass upon the conduct of Employee, or should the conduct of Employee be detrimental to the reputation, character, or standing of [Your Name];
   - Employee repeatedly fails to follow the directions of [Your Name];
   - Employee breaches any of the provisions of this Agreement;
   - Employee engages in any conduct harmful to [Your Name]'s practice;
   - Employee fails to work harmoniously with other office personnel or patients;
   - Employee is convicted of a felony or serious misdemeanor.

In the event that this Agreement is terminated pursuant to the provisions of this Agreement, Employee, at the sole and exclusive option of [Your Name], shall complete all general dentistry services on patients then under [his/her] care as expeditiously as reasonably possible.

In addition, in the event of a termination of this Agreement, the rights and obligations of the parties pursuant to this Agreement with regard to the compensation of Employee for general dentistry services previously rendered, indemnification, records, confidentiality, and the covenant against competition, shall continue in full force and effect.

7. **EMERGENCY SERVICES**: Employee shall share responsibility with [Your Name] and any other associate dentists, if any, for treating patients of [Your Name]'s practice on weekends and weekday evenings for emergency care. The "on call" schedule for [Your Name]'s practice shall be determined by [Your Name] in [Your Name]'s sole discretion.

8. **STANDARD OF PRACTICE**: Employee shall comply with all federal, state, and municipal laws, rules, and regulations, as well as the canons of ethics of the American Dental Association and the [Your State] Dental Association, that are now or may in the future become applicable to Employee, equipment, and personnel engaged in the practice of general dentistry.

9. **NO ASSIGNMENT**: Due to the professional and personal nature of the general dentistry services to be rendered pursuant to this Agreement, neither [Your Name] nor Employee will have the right to assign his/her rights or delegate [his/her] duties pursuant to this Agreement without the express written consent of the other. Such consent may be withheld in a party's sole, subjective discretion.

10. **INDEMNIFICATION**: Without limitation, Employee shall indemnify and hold harmless [Your Name] from any and all liabilities and defend [Your Name] against any losses, expenses, damages, attorney's fees and court costs, and costs that may arise as a result of any act or failure to act by Employee during the course of this Agreement.

11. **OTHER EMPLOYEES**: Owner may, during and after the term of this Agreement, engage other employee(s) or independent contractor dentist(s) to perform the same types of services to be performed by Employee pursuant to this Agreement.

12. **RECORDS**: Except as provided below, all present and future patient and business records of [Your Name]'s practice shall be the property of [Your Name] exclusively. However, patient records for patients brought into [Your Name]'s practice by Employee (i.e., any patients referred specifically to Employee by Employee's friends or family) shall become the property of Employee and may be taken by Employee at the termination of this Agreement. The parties shall maintain an ongoing list of such patients which shall be amended and initialed by both parties each time Employee brings a new patient into [Your Name]'s practice. Upon termination of this Agreement, all other patient records and all business records shall remain the property of [Your Name] exclusively. Upon reasonable notice and at reasonable times, Employee shall be entitled to review the business records of [Your Name]'s practice to the minimal extent reasonably necessary to resolve any dispute which may arise in connection with the compensation to be paid to Employee pursuant to this Agreement.

13. **RETREATMENT**: In the event that a patient's general dentistry work which was performed by Employee during the course of this Agreement proves to be defective within a period of one (1) year after the work was performed, Employee shall, subject to the patient's consent, correct the defective work without any additional compensation. If the patient decides that he or she does not wish to have Employee personally correct the defective work, Employee agrees to so advise [Your Name] and [Your Name] shall have the exclusive right to determine whether [Your Name] or any other employee dentist will treat the patient or refer the patient to another dentist. If [Your Name] determines that the patient should be referred to another dentist besides Employee, [Your Name] shall have the sole right to determine the other dentist to whom the patient shall be referred. If Employee performs the work necessary to correct the

problem, [Your Name] and Employee shall equally pay the cost of all supplies and actual expenses associated with the work and shall equally pay any gross salaries necessary to provide Employee with a chairside assistant if used by Employee. If [Your Name] or another employee dentist performs the work necessary to correct the problem, then Employee shall pay [Your Name] one-half (1/2) of [Your Name]'s usual and customary fee for the work being done and the full amount of any related laboratory fees. If [Your Name] refers the patient to another dentist for retreatment, then Employee shall pay the treating dentist's usual and customary fee for the work being done.

14. **CONFIDENTIALITY**: Employee specifically agrees that he/she will not at any time during the term of this Agreement or at any time thereafter divulge or disclose to any person, firm, or business entity of any nature, either directly or indirectly, any information of any kind concerning any matters affecting or relating to the general dentistry practice of [Your Name] including, without limitation, the names and addresses of any patients of the practice, the fee practices or the fee schedules maintained in the practice, the dental history or dental needs of any patients, or x-rays or other data relating to any patients. The parties agree that all such information is confidential and is important to the success of [Your Name]'s general dentistry practice and to the maintenance of [Your Name]'s goodwill.

15. **NATURE OF RELATIONSHIP**: The relationship between [Your Name] and Employee shall be strictly that of [Your Name] as an employer and Employee as an employee. [Your Name] and Employee shall not be considered partners or joint ventures, and shall not be considered to operate or have formed any sort of business entity. Employee shall not hold or acquire any proprietary interest of any nature in [Your Name]'s general dentistry practice.

16. **COVENANTS NOT TO COMPETE**: Employee agrees that [he/she] will not, during a period of two (2) years after the termination of this Agreement, solicit or treat any patients who have been or are then currently being treated within [Your Name]'s practice other than patients which Employee brought into [Your Name]'s practice, if any. Employee further covenants that [he/she] will not, during the term of this Agreement and for three (3) year after termination of this Agreement, directly or indirectly induce any patients of [Your Name]'s practice (other than patients which Employee brought into [Your Name]'s practice) or the referring sources of [Your Name]'s practice to patronize or recommend patronizing any dentist other than [Your Name]. In the event of any breach or threatened breach of the provisions of this Section 16, Employee agrees that [Your Name]'s remedy at law (e.g., money damages) shall be inadequate and [Your Name] shall be entitled, without limitation, to appropriate injunctive relief in addition to any legal remedies. Should the foregoing covenants contained in this Section 16 be adjudged to any extent invalid by a competent tribunal, such covenants shall be deemed modified to the minimum extent necessary to make them enforceable.

17. **ENTIRE AGREEMENT**: This Agreement constitutes the only agreement between the parties and supersedes any prior agreements, whether oral or written, between them. This Agreement can be amended only in writing.

18. **ATTORNEY'S FEES**: If any court or arbitration proceeding is brought by either party against the other party, the prevailing party in such court or arbitration proceeding shall be entitled to recover costs incurred and reasonable attorney's fees in addition to any other award.

19. **NOTICES**: All notices to be given under this Agreement shall be in writing and personally delivered or sent by (a) certified mail, return receipt requested, in which case notice shall be deemed delivered three (3) business days after deposit, postage prepaid, in the United States Mail, or (b) a nationally recognized overnight courier, in which case notice shall be deemed delivered one (1) business day after deposit with the courier, to the addresses set forth at the beginning of this Agreement. A party's address may be changed by written notice to the other party, provided that the change of address shall not be effective until actual receipt of that notice.

20. **SEVERABILITY**: If any term or provision of this Agreement is, to any extent, held invalid or unenforceable, the remainder of this Agreement shall not be affected.

21. **WAIVERS**: No waiver or any breach of any covenant or provision in this Agreement shall be deemed a waiver of any other covenant or provision in this Agreement, and no waiver shall be valid unless in writing and executed by the waiving party. No extension of time for performance of any obligation or act shall be deemed an extension of the time for performance of any other obligation or act.

22. **CONSTRUCTION**: Headings at the beginning of each paragraph are solely for the convenience of the parties and are not a part of nor should they be used to interpret this Agreement. The singular form shall include plural, and vice versa. This Agreement shall not be construed as if it had been prepared by one of the parties, but rather as if both parties had prepared it. Unless otherwise indicated, all references to paragraphs are to this Agreement.

23. **GOVERNING LAW**: This Agreement shall be governed and construed in accordance with laws of the State of [Your State].

24. **LEGAL REPRESENTATION**: Employee has either consulted with legal counsel of [his/her] own choosing prior to signing this Agreement, or has voluntarily decided to refrain from doing so. Executed and delivered as of the date of later execution hereof by [Your Name] and Employee.

______________________	______________
Employee	Date
______________________	______________
(Practice Owner's Name)	(Date)

Acknowledgements

Authoring this book is just another way of fulfilling my purpose. It's also a way to honor all those individuals who shaped who I have become.

I owe an immeasurable debt of gratitude to my chosen profession (or did it choose me?) and the patients I was honored to serve.

I was blessed to work beside some incredible professionals – assistants, hygienists, dentist associates, and business office personnel. One in particular, Ms. Mandy Wallin, made important contributions to the financial systems portion of this book.

Three esteemed colleagues of mine, Dr. Matt VanderMolen, Dr. Devin Hall, and Dr. Justin Bonaventure, graciously reviewed the original manuscript and recommended valuable edits. I am grateful for the time and expertise they brought to this project.

There were also mentors, some of whom I was fortunate enough to work with in person, and others whose books and video teachings had tremendous impact on my knowledge and how I viewed the world. They taught me how to think, and thoughts shape a person's destiny.

As a young dentist I was blessed to learn under Dr. Peter Dawson who taught me just how much I didn't know – the first step in the never-ending educational journey. I couldn't have had a better role model of how to live a high-quality life than Dr. Dawson.

Credit for the opportunity to author this book, as well as so many other amazing experiences in my professional life, goes to my good friend, Mark Ferber. As much as I've been the recipient of his talent and wisdom, it has been his unyielding belief in me that has allowed me to rise above my highest expectations.

I would not have met Mark if it weren't for my very good friend, Dr. Leslie Fang. Les has been a teacher, mentor, and the best possible example of what it means to be an educator at the highest level. Every educational endeavor I produce, including this one, cannot help but have his imprint on it.

This book would not be possible without all the many experiences I have had with dentists who trusted me enough to be their mentor, consultant, coach, and friend. Through supporting them on their journey to success, I learned more from them than they learned from me.

Some of my greatest pleasures in life were their successes, and some of my lowest points were their defeats, because I always treated their practices like they were my own. They will fulfill my professional legacy by teaching and coaching others to be more successful.

Finally, and most importantly, I owe my greatest debt of gratitude to my family. I could not have had a better soulmate than my wife Becky, who unselfishly allowed me to pursue my purpose and sacrificed and supported me on that quest. Any rewards resulting from that would be meaningless without her.

Meredith and Travis have been and remain loving reminders of how important it is to keep the main thing in life the main thing. They have brought real meaning to my life, and I am so proud to be their father. They've always been the "why" in my life.

And now I have another "why" – my granddaughter Logan. I hope and pray that she, like her "grumpy," finds her passionate purpose and lives a life full of joy, fulfillment, and, of course, prosperity.

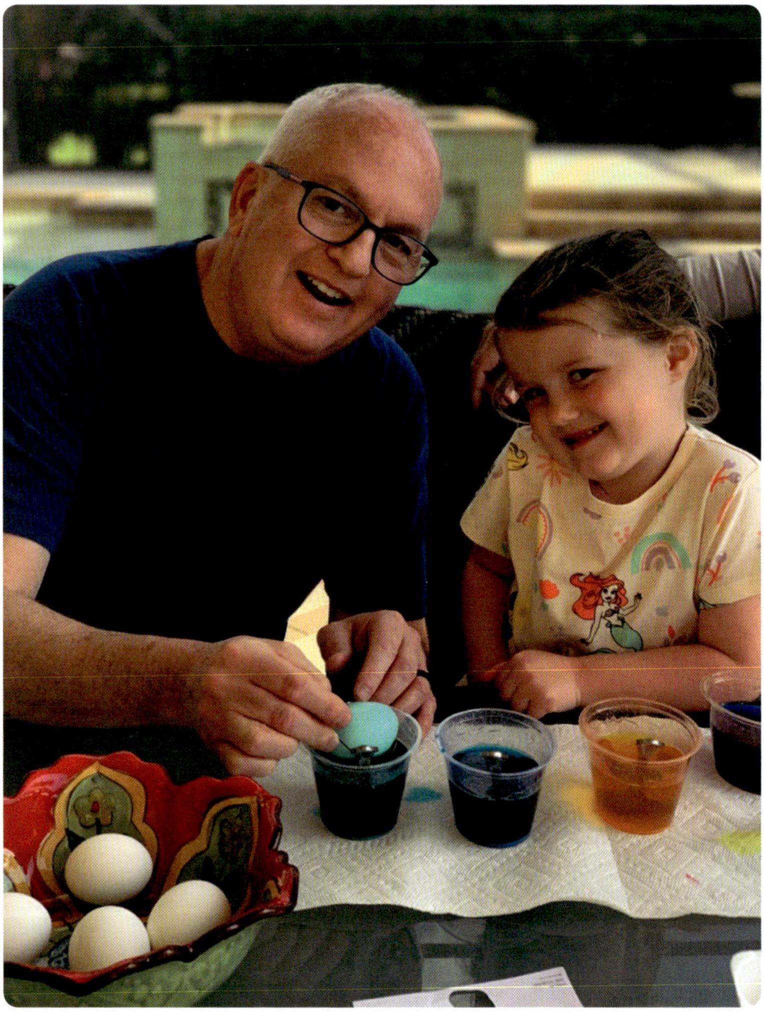

About the Author

Dr. Anthony Feck has 39 years of private practice experience and a long list of professional accomplishments. He is a sought-after speaker at professional events and has shared his methods of success with thousands of dentists and their teams.

Dr. Feck is widely recognized as a clinical educator, both a pioneer and an authority on the use of conscious sedation in dentistry. His teaching resumè includes an extensive list of other clinical topics aimed at the general practitioner who desires to be a Super GP.

Dr. Feck founded Sunrise Dental Solutions (SDS), a practice optimization company, in 2005. SDS is a community of highly successful, practicing dentists who have succeeded through different paths. SDS utilizes an innovative approach to creating financial and lifestyle freedom for its clients through coaching support, training, and networking.

Dr. Feck practices in a multi-doctor practice in Lexington, Kentucky, that concentrates on sedation dentistry, dental implantology, and dental-facial rehabilitation.

He can be reached at Tony@SunriseDentalSolutions.com.